DICTIONARY OF EYE TERMINOLOGY

THE EYE

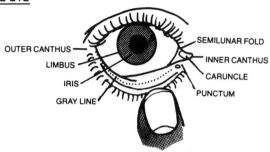

OUTER CANTHUS
LIMBUS
IRIS
GRAY LINE

SEMILUNAR FOLD
INNER CANTHUS
CARUNCLE
PUNCTUM

THE ORBIT

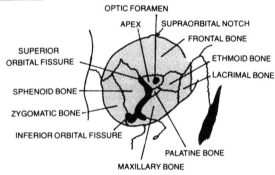

OPTIC FORAMEN
APEX
SUPRAORBITAL NOTCH
FRONTAL BONE
SUPERIOR ORBITAL FISSURE
ETHMOID BONE
LACRIMAL BONE
SPHENOID BONE
ZYGOMATIC BONE
INFERIOR ORBITAL FISSURE
PALATINE BONE
MAXILLARY BONE

THE VISUAL PATHWAY

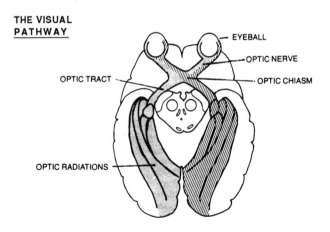

EYEBALL
OPTIC NERVE
OPTIC TRACT
OPTIC CHIASM
OPTIC RADIATIONS

DICTIONARY OF
EYE TERMINOLOGY

THIRD EDITION

Barbara Cassin

Sheila A.B. Solomon

Melvin L. Rubin, M.D.
Editor

 TRIAD PUBLISHING COMPANY   GAINESVILLE, FLORIDA

Library of Congress Cataloging-in-Publication Data

Cassin, Barbara, 1929–
    Dictionary of eye terminology / Barbara Cassin, Sheila A.B. Solomon ; Melvin L. Rubin, editor. -- 3rd ed.
        p.   cm.
    ISBN 0-937404-44-6 (pbk.)
    1. Ophthalmology--Dictionaries.   I. Solomon, Sheila, 1954–
II. Rubin, Melvin L.   III. Title.
    [DNLM: 1. Ophthalmology--dictionaries.   WW 13 C345d   1997]
RE21.C37   1997
617.7'003--dc20
DNLM/DLC
for Library of Congress   96-23368
                                             CIP

Published and distributed by
Triad Publishing Company
Post Office Box 13355
Gainesville, Florida 32604

Additional copies of the *Dictionary of Eye Terminology, 3rd edition,* may be obtained from the publisher by sending $24.95 per copy, plus shipping and handling ($6 1st book, $2 each addl.) plus Florida sales tax, if applicable. Foreign orders write for shipping.

CONTENTS

PREFACE

Much of the impetus for this third edition of the *Dictionary of Eye Terminology* came from comments and requests by readers. The requests centered on two major themes: (1) include more drugs, diseases, procedures, etc., BUT... (2) do not let the book become larger! Where to draw the line has been difficult. It's been a balancing act.

Based on the requests, a number of additions and modifications were decided upon. We have added plurals (those that are not obvious), new surgical techniques, new laser technology, many more drugs, and systemic diseases with ocular manifestations or those that frequently affect eye patients.

In addition, we've made revisions to improve original definitions and to reflect scientific advances and changes in terminology as disease entities have become better understood.

Since publication of the first edition in 1984, the *Dictionary* has received a universally enthusiastic response by providing a handy, easy-to-use guide for looking up unfamiliar terms and finding a definition that could be understood without a medical or science background.

Our sagacious editor, Melvin L. Rubin, M.D., has amplified, clarified and refined the definitions. I acknowledge his significant contributions with sincere gratitude.

As always, your comments and suggestions are most welcome.

Barbara Cassin

PREFACE
TO THE 2ND EDITION

This book grew out of necessity. The difficulty in deciphering eye "jargon" was a frustration constantly voiced by the personnel and trainees at the University of Florida's Shands Eye Center as well as by many non-ophthalmic physicians. A source to aid layment in decoding ophthalmic terminology was nonexistent.

With this in mind, and with the encouragement and enthusiasm of our ophthalmic technology students, we embarked upon compiling and writing a glossary geared to making ophthalmic terminology accessible and understandable to all who were not familiar with the field. Such a book would also simplify the task of learning about the eye and eye related problems.

Focusing on the needs of the ophthalmic technologist students, we tried to make looking up definitions a simple process, not requiring constant hunting for the meanings of words used in the definitions themselves. We also tried to create definitions that were clear and simple. But since precise defining of medical and scientific words does require the use of other medical and scientific words, and in many cases just cannot be defined simply, technical accuracy was occasionally sacrificed to maintain concept understandability.

Even though the scope of this second edition has been expanded, we feel it is necessary for the Dictionary to remain a manageable size. We have therefore, as before, excluded most general medical terms that can be found in standard medical dictionaries, except for those terms that have a specific ophthalmic application, such as systemic diseases that affect the eyes.

Much of the impetus for the project and almost half the words in the first edition were submitted by the following former ophthalmic technologist students: Nancy Caplan Solomon, Susan Corwin Mitchell, Virginia Carlson Hansen, Donna Leef, Stephanie Lenit Griffin, Donna Loupe, Paul Paresi, and Linda Stinnett Musfeldt.

To our editor and department chairman, Melvin L. Rubin, MD, we gratefully acknowledge his performing a monumental editorial task correcting, tightening, and polishing the definitions.

Finally, we express our appreciation to our respective spouses, Sidney Cassin, PhD, and Stanford R. Solomon, Esq, for their patient understanding of the time required for the compilation of the Dictionary.

Barbara Cassin
Sheila A.B. Solomon

GUIDE TO THE DICTIONARY

The *Dictionary of Eye Terminology* is written so that a science background is not necessary for understanding the terms or their definitions. Lay language has been used wherever possible, and throughout the dictionary scientific or medical terms are included (in parentheses) within the definitions. Sometimes, for clarity, this is reversed, with the medical word used in the definition and its clarification in parentheses.

MAIN ENTRIES, the word or phrase being defined, are printed in **bold** type and set out to the left of the margin.

ORDER OF MAIN ENTRIES: alphabetically letter-by-letter without regard to intervening spaces or hyphens. Thus, "background retinopathy" precedes "back vertex power."

SYNONYMS and words having the same application as the entry (though not necessarily the identical meaning) are printed in **bold** type alongside the entry. Each of these is also given its own listing.

CAPITALIZATION: upper case letters are used only when the word is normally capitalized, such as for a proper name.

An ABBREVIATION for an entry follows it (in parentheses). A complete listing of abbreviations and acronyms precedes the dictionary listings.

CATEGORY: most listings are followed by a word or phrase printed in *italics* (*pathologic condition, surgical procedure, test*) that will instantly categorize it.

COMMONLY MISSPELLED WORDS are alphabetized as main entries, though not in bold type, with the explanation (in *italics*): *"Incorrect spelling of (CORRECT SPELLING)."* This makes it easy to find a term without knowing its spelling.

When the PLURAL FORM is not apparent, it is included at the end of the definition.

CROSS REFERENCES are minimized: sufficient information to understand a definition is given within the definition, and to avoid guesswork, many entries are placed in more than one location—e.g., astigmatism (irregular), irregular astigmatism. "See also" is used to indicate related information. References to other terms in the dictionary are printed in SMALL CAPITAL LETTERS.

PRONUNCIATION: phonetic spelling follows (in parentheses) entries whose pronunciation is not readily apparent. No attempt has been made to indicate fine gradations of sound by diacritical marks. The pronunciation given may not be the only correct way; there is wide variation in pronouncing ophthalmic terms. When a word appears at the start of successive entries, pronunciation is given only at its first appearance.

PRONUNCIATION KEY:

Accented (stressed) syllables are indicated by CAPITAL LETTERS.

Vowel sounds are pronounced as follows:

A	as in day	ay
	as in map	a + consonant
	as in father	ah
E	as in see	ee
	as in net	e + consonant (at end of syllable: eh)
	as in term	ur
I	as in eye, site	i (or i + consonant + e)
	as in tin	i + consonant (at end of syllable: ih)
O	as in go	o, oh
	as in mother	uh
	as in dot	ah
	as in fog	aw
	as in do	u, oo
U	as in blue	u, oo
	as in cute	yu, yoo
	as in cut	uh
Y	as in family	ee
	as in myth	ih

ABBREVIATIONS & ACRONYMS

The use of shortcuts in medical notation has evolved over many years. So far, there is no universally accepted list, nor is there any consistency as to the use of periods and capitalized letters. This following have been collected from many sources and are all in common usage.

SYMBOLS

Δ	change
∞	infinity
$\triangle$	prism diopter
♀	female
♂	male
>	greater than
<	less than
↑	increased
↓	decreased
⊕	orthophoria
1°	primary
2°	secondary

DOUBLE-HEIGHT LETTERS

Measurements made on each eye are recorded next to a double-height letter, with the value for the right eye given first (on top or to the left), followed by the value for the left eye.

K	keratometry readings
L	lensometer
M	manifest refraction
NV	near vision
NVW	glasses worn by patient (near vision wear)
R	retinoscopic findings
Rx	prescription (for glasses)
T	tension (intraocular pressure)
T_a	tension by applanation
T_s	tension by Schiotz tonometry
V	visual acuity
W	glasses worn by patient (wear)

A

a	before
A	applanation tension
A 1	atropine 1%
AA	amplitude of accommodation
AACG	acute angle closure glaucoma
Ab	antibodies
ABK	aphakic bullous keratopathy
a.c.	before meals (ante cibum)
AC	anterior chamber
ACA	anterior cerebral artery
AC/A	accommodative convergence/ accommodation ratio
acc	accommodative
ACG	angle closure glaucoma
ACIOL	anterior chamber intraocular lens
ACLS	advanced cardiac life support
ACT	alternate cover test
ACTH	adrenocorticotropic hormone
AD	autosomal dominant
add	added power for near vision
ad. lib.	as desired (ad libitum)
ADV	adenovirus
AFB	acid-fast bacillus
AFGE	air fluid gas exchange
AFIP	Armed Forces Institute of Pathology
AHF	anterior hyaloid face
AHM	anterior hyaloid membrane
AI	auto-immune
AIDS	autoimmune deficiency syndrome
AION	anterior ischemic optic neuropathy
AK	actinic keratosis
aka	also known as
AL	axial length
ALK	automated lamellar keratoplasty
ALL	acute lymphocytic leukemia

ALT	argon laser trabeculoplasty	BCBS	Blue Cross–Blue Shield
AMD	age-related macular degeneration	BCC	basal cell carcinoma
AML	acute myelogenous leukemia	BD	base-down prism
AMPPE	acute multifocal placoid pigment epitheliopathy	BDR	background diabetic retinopathy
		BEB	benign essential blepharospasm
ANA	antinuclear antibodies test	BF	black female
ANCA	anti-neutrophil cytoplasmic antibodies	BFP	binocular fixation pattern
		BI	base-in prism
ANS	autonomic nervous system	b.i.d.	twice a day (bis in die)
AO	American Optical	bil	bilateral
AO-HRR	American Optical Hardy-Rand-Rittler color vision plates	BM	black male
		BM	bowel movement
AODM	adult onset diabetes mellitus	BMR	basal metabolic rate
APCT	alternate prism + cover test	BMR	bilateral medial rectus recession
APD	afferent pupillary defect	BO	base-out prism
Appl	applanation tension	BP	blood pressure
AR	autosomal recessive	BRAO	branch retinal artery occlusion
ARAM	acquired retinal arterial macro-aneurysm	BRVO	branch retinal vein occlusion
		BS	blind spot
ARC	abnormal retinal correspondence	BSS	balanced salt solution
ARC	AIDS-related complex	BSV	binocular single vision
ARDS	adult respiratory distress syndrome	BU	base-up prism
ArF	argon fluoride	BUN	blood urea nitrogen level
ARG	angle recession glaucoma	BUT	breakup time (of tear film)
ARM	age-related maculopathy	BVA	best-corrected visual acuity
ARMD	age-related macular degeneration	BVO	branch vein occlusion
ARN	acute retinal necrosis	Bx	biopsy
ARNS	atropine retinoscopy		

C

ASA	aspirin (acetylsalicylic acid)	c	with (cum)
ASAP	as soon as possible	C 1	cyclopentolate (Cyclogyl) 1% eyedrops
asb.	apostilb		
ASC	anterior subcapsular cataract	C	centigrade
ASCVD	atherosclerotic cardiovascular disease	C	cranial nerve
		C	cycloplegic
ASO_4	atropine (as the sulfate)	C	Cyclogyl
AT	applanation tension	Ca	calcium
A-T	ataxia telangiectasia	CA	carcinoma
ATR	against-the-rule astigmatism	CA	cancer, corneal abrasion
A-V	arterio-venous	CAB	cellulose acetate butyrate
AVM	arterio-venous malformation	CACG	chronic angle closure glaucoma
		CAD	coronary artery disease

B

B	betaxolol	CAG	closed angle glaucoma
B	Betoptic	CAI	carbonic anhydrase inhibitor
B	bilateral (+ EOM name)	CAT	computerized axial tomography
BAO	branch artery occlusion	cat.	cataract
BARN	bilateral acute retinal necrosis	cat. ext.	cataract extraction
BBB	blood brain barrier	Cat-Trab	combined cataract-trabeculectomy
BBB	bundle branch (heart) block	CBB	ciliary body bend
BC	base curve	CBC	complete blood count

cc	cubic centimeter	CNVM	choroidal neovascular membrane
cc	with correction *(cum correctio)*	c/o	complains of
CC	chief complaint	CO_2	carbon dioxide
C-C fistula	carotid (artery)-cavernous (sinus) fistula	COAD	chronic obstructive airway disease
		COAG	chronic open angle glaucoma
CCT	computed coronal tomography	COLD	chronic obstructive lung disease
CCT	cyclocryotherapy	COMA	congenital oculomotor apraxia
CCTV	closed circuit TV (magnifier)	conj	conjunctive, conjunctival
CCU	coronary care unit	COPD	chronic obstructive pulmonary disease
C/D	cup-to-disc ratio		
CE	cataract extraction	COWS	cold opposite, warm same
CEBMD	corneal epithelial basement membrane dystrophy	CPC	central posterior curve
		CPC	clinico-pathologic conference
CF	confrontation field	CPEO	chronic progressive external ophthalmoplegia
CF	counts fingers (vision)		
C&F	cell and flare	CPK	creatinine phosphokinase (lab test)
C_3F_3	perfluoropropane	CPR	cardio-pulmonary resuscitation
CFFF	critical flicker fusion frequency	CRA	central retinal artery
CG	ciliary ganglion	CRAO	central retinal artery occlusion
CHED	congenital hereditary endothelial dystrophy	CrCl	creatinine clearance
		CRF	chronic renal failure
CHF	congestive heart failure	CRF	corticotrophin releasing factor
CHRPE	congenital hypertrophy of the retinal pigment epithelium	CRV	central retinal vein
		CRVO	central retinal vein occlusion
CICU	cardiac intensive care unit	C + S	culture and sensitivity
CIE	*Commission Internationale de l'Eclairage*	CSF	cerebrospinal fluid
		CSM	central, steady and maintained fixation
CIN	corneoconjunctival intra-epithelial neoplasia		
		CSNB	congenital stationary night blindness
CIOM	closed intraocular microsurgery		
CL	contact lens	CSR	central serous (chorio)retinopathy
CLL	chronic lymphocytic leukemia	CSUM	central, steady, unmaintained fixation
CLEK	collaborative longitudinal eval-uation of keratoconus		
		CT	computerized axial tomography
cm	centimeter	CT	cover test
CME	cystoid macular edema	CTD	connective tissue disease
CMI	cell mediated immune response	CUSUM	central, unsteady, unmaintained fixation
CMI	cytomegalic inclusion disease		
CML	chronic myelogenous leukemia	CV	color vision
CMV	cytomegalovirus	CVA	cerebrovascular accident; stroke
CN	cranial nerve	CVD	cardiovascular disease
CN2	2nd cranial nerve (optic)	cyl	cylinder
CN3	3rd cranial nerve (oculomotor)	Cx	cylinder (in diopters), axis (in degrees)
CN4	4th cranial nerve (trochlear)	CXR	chest x-ray
CN5	5th cranial nerve (trigeminal)		
CN6	6th cranial nerve (abducens)		**D**
CNAG	chronic narrow angle glaucoma	D	diopter
CNDO	congenital nasolacrimal duct obstruction	D	distance, distance vision
		D	Diamox
CNS	central nervous system	D-15	Farnsworth D-15 color vision test

D-100	Farnsworth D-100 color vision test	EKC	epidemic keratoconjunctivitis
D 250	Diamox 250 mg	EKF	epikeratophakia
DA	dark adaptation	EKG	electrocardiogram
dB	decibel	ELISA	enzyme-linked immuno-absorbent assay
DC	discontinue		
DC, D/C	discharge (from hospital/clinic/care)	EMP	epimacular proliferation
		EOG	electro-oculogram
DCR	dacryocystorhinostomy	EOM	extraocular muscle
DD	(optic) disc diameter	EOMB	extraocular muscle balance
DDH	dissociated double hypertropia	epi	epithelium
DFP	diisopropyl fluorophosphate	EPI	epinephrine
diam	diameter	ERG	electroretinogram
dil	dilate	ERM	epiretinal membrane
DJD	degenerative joint disease	ERP	early receptor potential
dl	deciliter (100 cc)	ESR	erythrocyte sedimentation rate
DM	diabetes mellitus	ESRD	endstage renal disease
DMV	disc, macula, vessels	ESRF	endstage renal failure
D + N	distance and near	et	and
DNR	do not resuscitate	ET	esotropia at distance
DOA	dead on arrival	ET'	esotropia at near
DOB	date of birth	E(T)	intermittent esotropia at distance
DPE	dipivefrin		
DPT	diphtheria-pertussis-tetanus	E(T)'	intermittent esotropia at near
D&Q	deep and quiet	ETOH	elhanol; alcohol (in reference to alcohol abuse)
DR	diabetic retinopathy		
DT's	delirium tremens	EUA	examination under anesthesia
DTR	deep tendon reflexes	EVA	electronic visual aids
DUSN	diffuse unilateral subacute neuroretinitis	EW	Edinger-Westphal nucleus
		EW	extended wear contact lens
D&V	ductions and versions	EWSCL	extended-wear soft contact lens
DVD	dissociated vertical deviation		
DVM	optic disk, retinal vessels and macula		**F**
		FA, f/a	fluorescein angiogram/angiography
DVT	deep venous thrombosis		
DWSCL	daily-wear soft contact lens	FAV	foveal avascular zone
Dx	diagnosis	FB	foreign body
Dz	disease	FBS	fasting blood sugar test
		FBS	foreign body sensation
	E	FEF	frontal eye fields
E	esophoria at distance	FEM	fast eye movements
E'	esophoria at near	F + F	fix and follow vision
E	epinephrine	FEVR	familial exudative vitreal retinopathy
E 1	epinephrine 1%		
ECCE	extracapsular cataract extraction	FFA	fundus fluorescein angiography
ECD	endothelial cell density	FFF	flicker fusion frequency (fields)
ECG	electrocardiogram	FH	family history
EDMA	ethylene glyco-dy-methacrylate	FM 100	Farnsworth-Munsell 100-hue color vision test
EDTA	ethylene diamine tetra acetate		
EEG	electroencephalogram	FNA	fine needle aspiration
e.g.	for example *(exempligrata)*	FP	fixation preference

fpa	far point of accommodation		HK	herpes keratitis
FPL	forced preferential looking		HLA	human leukocyte antigen
FT	full-time		HM	hand motion/movement (vision)
F_3T	trifluorothymidine		h/o	history of
FTA	fluorescent treponema absorp- tion (test for syphilis)		HOTV	HOTV vision test
			H + P	history and physical
FTC	full to confrontation visual fields		HPI	history of present illness
FTFC	full to finger counting		HR	heart rate
FTG	full-time glasses		HRR	Hardy-Rand-Rittler (color plates)
FTO	full-time occlusion		h.s.	at bedtime *(hora somni)*
FTP	full-time patch		HS	herpes simplex
FTT	failure to thrive		HSK	herpes simplex keratitis
f/u	follow-up		HSV	herpes simplex virus
FUO	fever of unknown origin		hT	hypotropia at distance
Fx	fracture		hT'	hypotropia at near

G

H

I

			HT	hypertropia at distance
			HT'	hypertropia at near
GC	gonococcus (gonorrhea)		H(T)	intermittent hypertropia at distance
GCL	ganglion cell layer		H(T)'	intermittent hypertropia at near
GFR	glomerular filtration rate		HTN	hypertension
GHPC	giant helicoid peripapillary choroidopathy		HVF	Humphrey visual field
			Hx	history
GP	gas permeable (contact lens)		hypo	hypotropia
GPC	giant papillary conjunctivitis		HZ	herpes zoster
GSW	gun shot wound			
GTT	glucose tolerance test		I/A	infusion-aspiration (or) irrigation-aspiration
gtts	drops *(guttae)*			
GVF	Goldmann visual field		IC	inferior colliculus
Gy	Gray		IC	interstitial nucleus of Cajal
			ICCE	intracapsular cataract extraction
H	hyperphoria		ICD	intercanthal distance
HA	headache		ICE	iridocorneal epitheliopathy
HA	heart attack		ICG	indocyanine green (angiography)
HA 5	homatropine 5% eyedrops		ICP	intracranial pressure
HATTS	hemoagglutination treponema test for syphilis		ICR	intrastromal corneal ring
			ICU	intensive care unit
Hb	hemoglobin		IDDM	insulin-dependent diabetes mellitus
HBP	high blood pressure			
HCL	hard contact lens		IDU	idoxuridine
Hct	hematocrit		IgA	immunoglobulin A
HCTZ	hydrochlorthiazide		IgD	immunoglobulin D
HCVD	hypertensive cardiovascular disease		IgE	immunoglobulin E (hyper- sensitivity reactions)
HEMA	hydroxy ethyl methacrylate		IgG	immunoglobulin G (bacterial & viral infections)
Hgb	hemoglobin			
HGC	horizontal gaze center		IgM	immunoglobulin M (bacterial & viral infections)
HGLD3	test of the immune system			
HHC	home health care		IHD	ischemic heart disease
HIV	human immunodeficiency virus		IK	interstitial keratitis

ILM	internal limiting membrane	LCT	lateral canthal tendon
IM	intramuscular	LD	lattice degeneration
INL	inner nuclear layer	LE	left esophoria
INO	internuclear ophthalmoplegia	LE	left eye
IO	inferior oblique	LE	lupus erythematosus
IOFB	intraocular foreign body	LET	left esotropia
IOL	intraocular lens	LE(T)	intermittent left esotropia
ION	ischemic optic neuropathy	LFT	liver function test
IOP	intraocular pressure	LGB	lateral geniculate body
IPD	interpupillary distance/	LGN	lateral geniculate nucleus
	pupillary distance	LhT	left hypertropia
IPL	inner plexiform layer	LH(T)	intermittent left hypertropia
IR	inferior rectus	LHT	left hypotropia
IRMA	intraretinal microvascular	LID	left inferior oblique
	abnormalities	LIR	left inferior rectus
Ish.	Ishihara Plates (color vision test)	LKP	lamellar keratoplasty
ITT	induced topia test	LL	lower lid
IV	intravenous	LLL	left lower eyelid
IVFA	intravenous fluorescein	LLR	left lateral rectus
	angiography	LMG	lethal midline granuloma
		LMR	left medial rectus

J

		LOC	loss of consciousness
J1, J2...	Jaeger notation/size of type for	LOM	lens opacity meter
	near vision	LP	light perception
JODM	juvenile onset diabetes mellitus	LP	lumbar puncture
JRA	juvenile rheumatoid arthritis	LPCA	long posterior ciliary artery
JXG	juvenile xanthogranuloma	LPI	laser peripheral iridotomy
		LP + P	light perception and projection
		LPw/P	light perception with projection

K

K	curvature	LR	lateral rectus
K	flattest meridian of keratometry	LSO	left superior oblique
	reading	LSR	left superior rectus
K	potassium	LTG	low tension glaucoma
KCS	keratoconjunctivitis sicca	LTP	laser trabeculoplasty
KOH	potassium hydroxide	LUL	left upper eyelid
KPs	keratic precipitates	LVA	low vision aids
KrF	krypton fluoride	LVH	left ventricular hypertrophy
KS	keratitis sicca	L + W	living and well
K sicca	keratoconjunctivitis sicca	LXT	left exotropia
KUB	kidney, ureter, bladder	LX(T)	intermittent left exotropia

L

M

L	left	M	macula
L	lensometer	M	manifest refraction
LA	light adaptation	M	meter
LASER	light amplification by stimulated	M 1	tropicamide (Mydriacyl)
	emission of radiation		1% eyedrops
LASIK	laser in situ keratomileusis (or)	Max	maximum
	laser assisted intrastromal	Max	maxitrol
	keratoplasty	MCA	middle cerebral artery

MCE	microcystic edema	NMI	no manifest improvement
MCT	medial canthal tendon	nml	normal
MEWDS	multifocal evanescent white dot syndrome	NMR	nuclear magnetic resonance
MG	Marcus-Gunn pupil	NP	near point (punctum proximum)
MG	myasthenia gravis	npa	near point of accommodation
MGD	meibomian gland dysfunction	npc	near point of convergence
MI	myocardial infarction; heart attack	NPDR	non-proliferative diabetic retinopathy
MICU	medical intensive care unit	n.p.o.	nothing by mouth (nil per os)
MKM	myopic keratomileusis	NR	non-reactive
MLF	medial longitudinal fasciculus	NRC	normal retinal correspondence
mm.	millimeter	NS	Neosynephrine
MMC	mitomycin C	NS	normal saline
monos	monocytes	NS	nuclear sclerosis
MPP	massive preretinal proliferation	NSAID	non-steroidal anti-inflammatory drug
MPR	massive preretinal retraction	N + V	nausea and vomiting
MPS	mucopolysaccharidosis	NVD	neovascularization of the disc
MR	manifest refraction	NVE	neovascularization elsewhere
MR	medial rectus	NVG	neovascular glaucoma
MRD	marginal reflex distance	NVM	neovascular membrane
MRI	magnetic resonance imaging		
MRSA	methicillin-resistant staph aureus		
MS	multiple sclerosis		

N

N	near
N	near vision
N	Neptazane
N 2.5	phenylephrine HCl (Neosynephrine) 2.5% eyedrops
N 50	Neptazane 50 mg
NA	not applicable
Na	sodium
NaCl	sodium chloride; saline
NDF	neutral density filter test
NdYAG	neodymium yittrium-aluminum-garnet laser
Neo	neosynephrine
NFL	nerve fiber layer
NI	no improvement; not improvable
NICU	neonatal intensive care unit
NKA	no known allergies
NKDA	no known drug allergies
nl	normal
NLD	nasolacrimal duct
NLP	no light perception; total blindness
nm	nanometer

O

O_2	oxygen
OA	overactive muscle
OAG	open angle glaucoma
OA IO	overactive inferior oblique
OA IO OU	overactive inferior obliques, both eyes
OA SO	overactive superior oblique
OA SO OU	overactive superior obliques, both eyes
OD	right eye (oculus dexter)
OD	optic disc
OD	overdose
ODM	ophthalmodynamometry
ODN	ophthalmodynamometry
OHT	ocular hypertension
OKN	optokinetic nystagmus
ON	optic nerve
ONG	optic nerve glioma
ONL	outer plexiform layer
ONSD	optic nerve sheath decompression
ONSF	optic nerve sheath fenestration
ophth.	ophthalmology, ophthalmic, etc.
OPL	outer plexiform layer
OR	operating room
OR	over-refraction
Ortho.	orthophoria
OS	left eye (oculus sinister)

OT	ocular tension	PH	past history
OT	orthotropia	ph	pinhole (visual acuity)
OU	both eyes *(oculus uterque)*	PHF	posterior hyaloid face
OWS	overwear syndrome	PHM	posterior hyaloid membrane
		PHN	post herpetic neuralgia

P

p	after *(post)*	PHNI	pinhole, no improvement
P	pilocarpine	PHPV	persistent hyperplasia of the primary vitreous/persistent hyperplastic primary vitreous
P 1	Pilocarpine 1% eyedrops		
P	pupil	PI	peripheral iridectomy/iridotomy
PA	periarteritis nodosa	PI	phospholine iodide
PACG	primary angle closure glaucoma	PI	present illness
PACT	prism + alternate cover test	PICU	pediatric intensive care unit
PAM	primary acquired melanosis	PK	penetrating keratoplasty
PAM	potential acuity meter	PKP	penetrating keratoplasty
PAN	periarteritis nodosa	PKU	phenylketonuria
PAS	peripheral anterior synechia	pl	piano lens
PAT	prism adaptation test	PLS	posterior lip sclerectomy
PBI	protein bound iodine	PLT	preferential looking technique
PBK	pseudophakic bullous keratopathy	PMH	past medical history
p.c.	after meals *(post cibum)*	PMMA	polymethylmethacrylate
PC	peripheral curve	PMN	polymorphonuclear leukocyte
PC	post-cycloplegic	PN	periarteritis nodosa
PC	posterior capsule	PNS	peripheral nervous system
PC	posterior chamber	p.o.	by mouth *(per os)*
PC	posterior commissure	po	post-operative
PC	present correction	POAG	primary open angle glaucoma
P + C	prism and cover test	POHS	presumed ocular histoplasmosis syndrome
PCA	posterior cerebral artery		
PCIOL	posterior chamber intraocular lens	poly's	polymorphonuclear leukocytes
PCN	penicillin	POZ	posterior optical zone
PD	pupillary distance (or) interpupillary distance	p.p.	after eating *(post prandial)*
		PP	pars plana
PD	prism diopter	PP	pars plicata
PDR	Physicians Desk Reference	PP	near point *(punctum proximum)*
PDR	proliferative diabetc retinopathy	PPA	near point *(punctum proximum)* of accommodation
PE	physical exam		
PE	(retinal) pigment epithelium	PPC	near point *(punctum proximum)* of convergence
PE	pulmonary embolus		
PEO	progressive external ophthal-moplegia	PPD	purified protein derivative (tuberculin skin test)
PERRLA	pupils equal, round and reactive to light and accommodation	PPDR	preproliferative diabetic retinopathy
PET	partial excimer trabeculectomy	PPG	pilopine gel
PF	pred forte	PPL	pars plana lensectomy
PFCL	perfluorocarbon liquid	PPMD	posterior polymorphous dystrophy
PFT	pulmonary function test	PPRF	pontine paramedian reticular formation
PGC	pontine gaze center		
pH	measure of acidity/alkalinity of a solution	PPV	pars plane vitrectomy
		PR	far point *(punctum remotum)* of accommodation

PRK	photorefractive keratectomy	RA	react to accommodation
prn	when necessary, as the occasion arises *(pro re nata)*	RA	rheumatoid arthritis
		R & R	recess and resect (recess-resect)
PRP	panretinal photocoagulation		
PRRE	pupils round, regular & equal	RAPD	relative afferent pupillary defect
PSC	posterior subcapsular cataract	RB	retinoblastoma
PSCC	posterior subcapsular cataract	RBC	red blood cell (erythrocyte)
PSD	paving stone degeneration	RBC	red blood count
PSP	progressive supranuclear palsy	RD	retinal detachment
pt	patient	RDE	random dot E stereogram
PT	prothrombin time	RE	right esophoria
PTA	prior to admission	RE	right eye
PTC	pseudotumor cerebri	Ref	refraction
PTK	phototherapeutic keratectomy	REM	rapid eye movements
PTN	pre-tectal nucleus	RET	retinoscopy
PTO	part time occlusion (patch)	RET	right esotropia
PTP	part time patch	RE(T)	intermittent right esotropia
PTT	partial thromboplastin time	ret. pig.	retinitis pigmentosa
PVA	polyvinyl alcohol	RGP	rigid gas permeable (contact lens)
PVC	premature ventricular contraction		
PVD	posterior vitreous detachment	RHT	right hypertropia
PVD	principal visual direction	RH(T)	intermittent right hypertropia
PVR	proliferative vitreoretinopathy		
Px	prognosis	RhT	right hypotropia
PXE	pseudo-xanthoma elasticum	RIO	right inferior oblique
PXF	pseudo exfoliation	RIR	right inferior rectus
		RK	radial keratotomy

Q

q.a.m.	every day before noon *(quaque ante meridiem)*	RLF	retrolental fibroplasia
		RLL	right lower eyelid
q.d.	every day *(quaque die)*	RLR	right lateral rectus
q.h.	every hour *(quaque hora)*	RMR	right medial rectus
q.h.s.	every bedtime *(quaque hora somni)*	r/o	rule out
q.i.d.	4 times a day *(quater in die)*	ROP	retinopathy of prematurity
q.n.	every night *(quaque nocte)*	ROS	review of systems
q.n.s.	quantity not sufficient *(quantum non sufficiat)*	RP	retinitis pigmentosa
		RPA	retinitis punctata albescens
q.o.d.	every other day *(quaque die)*	RPE	retinal pigment epithelium
q.p.m.	every day after noon *(quaque postmeridiem)*	RPED	retinal pigment epithelium detachment
		RSO	right superior oblique
q.s.	sufficient quantity *(quantum sufficiat)*	RSR	right superior rectus
		RT	radiation therapy
q 3 h	every 3 hours *(quaque 3 hora)*	RTC	return to clinic
		RTO	return to office

R

R	recession (of extraocular muscle)	RUL	right upper eyelid
R	refraction	Rx	treatment: glasses, medicine, etc.
R	resection (of extraocular muscle)	RX	right exophoria
R	retinoscopy	RXT	right exotropia
R	right	RX(T)	intermittent right exotropia

S

s	without *(sin)*
S	spectacles
S	sphere
SB	scleral buckling procedure
SBC	sensory binocular cooperation
SBV	single binocular vision
sc	subcutaneous
sc	without correction *(sin correctio)*
SC	superior colliculus
SCC	squamous cell carcinoma
SCH	subconjunctival hemorrhage
SCH	suprachoroidal hemorrhage
SCL	soft contact lens
SCT	single cover test
SEM	slow eye movements
SEM	scanning electron microscope/ microscopy
SF_6	sulfur hexafluoride
SFG	sulfur hexafluoride gas
SFP	simultaneous foveal perception
SG	Sheridan-Gardner visual acuity test
SI	sector iridectomy
SICU	surgical intensive care unit
SLE	slit lamp exam
SLE	systemic lupus erythematosus
SMCD	senile macular and choroidal degeneration
SMD	senile macular degeneration
SMP	simultaneous macular perception
SO	superior oblique
SOB	shortness of breath
SOF	superior orbital fissure
soln	solution
SOV	superior ophthalmic vein
s/p	condition after *(status post)*
SPCA	short posterior ciliary artery
SPCT	simultaneous prism & cover test
Sph	sphere
SPK	superficial punctate keratitis
SQ	subcutaneous (under the skin)
SR	superior rectus
SRF	subretinal fluid
SRH	subretinal hemorrhage
SRK	Sanders, Retzlaff, Kraff formula (for IOL power)
SRM	subretinal membrane
SRN	subretinal neovascularization
SRNV	subretinal neovascularization
SRNVM	subretinal neovascular membrane
SS	scleral spur
S/S	signs and symptoms
SSPE	subacute sclerosing pan-encephalitis
ST	esotropia (at distance)
ST'	esotropia at near
S(T)	intermittent esotropia at distance
S(T)'	intermittent esotropia at near
stat.	immediately
subcut.	subcutaneous (under the skin)
sub q	subcutaneous (under the skin)
SVP	spontaneous venous pulsation
Sx	symptoms

T

T	tension
T 0.5	timolol maleate (Timoptic) 0.5% eyedrops
TA	tension by applanation
tab	tablet
TAC	Teller acuity cards
TAP	tension by applanation
Tapp	tension by applanation
TB	tuberculosis
TBT	tear break-up time
TBUT	tear break-up time
TFT	thyroid function test
TFT	trifluorothymidine
TIA	transient ischemic attack
t.i.d.	3 times a day *(ter in die)*
TM	trabecular meshwork
TN	tension
TNF	tension normal by finger (palpation)
TNO	TNO stereopsis test
TNTC	too numerous to count
TORCH	toxoplasmosis, rubella, cyto-megalovirus, herpes
TOV	transcient obscuration of vision
Tp	tension by pneumotonometry
Tp	toxoplasmosis
TPI	treponema pallidum immobili-zation test
Tpn	tension by pneumotonometer
TPPL	trans pars plana lensectomy
TPPV	trans pars plana vitrectomy
Trab.	trabeculectomy

TRD	total retinal detachment
TRD	traction retinal detachment
TRIC	trachoma or inclusion conjunctivitis (agent)
Ts	tension by Schiotz
Tx	treatment

U

UA	underactive (muscle)
U/A	urinalysis
UA IO	underactive inferior oblique
UA IO OU	underactive inferior obliques, both eyes
UA SO	underactve superior obliques
UA SO OU	underactive superior obliques, both eyes
UCUSUM	uncentral unsteady unmaintained fixation
UGH	uveitis glaucoma hyphema syndrome
UL	upper lid
ung	ointment
UPECCE	unplanned extracapsular cataract extraction
URTI	upper respiratory tract infection
URI	upper respiratory tract infection
US	ultrasound
UTI	urinary tract infection

V

V	vessels
V	visual acuity
V	vitreous
VA	visual acuity
VDRL	venereal disease research lab
VECP	visual evoked cortical potential
VEP	visual evoked potential
VER	visual evoked response
VF	visual field

VGC	vertical gaze center
VISC	vitreous infusion suction cutter
Vit.	vitreous
VKH	Vogt-Koyanagi-Harada syndrome
VOD	vision right eye
VOR	vestibulo-ocular reflex
VOS	vision left eye
VOU	vision both eyes
VS, V/S	vital signs
VSS	vital signs stable

W

WBC	white blood cells or count
WD WN	well developed, well nourished
WEBINO	wall-eyed bilateral internuclear ophthalmoplegia
WF	white female
W4D	Worth 4-dot test
WGOA	wearing glasses on arrival
WM	white male
WNL	within normal limits
WPOA	wearing patch on arrival
WTR	with-the-rule astigmatism
w/u	work-up

X

x	axis
X	exophoria at distance
X'	exophoria at near
XLR	X-linked recessive
XT	exotropia at distance
XT'	exotropia at near
X(T)	intermittent exotropia at distance
X(T)'	intermittent exotropia at near

Y

YAG	yittrium-aluminum-garnet laser
y/o	years old

abducens (ab-DU-senz). *Anatomy.* Sixth cranial nerve. Motor nerve that in-nervates the lateral rectus muscle, enabling each eye to rotate outward (away from nose). Originates in lower pons area of the brainstem; enters the orbit through the superior orbital fissure.

abducens palsy, lateral rectus *(or)* **6th nerve palsy.** *Pathologic condition.* Partial or total loss of function of the 6th (abducens) cranial nerve. The affected eye deviates inward (esotropia) and has defective ability to turn out beyond the midline (abduct) since it no longer receives adequate innervation; thus the deviation becomes greater and more apparent when both eyes rotate toward the affected side.

abduct (ab-DUKT). *Function.* To move away from the midline. See also ADDUCT.

abduction (ab-DUK-shun). *Function.* Movement away from the midline, e.g., outward rotation of an eye from the straight-ahead position. See also ADDUC-TION.

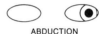

abductor (ad-DUK-tur). *Anatomy.* Muscle that moves a part of the body away from the midline. In the eye, the abductor muscles move the eyeball out-ward (away from nose) from the straight-ahead position; primary abduc-tor is the lateral rectus.

aberrant regeneration (ab-EHR-unt). *Functional defect.* Abnormal regrowth of damaged nerve fibers along preexisting pathways; e.g., following injury to the 3rd cranial nerve, regenerated nerve fibers to the inferior rectus muscle may grow into the upper eyelid and cause it to rise (instead of lower) when the eye looks down. See also PSEUDO-VON GRAEFE'S SIGN.

aberration ab-ur-AY-shun). *Optics.* Blurred or distorted image quality that re-sults from inherent physical properties (shape, curvature, density) of an optical device (lens or prism).

   chromatic (kroh-MAT-ik): distortion of an image into images with fuzzy and colored edges; occurs because different wavelengths of light are re-fracted to different extents.

   spherical: type of blur caused by light rays (from an object point) strik-ing the lens periphery where they are bent too much (overrefracted).

abetalipoproteinemia (ay-BAY-tuh-LI-poh-PROH-teen-EE-mee-uh), **Bassen-Kornzweig syndrome.** *Pathologic condition.* Characterized by inability of the body to absorb fats (lipids), malformed red blood cells, progressive nervous system defects, and retinitis pigmentosa. Retinal changes re-semble those in vitamin A deficiency (rod vision deteriorates before cone vision). Congenital; hereditary.

ablate (ab-LATE). *Procedure.* To remove or destroy tissue, as by radiation or photocoagulation.

ablation (ab-LAY-shun). *Procedure.* Removal or destruction of tissue, as by radiation or photocoagulation.

ablepharon (ay-BLEF-ur-ahn). *Congenital anomaly.* Absence of eyelids.

abnormal retinal correspondence (ARC). See ANOMALOUS RETINAL CORRES-PONDENCE.

abrade. To scrape or rub away a surface; chafe. See also ABRASION.

abrasion, corneal abrasion. *Injury.* Scraped area of corneal surface; ac-companied by loss of superficial tissue (epithelium).

absolute glaucoma (glaw-KOH-muh). *Pathologic condition.* End-stage of glaucoma, in which intraocular pressure remains elevated and vision is completely lost.

absolute hyperopia (hi-pur-OH-pee-uh). *Refractive error.* Refers to an eye with insufficient optical power, whose natural lens does not automatically compensate by increasing its plus power. Corrected by a plus lens (spectacle or contact) of the smallest optical power that enables the patient to see clearly. See also HYPEROPIA.

absolute scotoma (skuh-TOH-muh). *Functional defect.* Blind area within the visual field where any target, regardless of size or brightness, is invisible. See also BLIND SPOT, RELATIVE SCOTOMA.

Absorbonac. *Drug.* Trade name of hypertonic sodium chloride eyedrops.

absorptive lenses, sunglasses. *Optical device.* Spectacles whose lenses absorb a high percentage of light, thus reducing the amount of light transmitted to the eye. Worn in bright sunlight for comfort and for protection from light damage.

Acanthamoeba (ay-kan-thuh-MEE-buh). *Organism.* Single-celled organism (protozoan) found in soil and contaminated water. Can cause a severe corneal infection (keratitis) after improperly sterilized extended wear contact lenses are worn.

AC/A ratio (accommodative convergence/accommodation ratio). *Function.* Numerical expression for the relationship between the amount both eyes simultaneously turn inward (converge) and the amount their lenses increase in power (accommodate). In normal individuals this ratio averages 5:1. Accommodative convergence is expressed in prism diopters (Δ), and accommodation is expressed in diopters (D).

accommadation. Incorrect spelling of ACCOMMODATION.

accommodation (uh-kah-muh-DAY-shun). *Function.* Increase in optical power by the eye in order to maintain a clear image (focus) as objects are moved closer. Occurs through a process of ciliary muscle contraction and zonular relaxation that causes the elastic-like lens to "round up" and increase its optical power. See also PRESBYOPIA.

    amplitude of a: maximum increase in optical power produced by a change in shape of the lens; maximal (18 diopters) at birth, decreasing to almost zero by age 60.

    far-point of a: most distant point from the eye at which an object can be seen clearly.

    near point of a: position closest to the eye where a small object (usually small print) can be kept in sharp focus by maximal accommodation. See also PRINCE RULE.

    range of a: distance (from eye) between the nearest and farthest points at which clear vision can be maintained.

accommodative convergence. *Function.* Portion of the range of inward rotation (toward nose) of both eyes that occurs in response to an increase in optical power for focusing (accommodation) by the eyes' lenses.

accommodative convergence/accommodation ratio. See AC/A RATIO.

accommodative effort syndrome. *Functional defect.* Eyestrain and blurred vision at near that results from excessive focusing effort of the eye's crystalline lens, to see near objects clearly.

accommodative esotropia (ee-soh-TROH-pee-uh). *Functional defect.* Excessive inward (toward nose) turning of an eye caused by an overactive convergence response to the accommodative effort necessary to keep vision clear. More common in farsighted (hyperopic) children. Eyeglass correction for the hyperopia relaxes accommodation, allowing the eyes to remain properly aligned. Sometimes bifocals are necessary to correct the excessive inturning at near. See also AC/A RATIO, ACQUIRED ESOTROPIA, NON-ACCOMMODATIVE ESOTROPIA.

accommodative palsy. *Functional defect.* Inability to focus the eyes for near objects (accommodation). Usually occurs after concussion or whiplash injury. Gradual recovery may occur in weeks to years.

accommodative spasm. *Functional defect*. The eye's crystalline lens does not relax after accommodating (increasing optical power for focusing), resulting in vision that is sharp for near but not for distance. The entire near-reflex is also in spasm, with pupils constricted and eyes overconverged (esotropia). Associated with hysteria. Responds to atropine, eye exercises, or time. See also CONVERGENCE SPASM, PSEUDOMYOPIA.

accommodative target. *Test object*. Small object, held at a standard distance (16 in. or 20 ft.); requires visual acuity of 20/40 or better and maximal focusing (accommodative) effort to be seen clearly. Used during refraction or motility testing.

accommodometer (uh-kah-moh-DAH-muh-tur). *Instrument*. Hand-held paddle with a window for presenting size-graded symbols; used for measuring convergence control as patient focuses (accommodates).

accomodation. Incorrect spelling of ACCOMMODATION.

acetazolamide (uh-see-tuh-ZOH-luh-mide). *Drug*. Oral medication that decreases aqueous fluid production by the ciliary body, lowering intraocular pressure. Used for treating glaucoma. Trade name: Diamox. See also CARBONIC ANHYDRASE INHIBITOR.

acetylcholine (uh-see-til-KOH-leen). *Chemical*. Occurs natually in the body; transmits impulses across nerve junctions throughout the nervous system. Administered into the eye during surgery as a cholinergic stimulator, to induce pupillary constriction (miosis). Trade name: Miochol.

achromatic lens (ay-kroh-MAT-ik). *Optics*. Lens that combines a plus lens (of one refractive index) and a minus lens (different refractive index); minimizes fuzziness and colored edges of images (chromatic aberration) by reducing the dispersion of white light into its spectral colors.

achromatic perimetry (puh-RIM-uh-tree). *Test*. Visual field examination with white targets.

achromatopsia (ay-kroh-muh-TAHP-see-uh), **monochromacy**. *Congenital defect*. Rare inability to distinguish colors. Nonprogressive; hereditary. See also CONE MONOCHROMACY, ROD MONOCHROMACY.

Achromycin. *Drug*. Trade name of tetracycline, an antibiotic.

acid burns. *Injury*. Conjunctival and corneal burns from contact with acid, which can result in severe, irreversible vision loss. Immediate, copious irrigation with water for up to 30 minutes is mandatory to dilute and wash away the acid. If a corneal scar forms, a corneal graft may be necessary to restore vision.

acidophilic adenoma (uh-sid-oh-FIL-ik ad-in-OH-muh). *Pathologic condition*. Tumor of the anterior lobe of the pituitary gland (so named because its cells absorb stain from acid dyes). Systemic effects caused by presence of excessive hormones are conspicuous, but vision and visual field losses do not tend to be severe.

acommodation. Incorrect spelling of ACCOMMODATION.

acquired esotropia (ee-soh-TROH-pee-uh). *Functional defect*. Inward (toward nose) eye deviation that appears after the age of 6 months. Often helped by eyeglasses.

acquired retinal arterial macroaneurysm (ARAM). *Pathologic condition*. Sac-like outpouching of the retinal artery that can lead to leakage of fluid or blood, most commonly from the superotemporal artery. Occurs after age 60; associated with high blood pressure. Usually self-limited, with resolution of the leakage. See also BRANCH VEIN OCCLUSION, DIABETIC RETINOPATHY.

acrocephalosyndactylia of Apert (ak-roh-SEF-uh-loh-sin-dak-TEE-lee-uh), **Apert's syndrome**. *Congenital anomaly*. Characterized by severe mental retardation, heart and kidney malformations, underdevelopment of mid-portion of face, and webbed fingers and toes. Eye defects may include shallow orbits, protruding eyes, exposed corneas, widely spaced eyes, outward deviation (exotropia), optic nerve damage, and visual field disorders. See also CROUZON'S SYNDROME.

actinic keratosis (ak-TIN-ik kehr-uh-TOH-sis), **solar keratosis**. *Pathologic condition*. Flat, scaly precancerous skin lesion(s) that appear on skin that is dry and wrinkled from years of sun exposure, usually in fair-skinned persons. May occur on eyelids. See also CUTANEOUS HORN.

acuity, visual acuity. *Measurement*. Measure of an eye's ability to distinguish object details and shape. Assessed by the smallest identifiable object that can be seen at a specified distance (usually 20 ft. or 16 in.).

Acular. *Drug*. Trade name of ketorolac tromethamine eyedrops; for treating allergic conjuctivitis.

acute. Of sudden, rapid onset, usually with notable symptoms. See also CHRONIC.

acute angle closure glaucoma (AACG) (glaw-KOH-muh), **angle closure *(or)* closed angle *(or)* narrow angle glaucoma**. *Pathologic condition*. Sudden rise in intraocular pressure. Aqueous fluid behind the iris cannot pass through the pupil and pushes the iris forward, preventing drainage through the angle (pupillary block mechanism). Occurs in patients with narrow anterior chamber angles. See also OPEN-ANGLE GLAUCOMA.

acute multifocal placoid pigment epitheliopathy (PLAK-oyd, ep-uh-thee-lee-AH-puh-thee). See AMPPE.

acute retinal necrosis. See ARN.

acute spastic entropion. *Pathologic condition*. Inward turning of an eyelid following acute lid infections or long-term patching of the eye.

acyclovir (ay-SI-kloh-veer). *Drug*. Antiviral agent used for treating herpetic eye infections. See also ACUTE RETINAL NECROSIS, CMV RETINITIS, FOSCARNET SODIUM, GANCICLOVIR.

add. 1. *Optics*. Amount of plus power required for near use (over eyeglass correction for distance). 2. *Optical device*. Plus lens fused to corrective eyeglasses (usually lower part); used for near work to compensate for the decrease in focusing ability (accommodation) that occurs normally with age. See also BIFOCALS, PRESBYOPIA.

Addison's disease. *Pathologic condition*. Destructive disease marked by deficient adrenocortical secretion and characterized by extreme weakness, loss of weight, low blood pressure, gastrointestinal disturbances, and brownish pigmentation of the skin and mucous membranes.

adduct (ad-DUKT). *Function*. To move toward the midline. See also ABDUCT.

adduction (ad-DUK-shun). *Function*. Movement toward the midline; inward rotation of an eye from the straight-ahead position. See also ABDUCTION.

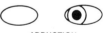
ADDUCTION

adductor (ad-DUK-tur). *Anatomy*. Muscle that moves a part of the body toward the midline. In the eye, the adductor muscles rotate the eyeball inward (toward the nose) from the straight-ahead position; the primary adductor is the medial rectus. See also ABDUCTOR.

adenoma. *Pathologic condition*. Benign tumor of a glandular structure or of glandular origin. Plural: adenomas, adenomata.

adenopathy (ad-en-AHP-uh-thee). *Pathologic condition*. Enlargement or involvement of glands, especially lymph nodes.

adenovirus (ADV) (AD-en-oh-vi-rus). *Microorganism*. Family of more than 30 viruses that can cause upper respiratory infections, conjunctivitis, and inflammation of the mucous membranes.

adherence syndrome, Johnson syndrome. *Congenital anomaly*. Limitation of outward eye movement (abduction) caused by adhesions between the lateral rectus and inferior oblique muscle sheaths, or limitation of upward eye movement caused by adhesions between the superior rectus and superior oblique muscle sheaths.

adherent leukoma (lu-KOH-muh). *Anatomic defect.* Dense corneal opacity to which the iris is attached.

adhesive syndrome, cicatricial strabismus. *Functional defect.* Limitation of eye movement with damage and scarring of muscle cone or supportive tissue (e.g., Tenon's capsule and fat); found after orbital trauma or surgery. See also RESTRICTIVE SYNDROME.

Adie's pupil (AY-deez), **pupillotonia, tonic pupil**. *Pathologic condition.* Characterized by slow pupillary constriction to light, with sluggish redilation and decreased focusing ability for near (accommodation). Unilateral; at first the affected pupil is larger, later smaller than in the fellow eye. Seen with diseases of, or injury to, the ciliary ganglion, often in young women. See also MECHOLYL TEST.

adjustable sutures. *Surgical technique.* Surgical stitches that can be shortened or lengthened after surgery to obtain better eye alignment. May be used in reattaching an extraocular muscle.

adnexa oculi (ad-NEKS-uh AH-kyu-li), **appendages of the eye, ocular adnexa**. *Anatomy.* Structures surrounding the eyeball; includes eyelids, eyebrows, tear drainage system, orbital walls, and orbital contents.

adrenergic blocking agent, beta blocker, sympatholytic drug. *Drug.* 1. Used topically for treating glaucoma. Blocks action of sympathetic nerve fibers by blocking beta adrenergic receptor sites for nerve impulse transmission; sometimes causes pupillary constriction. Betaxolol is a beta-one blocker; carteolol, levobunolol, metipranolol and timolol are beta-one and beta-two blockers. 2. Used systemically as heart medication to treat rapid arrhythmia and hypertension. Discontinuation may decrease intraocular pressure control.

adrenergic stimulating agent, sympathomimetic drug (sim-path-oh-mim-ET-ik). *Drug.* Mimics action of sympathetic nerves. Used (1) to control glaucoma by opening the anterior chamber angle to increase aqueous outflow, decrease aqueous secretion and help nerve transmission (beta-two receptors); examples: aproclonidine, dipivefrin, epinephrine, isoproterenol; (2) to dilate the pupil without affecting accommodation; examples: hydroxyamphetamine, phenylephrine; (3) to "whiten" the eye by constricting dilated conjunctival blood vessels; examples: naphazoline, phenylephrine, tetrahydrozaline.

Adsorbocarpine (ad-zor-boh-KAHR-peen). *Drug.* Trade name of pilocarpine eyedrops; for treating glaucoma.

Adsorbotear (ad-ZOR-boh-tir). *Drug.* Trade name of eyedrop containing methylcellulose and polyvinyl alcohol; for treating dry eyes.

advancement. *Surgical procedure.* Movement of an eye muscle from its attachment on the eyeball to a more forward position, to strengthen its action.

advancement flap. *Surgical procedure.* Type of conjunctival or skin flap used for covering a defect or for reconstructing eyelids.

aerial haze. Atmospheric conditions that give distant objects a bluish haze; provides a monocular cue to depth perception. See also MONOCULAR DEPTH PERCEPTION.

afakia. Incorrect spelling of APHAKIA.

afebrile (ay-FEH-brile). Without fever.

afferent nerve, input *(or)* **sensory nerve**. *Anatomy.* Any nerve that carries sensory information (impulses) toward the brain or spinal cord, e.g., 2nd cranial (optic) nerve. See also EFFERENT NERVE.

afferent pupillary defect (AF-ur-unt). See MARCUS-GUNN PUPIL.

afocal. *Optics.* Without a focal point.

after-cataract, secondary cataract. *Pathologic condition.* Remnants of an opaque lens remaining in the eye or opacities forming after extracapsular cataract removal. See also ELSCHNIG PEARLS.

after-image. *Illusion.* Image that continues to be seen following exposure of one or both eyes to a bright light. See also ENTOPIC PHENOMENON.

after-image test. A horizontal and a vertical streak of light, one before each eye, are used for determining whether retinal correspondence is normal or anomalous.

"against" motion. *Optics.* Image movement in the opposite direction from the movement of the instrument, light, or lens that creates it, e.g., image seen in the patient's pupil moves in the opposite direction from light from a retinoscope; can be neutralized with minus lenses. See also RETINOS-COPY, "WITH" MOTION.

"against-the-rule" astigmatism. *Refractive error.* Optical power that is greater (more plus power) in the horizontal meridian of an eye than in the vertical meridian. See also "WITH-THE-RULE" ASTIGMATISM.

age-related macular degeneration (AMD, ARMD) (MAK-yu-lur), **macular** *(or)* **senile macular degeneration**. *Pathologic condition.* Group of conditions that include deterioration of the macula, resulting in a loss of sharp central vision. Two general types: "dry," which is usually evident as a disturbance of macular pigmentation and deposits of yellowish material under the pigment epithelial layer in the central retinal zone; "wet," (sometimes called Kuhnt-Junius disease) in which abnormal new blood vessels grow under the retina and leak fluid and blood, further disturbing macular function. Most common cause of decreased vision after age 60.

agnosia (ag-NOH-zhuh). *Functional defect.* Inability to recognize common objects regardless of visual acuity.

agonist, primary mover. *Function.* Extraocular muscle primarily responsible for moving eye into desired position. See also ANTAGONIST.

Aicardi syndrome (ay-KAR-dee). *Pathologic condition.* Cerebroretinal disorder that includes central nervous system malformations and absence of the corpus callosum. Ocular findings include retinal malformation with non-pigmented chorioretinal spots, especially near the optic disc. Hereditary.

air fluid gas exchange (AFGE). *Surgical procedure.* Replacement of vitreal fluid with air or gas; sometimes used with vitrectomy and retinal detachment surgery. Liquid is drawn from the vitreous through one port of the vitrectomy instrument as air is injected through another port. See also PERFLUOROPROPANE, SULPHUR HEXAFLUORIDE.

Airvin-Gass syndrome. Incorrect spelling of IRVINE-GASS SYNDROME.

AK-Chlor. *Drug.* Trade name of chloramphenicol, broad-spectrum antibiotic eyedrops or ointment.

AK-Con. *Drug.* Trade name of naphazoline decongestant eyedrop; "whitens" the eyes.

AK-Dilate. *Drug.* Trade name of phenylephrine; for dilating the pupil.

akinesia (ah-kin-EE-shuh). *Functional loss.* Loss or impairment of voluntary muscle activity leading to immobility, as with the injection of a local anesthetic before surgery.

alacrima (uh-LAK-ruh-muh). *Functional defect.* Lack of tear production. See also RILEY-DAY SYNDROME.

AK-Mycin. *Drug.* Trade name of erythromycin, an antibiotic ointment.

AK-Mydfrin. *Drug.* Trade name of phenylephrine; for dilating the pupil.

AK-NaCl. *Drug.* Trade name of hypertonic sodium chloride ointment.

AK-Nefrin. *Drug.* Trade name of phenylephrine eyedrops; "whitens" the eyes.

AK-Pred. *Drug.* Trade name of prednisolone, anti-inflammatory steroid eyedrops.

AK-Taine. *Drug*. Trade name of proparacaine, a local anesthetic for the eye.

AK-Tracin. *Drug*. Trade name of bacitracin, an antibiotic used for treating mild external eye infections.

AKWA Tears. *Drug*. Trade name of polyvinyl alcohol eyedrops or ointment; for treating dry eyes.

Albalon (AL-buh-lahn). *Drug*. Trade name of naphazoline decongestant eyedrops; "whitens" the eyes.

albinism (AL-bin-izm). *Congenital defect*. Lack of pigment in eyes, hair and skin. Usually associated with decreased visual acuity, rhythmic side-to-side eye movements (nystagmus) and light sensitivity (photophobia).

　　ocular: lack of pigment in iris and choroid; results in reddish pupils and iris (from choroidal vessels seen through overlying retina). Usually accompanied by poor vision, photophobia, and nystagmus.

Albright's disease, polyostotic fibrous dysplasia. *Pathologic condition*. Characterized by pigmented skin lesions, early puberty, and bone abnormalities. Eye findings include protrusion of the eye (proptosis) and visual field defects resulting from compression of the optic nerve.

Alcaine. *Drug*. Trade name of proparacaine anesthetic eyedrops.

alcohol amblyopia. *Functional defect*. Bilateral vision loss with central field defects, presumably caused by poisoning from drinking ethyl or methyl alcohol or by poor nutrition. See also TOXIC AMBLYOPIA.

Alexander's law. *Abnormal function*. Rhythmic side-to-side eye movements (nystagmus) increase when the eyes look in the direction of the faster phase of the movement.

alexia (uh-LEK-see-uh). *Functional defect*. Total inability to read despite normal vision. Caused by brain damage.

alkali burns. *Injury*. Chemical burns from contact with an alkali substance; can cause severe ocular scarring and permanent vision loss. Immediate, copious irrigation with water for 30 minutes is mandatory to dilute and wash away alkali liquid or particles. Meticulous inspection for residual alkali should be followed with prolonged saline solution irrigation. See also ACID BURNS.

alkaptonuria (al-kap-tun-YUR-ee-uh). *Pathologic condition*. Metabolic disorder characterized by dark urine, tendency to heart and blood vessel diseases, and pigmentation of connective tissue, cornea, sclera and conjunctiva. Rare; hereditary.

Allen cards. *Test object*. Set of picture cards used for testing vision in preschool children.

allergic conjunctivitis. *Pathologic condition*. Hypersensitivity of the conjunctiva (membrane covering white of eyes and inner lids) to foreign substances. Characterized by discharge, itching, irritation, swelling, tearing, redness, and light sensitivity. The discharge contains a large number of white blood cells (eosinophils).

alloplastic intrastromal lens. *Optical device*. Intracorneal implant of rigid impermeable plastic. See also HYDROGEL, KERATOPHAKIA.

Alomide. *Drug*. Trade name of lodoxamide eyedrops; for treating allergic and vernal conjunctivitis.

alpha (angle). *Optics*. Angle formed at the nodal point of an eye between the visual axis and the optic axis.

alpha adrenergic. *Drug*. Compound that enhances the action of the sympathetic nerve fibers. See also PHENYLEPHRINE.

alpha-chymotrypsin (kime-uh-TRIP-sun). *Drug*. Enzyme injected into the anterior chamber during intracapsular cataract surgery; breaks tough zonular fibers supporting the lens, allowing easier lens removal. Trade names: Catarase, Zolyse. See also ZONULYSIS.

alpha hemolytic (hee-muh-LIT-ik). *Microorganism*. Type of bacteria that partially destroys red blood cells, changing blood agar plate culture zone from red to green. See also BETA HEMOLYTIC.

Alport's syndrome. *Pathologic condition.* Characterized by kidney disease and deafness. Eye defects involve lens abnormalities: anterior lenticonus, cataracts, small, round lenses. Hereditary.

alternate cover test (ACT), cross cover test. For determining inward, outward, upward or downward eye deviations. Target is viewed while a cover is moved from eye to eye and the direction of eye movement is noted.

alternate prism + cover test (APCT), prism + alternate cover test, screen + cover test. For measuring inward, outward, upward or downward eye deviations. As target is viewed, a prism is placed over one eye and a cover over the other eye; the cover is moved from eye to eye. Eye movement is noted as prism power is changed; power used when movement stops is the deviation measurement. See also SIMULTANEOUS PRISM AND ALTERNATE COVER TEST.

alternate day esotropia (ee-suh-TROH-pee-uh), **circadian heterotropia, clock-mechanism esotropia, cyclic strabismus**. *Functional defect.* Eye deviation that follows 48-hour cycle, alternating 24 hours of normal binocularity with 24 hours of one eye turning inward (toward nose).

alternating esotropia (ee-suh-TROH-pee-uh). *Functional defect.* Eye deviation that continuously changes between an inturning (toward nose) right eye and straight left eye, and an inturning left eye and straight right eye.

alternating strabismus (struh-BIZ-mus). See STRABISMUS.

alternating sursumduction, double *(or)* **dissociated double hypertropia, dissociated vertical deviation**. *Functional defect.* Eye deviation in which one eye floats upward and rolls outward (extorsion) whenever the two eyes are not working together, e.g., when one eye is covered.

altitudinal hemianopsia (hem-ee-uh-NAHP-see-uh). *Functional defect.* Bilateral visual field loss (blind area) involving either the lower or upper half. See also SCOTOMA.

amacrine cells (AM-uh-krin). *Anatomy.* Retinal nerve cells in the inner nuclear layer that interconnect bipolar cells and ganglion cells, and spread neural information within the retina.

amaurosis (am-uh-ROH-sus). *Functional defect.* Blindness.

amaurosis fugax (FYU-jaks). *Pathologic condition.* Sudden, transient, decrease in vision of one eye; varies from visual field constriction to total blindness. Usually caused by insufficient blood flow to the ophthalmic artery. See also TRANSIENT ISCHEMIC ATTACK.

amaurotic family idiocy (am-uh-RAH-tik). *Pathologic condition.* Hereditary disorder characterized by nervous system and retinal deposits that eventually destroy visual function. Lesions appear in the macula (area of central vision) and the optic nerve degenerates. Closely related conditions vary with age of onset: Jansky-Bielshowsky syndrome, Kufs' disease, Norman-Wood syndrome, Tay-Sachs disease, Vogt-Spielmeyer syndrome.

amaurotic nystagmus (ni-STAG-mus), **sensory nystagmus**. *Pathologic condition.* Involuntary, rhythmic eye movements in both eyes, caused by severe visual loss in early childhood. See also ALBINISM, ANIRIDIA, CONGENITAL CATARACT.

amaurotic pupil. *Functional defect.* Enlarged pupil that does not change size with direct light stimulation, but responds to light stimulus in the other eye. Occurs in a blind eye with a retinal or optic nerve problem.

amblyopia (am-blee-OH-pee-uh), "**lazy eye.**" *Functional defect.* Decreased vision in one or both eyes without detectable anatomic damage in the eye or visual pathways. Usually uncorrectable by optical means (e.g., eyeglasses).

   alcohol a: bilateral vision loss with central field defects; may be caused by poisoning from drinking ethyl or methyl alcohol or by poor nutrition.

ametropic a: (am-uh-TROH-pik): amblyopic eye that has a high uncorrected refractive error (usually hyperopia or astigmatism). Vision may improve after several months of eyeglass correction.

anisometropic a: (an-ni-suh-muh-TROH-pik): decreased vision in the eye with the greater optical error; occurs when the eyes have a significant difference in refraction. Vision may improve after several months of eyeglass correction. See also REFRACTIVE (below).

deprivation a: follows central fixation disuse (due to cloudy cornea, cataract, droopy lid, etc.).

a. ex anopsia: same as DISUSE (below). Term becoming obsolete.

functional a: can be corrected by occlusion and/or corrective eyeglasses worn during the first decade of life.

hysterical a: psychological disorder; apparent vision loss in eye(s) that have normal visual potential. Patient believes he cannot see. See also MALINGERER.

irreversible a: same as ORGANIC (below).

nutritional a: vision loss accompanied by dense central visual field defects in both eyes. Caused by B vitamin deficiency, usually in patients who consume excessive tobacco and alcohol.

occlusion a: 1. Caused by prolonged patching of the better eye to promote use of the weaker eye. 2. Same as DEPRIVATION (above).

a. of arrest: decreased vision in one eye leading to arrested development of visual acuity; believed to follow onset of childhood eye deviation. Obsolete term.

a. of disuse: amblyopic eye that has lost form discrimination after central fixation disuse (due to cloudy cornea, cataract, droopy lid, etc.).

organic a: caused by non-apparent damage to visual system. No effective therapy. Includes alcohol, nutritional and toxic amblyopia.

refractive a: associated with large uncorrected refractive error (ametropic) or difference in refraction between the two eyes (anisometropic). Vision may improve after several months of eyeglass correction.

relative a: partly functional (reversible) and partly organic (irreversible).

reversible a: same as FUNCTIONAL (above).

strabismic a: associated with a continuous eye deviation (usually inward) beginning in childhood before visual acuity stabilizes. Usually reversible during first 9 years of life by total occlusion of the non-affected eye (often for months).

suppression a: results from a physiologic process in childhood: one eye's retinal image is subconsciously ignored.

toxic a: reduced vision with visual field defect, usually in both eyes, from excessive consumption of tobacco, alcohol or poisonous substance.

ametropia (am-uh-TROH-pee-uh). *Refractive error.* Any optical error (e.g., myopia) that can be corrected by eyeglasses or contact lenses.

ametropic amblyopia. See AMBLYOPIA.

amikacin. *Drug.* Antibiotic agent used for treating severe eye infections.

AmoVitrax. *Drug.* Trade name of sodium hyaluronate viscoelastic agent.

amphotericin B (am-foh-TEHR-uh-sin). *Drug.* For treating fungal eye infections. Trade name: Fungizone. See also CANDIDA ALBICANS, CLOTRIMAZOLE, FLUCYTOSINE, KETOCONAZOLE, MICONAZOLE, NATAMYCIN.

ampicillin. *Drug.* Antibiotic agent used for treating eye infections.

amplitude of accommodation (AA). *Measurement.* Maximum increase in the eye's optical power produced by a change in the shape of its lens; maximal (18 diopters) at birth, decreasing to almost zero by age 60. See also RANGE OF ACCOMMODATION.

amplitudes, fusional amplitudes, vergence ability. *Measurement.* Amount (in diopters) the eyes can move inward (converge) added to the amount they can move outward (diverge) while maintaining single vision.

AMPPE (acute multifocal placoid pigment epitheliopathy). *Pathologic condition*. Rare retinal disease characterized by irregularly shaped, creamy yellow opacities (exudates) at the level of the pigment epithelium. Usually in young females. Generally does not cause a long-term adverse visual effect.

Amsler grid (AM-slur). *Test card*. Grid (black lines on white background or white lines on black background) used for detecting central visual field distortions or defects, e.g., in macular degeneration. See also METAMORPHOPSIA.

Amvisc, AmviscPlus. *Drug*. Trade names of sodium hyaluronate viscoelastic agents.

AMSLER GRID

amyloidosis (am-ih-loy-DOH-sis). *Pathologic condition*. Group of rare systemic disorders characterized by amyloid (protein-polysaccharide substance) deposits in the eyes. Causes optic nerve damage, blood vessel blockage and vitreous opacification; often accompanied by eye protrusion, droopy eyelids, ocular muscle weakness, pupil abnormality, glaucoma, pain, and thickening of eyelid, conjunctiva, sclera and retina.

anabolic (an-uh-BAH-lik. *Description*. Aspect of metabolism relating to processes that build up chemical bonds. See also CATABOLIC.

anaglyph (AN-uh-glif). *Test card*. Green and red images are viewed through red and green filters so each eye sees a different picture. Tests for fusion and stereoscopic ability. See also TNO STEREO TEST, WORTH 4-DOT TEST.

analgesia (an-ul-JEE-zhuh). *Condition*. Reduced sensitivity to pain while conscious.

analgesic, analgetic (an-ul-JEE-sik, an-ul-JEH-tik). *Drug*. Medication that reduces pain, e.g., acetaminophen.

anaphylaxis (an-uh-fuh-LAK-sus). *Pathologic condition*. Extreme allergic reaction to an antigen (foreign substance); results from sensitization following prior contact with the substance. Potentially fatal.

anastomosis. 1. *Surgical procedure*. Connecting (or re-connecting) of severed tissues, e.g., blood vessels, nerves, tear ducts. 2. The result of the procedure. 3. *Pathologic condition*. Abnormal connection between two blood vessels. Plural: anastomoses.

anatomic equator. Imaginary line around the circumference of an eyeball, equidistant from its anterior and posterior poles. See also GEOMETRIC EQUATOR.

Ancef. *Drug*. Trade name of cephazolin, an antibiotic.

Ancobon. *Drug*. Trade name of flucytosine, an anti-fungal medication (oral or topical) used for serious eye infections.

anencephaly (an-un-SEF-uh-lee). *Congenital anomaly*. Skull malformation with severe failure of brain development; infant dies within days. Eyes appear normal despite absence of retinal nerve fiber layer and underdeveloped retinal ganglion cell layer and optic nerves.

anesthesia. *Condition*. Total or partial loss of feeling, usually from disease or from drugs that decrease sensitivity to pain.

  general: affects entire body, with loss of consciousness.

  local: regional or topical anesthetic that affects a part of the body, without loss of consciousness.

  regional: affects an area of the body.

  topical: applied directly to the surface of an area and affects only that area (example: eyedrop).

anesthetic. *Drug*. Medication that removes all sensation, including pain. Examples: bupivacaine, procaine, lidocaine, mepivacaine, tetracaine, proparacaine.

aneurysm (AN-yuh-rizm). *Pathologic condition*. Ballooned-out section of a tubelike body part, such as a blood vessel, caused by a weakened area in the tube wall. Possibility of rupture.

Angelucci's syndrome (an-jeh-LU-cheez). *Pathologic condition.* Characterized by excitable temperament, heart palpitations, and blood vessel disturbance; may be associated with allergic (vernal) conjunctivitis.

angiitis (an-jee-I-tis). *Pathologic condition.* Inflammation of a blood vessel.

angiogenic. *Characteristic.* Stimulating the growth of new blood vessels.

angiogram (AN-jee-oh-gram). *Test.* Photographic image of blood vessels. See also ANGIOGRAPHY.

angiography (an-jee-AH-gruh-fee). *Test.* Technique used for visualizing and recording location and size of blood vessels, e.g., with radio-opaque dyes.

    fluorescein (FLOR-uh-seen): for evaluating retinal, choroidal and iris blood vessels and any eye problems affecting them; fluorescein dye is injected into an arm vein, then rapid, sequential photographs are taken of the eye as the dye circulates.

    indocyanine green (ICG): for evaluating retinal, choroidal and iris blood vessels and any eye problems affecting them; indocyanine green dye is injected into an arm vein, then rapid, sequential photographs are taken of the eye as the dye circulates. Allows visualization of leaks under a layer of blood, which is opaque to fluorescein.

angioid streaks (AN-jee-oyd). *Pathologic defect.* Irregular linear cracks in Bruch's membrane (layer separating the choriocapillaris from the retinal pigment epithelium); appear as reddish-brownish streaks radiating outward from the optic disc. Seen in pseudoxanthoma elasticum, Paget's disease and sickle cell disease.

angiokeratoma corporis diffusum universale (AN-jee-oh-kehr-uh-TOH-muh, yu-nih-vur-SAL-ee), **diffuse angiokeratoma, Fabry's disease**. *Pathologic condition.* Enzyme deficiency disease affecting fat (lipid) metabolism. Eye signs include whorl-like corneal opacities, star-shaped lens haze, and tortuous conjunctival and retinal veins. Hereditary, X-linked. See also SPHINGOLIPIDOSES.

angioma. *Pathologic condition.* Tumor of the blood or lymph vessels. Usually benign.

angiomatosis retinae (an-jee-oh-muh-TOH-sis RET-ih-nee), **Lindau's disease, von Hippel-Lindau disease**. *Pathologic condition.* One of several hereditary disorders called phakomatoses; characterized by tumors of the retina, central nervous system and visceral organs. Primary eye findings are blood-filled retinal tumors (hemangiomas) fed by large, tortuous blood vessels. May also be associated with exudate leakage into the retina and retinal detachment.

angiopathia retinae juvenilis (an-jee-oh-PATH-ee-uh RET-ih-nee ju-ven-IL-is), **Eales' disease, periphlebitis retinae, primary perivasculitis of the retina**. *Pathologic condition.* Characterized by inflammation and possible blockage of retinal blood vessels, abnormal growth of new blood vessels (neovascularization), and recurrent retinal and vitreal hemorrhages. Seen in young men. Cause unknown.

angioscotoma (an-jee-oh-skuh-TOH-muh). *Functional defect.* Small blind area in the visual field caused by the shadow of a retinal blood vessel.

angle alpha. *Optics.* Angle formed at the nodal point of an eye between the visual axis and the optic axis.

angle gamma. *Optics.* Angle formed at the center of rotation of an eye between the optic axis and the fixation axis.

angle kappa. *Optics.* Angle formed at the nodal point of an eye between the visual axis and the mid-pupillary line.

angle lambda. *Optics.* Angle formed at the center of a pupil between the visual axis and the optic axis.

angle, anterior chamber angle. *Anatomy.* Junction of the front surface of the iris and back surface of the cornea, where aqueous fluid filters out of the eye. Incorporates nearby structures, which include Schlemm's canal, scleral spur, trabecular meshwork, Schwalbe's line, and iris processes.

angle closure glaucoma (ACG) (glaw-KOH-muh), **acute angle closure** *(or)* **narrow angle glaucoma**. *Pathologic condition.* Sudden rise in intraocular pressure. Aqueous fluid behind the iris cannot pass through the pupil and pushes the iris forward, preventing aqueous drainage through the angle (pupillary block mechanism). Occurs in patients with narrow anterior chamber angles. See also OPEN-ANGLE GLAUCOMA.

    chronic: repeated attacks of angle obstruction over a long period (months to years), sometimes asymptomatically. The normal drainage channels are eventually blocked permanently.

angle of anomaly. *Functional defect.* Difference between the examiner's measurements of an eye deviation and the patient's response. Occurs in longstanding strabismus that has developed abnormal retinal correspondence. See also ANOMALOUS RETINAL CORRESPONDENCE.

angle of the anterior chamber. See ANGLE.

angle of deviation. *Measurement.* Amount an eye deviates from the straight-ahead position as the other eye remains straight and fixates normally.

angle of incidence. *Optics.* Angle formed between an incoming light ray and a perpendicular ("normal") to the surface, at the point where the ray encounters a refractive surface.

angle of refraction. *Optics.* Angle formed between a light ray and a perpendicular ("normal") to the surface after the ray crosses a refractive surface.

angular blepharitis (blef-ur-I-tis). *Pathologic condition.* Infection (usually staphylococcus) of the eyelid margin near the canthus (angle where upper and lower eyelids meet).

anhidrosis (an-hi-DROH-sis). *Pathologic condition.* Lack of normal sweating.

anhydrous. *Description.* Without water. Usually refers to a chemical.

aniridia (an-uh-RID-ee-uh). *Congenital anomaly.* Incomplete formation of the iris. Associated with glaucoma, nystagmus, sensitivity to light, and poor vision. See also REIGER'S ANOMALY.

aniseikonia (an-i-suh-KOH-nee-uh). *Optics.* Unequal retinal image sizes in the two eyes, usually from different refractive errors. See also ISEIKONIC LENS.

anisocoria (an-i-suh-KOR-ee-uh). *Anatomic defect.* Unequal pupil size (difference of 1 mm or more). See also ADIE'S PUPIL, HORNER'S SYNDROME.

anisometropia (an-i-suh-meh-TROH-pee-uh). *Functional defect.* Unequal refractive errors in the two eyes; usually at least 1 diopter different.

anisometropic amblyopia (an-i-suh-meh-TROH-pik am-blee-OH-pee-uh). *Functional defect.* Type of functional amblyopia in which the eyes have significantly unequal refractive errors and the eye with the larger error has lost visual acuity. See also HEIMANN-BIELSCHOWSKY PHENOMENON.

anisopia (an-ni-SOH-pee-uh). *Functional defect.* Unequal vision in the two eyes.

anisophoria (induced) (an-i-soh-FOR-ee-uh). *Optics.* Unequal displacement of images by the two eyes; occurs when looking through the periphery of different power lenses, which forces the eyes to move unequally to see the corresponding images. See also PRENTICE'S RULE.

ankyloblepharon (AN-kil-oh-BLEF-ur-ahn). *Anatomic defect.* Fusion (partial or complete) of upper to lower eyelids, often with scarring of the conjunctiva. See also SYMBLEPHARON.

ankylosing spondylitis (an-kil-OH-sing spahn-dih-LI-tis). *Pathologic condition.* Connective tissue disorder associated with iritis or scleritis; most commonly affects young men with arthritis of the sacroiliac joint.

annular scotoma, ring scotoma. *Functional defect.* Ring-shaped blind area in the visual field, usually located 20°-40° from central fixation. Associated with some retinal degenerations, e.g., retinitis pigmentosa. Can also occur as an optical phenomenon with high plus-powered eyeglasses.

annulus of Zinn. *Anatomy.* Ring of fibrous tissue surrounding the optic nerve at its entrance to the eye; consists of the origins of five extraocular muscles (lateral, medial, superior and inferior recti, and superior oblique).

anomaloscope (an-AHM-uh-luh-skohp), **Nagel anomaloscope**. *Instrument.* Used for sensitive color vision evaluation and diagnosis; patient mixes red and green in an attempt to match hue and brightness of a yellow standard.

anomalous. *Description.* Deviating from normal, especially of a body part or function.

anomalous retinal correspondence (ARC) (an-AHM-uh-lus), **abnormal retinal correspondence**. *Functional defect.* Binocular sensory adaptation to compensate for a long-standing eye deviation; fovea of the straight (non-deviated) eye and a non-foveal retinal point of the deviated eye work together, sometimes permitting single binocular vision despite the misalignment.

    harmonious ARC: fovea of the straight eye and a non-foveal point of the deviated eye (that corresponds to the deviation) work together, permitting single binocular vision of poor quality.

    unharmonious ARC: fovea of the straight eye and a non-foveal point of the deviated eye (but not one that corresponds to the angle of deviation) work together.

anomalous trichromacy (tri-KROH-muh-si). *Congenital defect.* Common type of color vision deficiency. Caused by lower-than-normal quantity (not absence) of one of the three types of cone photopigments. See also DICHROMATISM, MONOCHROMATISM.

anomaly. A deviation from normal, especially of a body part.

anophthalmia (an-ahf-THAL-mee-uh), **anophthalmos**. *Congenital anomaly.* Absence of the eyeball.

anopsia (an-AHP-see-uh). *Functional defect.* Loss of vision; usually refers to loss of part of the visual field.

anoxia (uh-NAHK-see-uh). *Pathologic condition.* Lack of oxygen. See also HYPOXIA.

antagonist. Extraocular muscle whose action opposes that of the contracting muscle that moves the eye. See also AGONIST.

    contralateral: action opposes that of a contracting muscle on the fellow eye (e.g., right superior rectus and left superior oblique).

    ipsilateral: action opposes that of another muscle on the same eye (e.g., medial rectus and lateral rectus).

anterior. *Location.* The front of the body or body part. See also POSTERIOR.

anterior capsule. *Anatomy.* Front of the capsule enclosing the crystalline lens; lies in the posterior chamber just behind the iris. See also POSTERIOR CAPSULE.

anterior capsulotomy (kap-sul-AH-tuh-mee). *Surgical procedure.* Opening the front lens capsule for extracapsular cataract extraction. See also CAPSULE, CAPSULORHEXIS, POSTERIOR CAPSULOTOMY.

anterior chamber (AC). *Anatomy.* Fluid-filled space inside the eye between the iris and the innermost corneal surface (endothelium).

anterior chamber angle, angle. *Anatomy.* Junction of the front surface of the iris and back surface of the cornea, where aqueous fluid filters out of the eye. Incorporates nearby structures, which include Schlemm's canal, scleral spur, trabecular meshwork, Schwalbe's line, and iris processes.

anterior chamber cleavage syndrome, mesodermal dysgenesis of cornea, Peter's anomaly. *Congenital anomaly.* Central cornea malformation characterized by adherence of the iris to Descemet's membrane and the endothelium (innermost corneal layer). May be associated with iridocorneal angle abnormalities and cataract.

anterior chamber intraocular lens (ACIOL). *Optical device.* Plastic lens surgically implanted into the anterior chamber in front of the iris, to replace the eye's natural lens after cataract extraction. See also POSTERIOR CHAMBER INTRAOCULAR LENS.

anterior chamber tap, keratocentesis, paracentesis. *Surgical procedure.* Corneal puncture with removal of some aqueous fluid, for analysis or to temporarily lower eye pressure.

anterior ciliary arteries (SIL-ee-ehr-ee). *Anatomy.* Seven blood vessels that supply blood to the limbus, iris, ciliary body, and ciliary processes; the forward extensions of the muscular arteries that join the long posterior ciliary arteries to form the greater arterial circle. See also POSTERIOR CILIARY ARTERIES.

anterior corneal staphyloma (staf-uh-LOH-muh). *Pathologic condition.* Malformation of the cornea (opaque, irregular, bulging). Commonly accompanied by congenital glaucoma.

anterior focal point. *Optics.* Point on the optical axis in front of a lens. Light rays passing through this point will strike the lens system and emerge parallel to the axis. In the eye, located 17 mm in front of the cornea.

anterior hyaloid membrane (AHM) (HI-uh-loyd). *Anatomy.* Front layer of vitreous; extends from the ora serrata to a ring-like insertion on the back of the lens. Separates the jelly-like vitreous from the watery aqueous in the posterior chamber. See also VITREOUS FACE, WEIGER'S LIGAMENT.

anterior ischemic optic neuropathy (AION) (iss-KEE-mik, nur-AHP-uh-thee). *Pathologic condition.* Damage to the part of the optic nerve closest to the eye, from insufficient blood supply. Causes an abrupt decrease in vision and optic disc pallor and swelling. See also CENTROCECAL SCOTOMA, INFERIOR ALTITUDINAL DEFECT.

anterior lacrimal crest. *Anatomy.* Front lower border of the orbital margin near the nose; formed by part of the maxillary bone.

anterior megalophthalmos (meg-uh-lahf-THAL-mus). *Congenital anomaly.* Symmetrical enlargement of the front third of the eyeball, accompanied by an abnormally deep anterior chamber. Rear two-thirds of eye, intraocular pressure, and cup-to-disc ratio all remain normal. Occurs mostly in males. See also BUPHTHALMOS, MEGALOCORNEA.

anterior pole. *Anatomy.* Center of the front surface of the cornea. See also GEOMETRIC AXIS, POSTERIOR POLE.

anterior sclerectomy (skler-EK-tuh-mee). *Surgical procedure.* Removal of a small tongue-shaped section from the front of the sclera, to form an alternate exit site for aqueous drainage. Treatment for glaucoma.

anterior segment. *Anatomy.* Front third of the eyeball; includes structures located between the front surface of the cornea and the vitreous. See also POSTERIOR SEGMENT.

anterior synechia (sin-EE-kee-uh). *Pathologic condition.* Adhesions binding the front of the iris to the innermost corneal surface. See also PERIPHERAL ANTERIOR SYNECHIA, POSTERIOR SYNECHIA.

anterior uveitis (yu-vee-I-tis), **iridocyclitis**. *Pathologic condition.* Inflammation of iris, anterior chamber or ciliary body. Causes pain, tearing, blurred vision, constricted pupil and a red (congested) eye. See also CILIARY INJECTION, POSTERIOR UVEITIS.

anterior vitrectomy. *Surgical procedure.* Removal of front portion of vitreous tissue. Used for preventing or treating vitreous loss during cataract or corneal surgery, or to remove misplaced vitreous, as in aphakic pupillary block glaucoma.

anteroposterior axis of Fick, longitudinal *(or)* **sagittal** *(or)* **y axis of Fick.** Imaginary line running through an eye's center of rotation, connecting the geometric center of the cornea (anterior pole) with the geometric center of the back of the eye (posterior pole). Tilting (torsional) eye rotations occur around this axis.

antibiotics. *Drug.* Chemical compounds (generally derived from bacteria or molds) that kill or inhibit growth of other bacteria. Used for treating bacterial infections. Examples: ampicillin, bacitracin, cefachlor, clindamycin, chloramphenicol, erythromycin, gentamicin, neomycin, tobramycin, vancomycin.

antibody. Immune system protein (immunoglobulin) produced by the body in response to a specific foreign antigen, which is then available to neutralize, inhibit or destroy that antigen. Plural: antibodies.

anti-cancer agents, anti-neoplastic agents. *Drug.* Highly toxic chemical compounds that kill all actively growing cells, including cancer cells, by affecting their growth and development. Many cause temporary hair loss; some produce severe reactions or reduce the body's resistance to infection. Examples: azathioprine, chlorambucil, cyclophosphamide, cytosine arabinoside, fluorouracil, mechlorethamine, methotrexate, prednisone, tamoxifen, vincristine.

anticholinesterase (an-tee-koh-lin-ES-tur-ayz). *Drug.* Eyedrop that mimics the action of parasympathetic nerves by inactivating cholinesterase, allowing prolonged activity of acetylcholine. Causes contraction of the iris sphincter, resulting in pupil constriction (miosis), and ciliary muscle contraction, which increases accommodation. Examples: carbachol, echothiophate iodide, phospholine iodide, physostigmine. See also CHOLINERGIC STIMULATING DRUGS.

anticoagulant. *Drug.* Substance that slows or prevents blood clotting.

antifungals. *Drug.* Class of drugs used for treating fungal infections, which are usually serious and severe in the eye, especially in immunocompromised patients. Examples: amphotericin B, clotrimazole, flucytosine, ketoconazole, miconazole, natamycin.

antigen (AN-tih-jun). Any substance that stimulates production of antibodies; part of the body's immune system.

antihistamines. *Drug.* Class of drugs that lessen the effects of histamine, which is released when some body tissues are irritated. For treating allergic and hypersensitivity reactions. Examples: Benadryl, Chlortrimeton.

anti-inflammatory agent. *Drug.* Reduces redness and swelling associated with inflammation. May be a (cortico)steroid, e.g., dexamethasone, fluorometholone, prednisolone, or a non-steroidal anti-inflammatory drug (NSAID), e.g., acetaminophen, aspirin, flurbiprofen, ibuprofen, ketorolac, naproxen.

antimetabolite. *Drug.* Any chemical that interferes with the normal metabolism and growth of a cell. Used for reducing scarring and for treating some forms of cancer.

antimetropia (an-tee-meh-TROH-pee-uh). "Opposite" refractive errors in the eyes: one nearsighted (myopic), one farsighted (hyperopic).

anti-mongoloid slant. *Anatomy.* Eyelids whose inner (near nose) corners are higher than the outer corners. See also MONGOLOID SLANT.

ANTI-MONGOLOID SLANT

anti-neoplastic agents. See ANTI-CANCER AGENTS.

antinuclear antibody test (ANA). *Lab test.* Blood test for detecting the presence of proteins associated with certain autoimmune disorders (in which the immune system directs an attack on normal body tissues), e.g., rheumatoid arthritis, uveitis.

antipodean strabismus (an-tee-POH-dee-un struh-BIZ-mus). *Functional defect.* Eye misalignment in which one eye turns inward (esotropia) while the other fixates normally; when the deviated eye straightens to fixate normally, the other turns outward (exotropia).

anti-reflective coating. *Optical device.* Magnesium fluoride applied to lenses in a thin layer to decrease surface reflections and glare.

anti-suppression exercise. *Treatment*. Technique that heightens awareness of double vision (diplopia), to enhance the possibility of fusion when one eye is deviated.

anti-viral agents. *Drug*. Class of drugs that interfere with DNA production in specific viruses, making them effective for treating viral infections. Examples: acyclovir, ganciclovir, idoxuridine, trifluridine, vidarabine.

Anton's syndrome. *Pathologic condition*. Patient believes he can see despite total blindness due to destruction of the visual cortex. See also CORTICAL BLINDNESS.

A-pattern. *Functional defect*. Horizontal eye misalignment in which an inward turning (esotropic) eye deviates more on up-gaze than on down-gaze, or an outward turning (exotropic) eye deviates more on down-gaze than up-gaze. See also STRABISMUS, V-PATTERN.

A-PATTERN EXOTROPIA

Apert's syndrome (AY-purtz), **acrocephalosyndactylia of Apert**. *Congenital anomaly*. Characterized by severe mental retardation, heart and kidney malformations, underdevelopment of mid-portion of the face, and webbed fingers and toes. Eye defects may include shallow orbits, protruding eyes, exposed corneas, widely spaced eyes, outward deviation (exotropia), optic nerve damage, and visual field disorders. See also CROUZON'S SYNDROME.

apex. 1. *Anatomy*. Innermost point of the pyramid-shaped bony orbit, near the optic foramen and superior orbital fissure. Also called the orbital apex. 2. *Optics*. Narrowest edge of a prism, where the two optical surfaces meet.

apex (corneal), apical zone, corneal cap. *Anatomy*. Central 3–5 mm of cornea, where the surface has greatest curvature; yields highest K-readings (steepest meridian) by keratometry.

Apgar score. *Test*. Evaluation of a newborn's clinical condition; based on five factors: heart rate, respiration effort, muscle tone, color, and response to a catheter in the nostrals.

aphake (AY-fayk). *Slang*. Patient whose crystalline lens has been removed, e.g., after cataract extraction.

aphakia (ay-FAY-kee-uh). *Anatomic defect*. Absence of the eye's crystalline lens, e.g., after cataract extraction. See also PSEUDOPHAKIA.

aphakic correction (ay-FAY-kik). *Optical device*. Contact or eyeglass lens that replaces optical power lost after cataract extraction, or lens loss from any cause.

aphakic pupillary block. *Pathologic condition*. Type of angle-closure glaucoma occuring at some time after cataract extraction. Caused by adhesions of the pupillary margin to the vitreous or to an intraocular lens. See also PUPILLARY BLOCK.

aphakic spectacles, cataract glasses. *Optical device*. Thick, plus-powered eyeglasses that replace optical power lost after cataract extraction, when no intraocular lens has been inserted. See also ASPHERIC LENTICULAR SPECTACLES.

apical clearance (AY-pih-kul). Space between the back of a contact lens and the corneal surface, at their centers.

apical disease. *Pathologic condition*. Any disorder localized to the apex (rear part) of the orbit, e.g., optic nerve compression.

apical radius. *Measurement*. Base curve of a contact lens; measured as a radius of curvature (in mm) rather than dioptric power.

aplasia (ay-PLAY-zhuh). *Congenital anomaly*. Absense or defective development of a tissue or organ.

apnea (AP-nee-uh). *Pathologic condition*. Cessation of breathing; usually temporary.

aponeurosis of the eyelid (ap-ahn-yu-ROH-sis), **levator aponeurosis**. *Anatomy.* Fan-shaped membranous expansion of the end of the levator muscle (its two extremities are called horns). Spans entire width of the upper orbit and attaches to the skin of the upper eyelid and to the tarsal plate. See also LATERAL HORN, MEDIAL HORN.

apoptosis (ah-pahp-TOH-sis). *Concept.* Naturally occuring programmed cell death, with every cell type having a different life expectancy.

apostilb (asb.) (AY-poh-stilb). *Measurement.* Light intensity (brightness) per unit area; used for describing target and background luminance in perimetry testing. Standard background for Goldmann and Humphrey perimeters is 31.5 asb.

appendages of the eye, adnexa oculi, ocular adnexa. *Anatomy.* Structures surrounding the eyeball; includes eyelids, eyebrows, tear drainage system, orbital walls and orbital contents.

applanation. Method of flattening the cornea. Used for measuring intraocular pressure. See APPLANATION TONOMETER.

applanation tonometer (tuh-NAHM-ih-tur). *Instrument.* Determines intraocular pressure by measuring the force required to flatten a small area of central cornea. Usually attaches to slit lamp. Examples: Draeger and Goldmann tonometers.

applanation tonometry. *Test.* Determinination of intraocular pressure by measuring the force required to flatten a small area of central cornea. See also TONOMETRY.

apraclonidine (ahp-ruh-CLOH-nuh-deen). *Drug.* Acts directly on alpha receptors in the sympathetic nerve fibers to reduce production of aqueous. Used in treating glaucoma. See also IOPIDINE.

aqueous (AY-kwee-us), **aqueous humor**. *Anatomy.* Clear, watery fluid that fills the space between the back surface of the cornea and the front surface of the vitreous, bathing the lens. Produced by the ciliary processes. Nourishes the cornea, iris, and lens and maintains intraocular pressure. See also ANTERIOR CHAMBER, POSTERIOR CHAMBER.

aqueous flare, flare, Tyndall effect. *Clinical sign.* Scattering of a slit lamp light beam when it is directed into the anterior chamber; occurs when aqueous has increased protein. Sign of iris or ciliary body inflammation (iritis).

aqueous humor. Less common term for AQUEOUS.

aqueous mis-direction syndrome, ciliary block *(or)* **malignant glaucoma**. *Pathologic condition.* Increase in intraocular pressure accompanied by a shallow anterior chamber and forward displacement of the iris and lens. Complication following surgery for acute angle closure glaucoma; may be caused by aqueous trapped behind vitreous.

aqueous outflow. *Function.* Passage of aqueous fluid from the eye, through anterior chamber angle structures.

Ara-A. *Drug.* Trade name of vidarabine, anti-viral eye ointment, for treating herpetic keratitis.

arachnodactyly (uh-rak-noh-DAK-til-ee), **Marfan's syndrome**. *Pathologic condition.* Connective tissue disease characterized by "spidery" fingers and toes (due to extra-long, slender bones), relaxed ligaments, spine and joint deformities, congenital heart disease, and dislocated lenses. Associated with a high nearsighted (myopic) refractive error, large corneas, cataracts, droopy eyelids (ptosis), eye deviation (strabismus), and incomplete choroid formation. Rare; hereditary.

arcades (temporal). *Description.* Normal pattern of retinal blood vessels as they leave the optic nerve head and arch around the macula.

arc of contact, contact arc. *Anatomy.* Distance between an extraocular muscle's initial point of contact with the sclera and its true insertion on the eyeball.

arc perimeter. *Instrument*. Used for plotting peripheral field of vision. Obsolete.

arcuate keratotomy. *Surgical procedure*. Method of flattening the steeper corneal meridian with a curved corneal incision, to reduce astigmatism after corneal surgery. See also KERATOREFRACTIVE SURGERY.

arcuate scotoma (AHR-kyu-it skuh-TOH-muh), **Bjerrum** *(or)* **comet** *(or)* **scimitar scotoma**. *Functional defect*. Arc-shaped blind area in the visual field, caused by damage to retinal nerve fiber bundles. Common in patients with glaucoma.

arcus juvenilis. See ARCUS SENILIS.

arcus senilis, gerontoxon. *Degenerative change*. Ring-shaped grayish deposit of fat near the peripheral edge of the cornea (limbus). Typically occurs after age 60; also in young patients with abnormally high blood fat levels (arcus juvenilis).

Arden plates. *Test*. For contrast sensitivity; tests the ability to detect subtle gradations in grayness between a test target and the background.

argon laser. *Surgical instrument*. Argon gas–filled laser used for placing minute burns, to selectively destroy bits of iris, retina, abnormal blood vessel tissue (neovascularization), tumors, etc. See also LASER IRIDOTOMY, PHOTOCOAGULATION, TRABECULOPLASTY.

argon laser trabeculoplasty (ALT). *Surgical procedure*. Using an argon gas-filled laser to selectively burn the trabecular meshwork area, to lower intraocular pressure. See also TRABECULOPLASTY.

Argyll-Robertson pupils (AHR-ghile). *Abnormal function*. Small, unequal, irregularly shaped pupils that constrict with near focus but do not respond to light stimulation. Often associated with syphilis. See also LIGHT-NEAR DISSOCIATION.

argyrosis (ahr-juh-ROH-sis). *Pathologic condition*. Silver deposits in conjunctiva, corneal epithelium, stroma, and Descemet's membrane after long-term use of silver-containing eyedrops, e.g., Argyrol. See also CHRYSIASIS.

Arion prosthesis (AIR-ee-un). *Surgical device*. Silastic rod(s) inserted through the tarsal plate of the upper and lower eyelids, to support lids that are malpositioned due to 7th (facial) cranial nerve weakness. See also PARALYTIC ECTROPION.

Arlt's line. *Anatomic defect*. Horizontal conjunctival scar on undersurface of the upper eyelid, seen in late stage after trachoma infection.

ARN (acute retinal necrosis). *Pathologic condition*. Severe retinal inflammation that leads to patchy retinal thinning, hole formation, retinal detachment and, usually, profound visual loss. Associated with herpes viruses, usually in healthy people. See also CMV RETINITIS, TOXOPLASMOSIS.

Arnold-Chiari malformation. *Pathologic condition*. Congenital maldevelopment of the pons, medulla and cerebellum. Associated with hydrocephalus, spina bifida, and herniation (protrusion) of central nervous tissue through the foramen magnum (bony opening at base of skull).

arrhythmia (ay-RITH-mee-uh). *Functional defect*. Abnormal heart rhythm, usually due to a disturbance in the heart's electrical impulses.

arterial circle of the iris (major). *Anatomy*. Primary blood distribution system to the front half of the eye; seven anterior ciliary arteries and two long posterior ciliary arteries form a circular configuration at the junction of the iris and ciliary body.

arterial phase. *Clinical sign*. Early phase of fluorescein angiography, when retinal arteries fill with dye. Follows choroidal flush.

arteriosclerosis. *Pathologic condition*. Chronic disease characterized by hardening and thickening of the walls of the smaller arteries. Tends to interfere with blood flow. See also ATHEROSCLEROSIS.

arteriovenous malformation (AVM). *Pathologic condition.* Localized group of abnormal connections between an artery and vein. May be congenital or developmental.

artery. *Anatomy.* Blood vessel that carries blood away from the heart. See also VEIN.

artificial tears. *Drug.* Eyedrop that approximates the consistency of normal tears, e.g., weak methylcellulose solution or polyvinyl alcohol. Alleviates dry eye symptoms; some products are used for treating recurrent corneal erosion. See also TEAR FILM BREAKUP TIME.

A-scan. *Instrument.* Type of ultrasound, radar-like device that emits very high frequency waves that are reflected by the ocular structures and converted into electrical impulses and displayed on a screen as a series of echo spikes. Used for differentiating normal and abnormal eye tissue or for measuring length of eyeball (axial length). See also B-SCAN, ECHOGRAPHY.

aseptic (ay-SEP-tik). *Description.* Sterile; free from pathogenic organisms.

Aspergillus (as-pur-JIL-us). *Microorganism.* Fungus that causes some eye infections. Identified by spores with bristly, knob-like tops.

aspheric (ay-SFIR-ik). *Description.* Refers to a surface that is not curved as part of a sphere.

asphericity (ay-sfir-ISS-ih-tee). *Characteristic.* Describes a surface that is not curved as part of a sphere.

aspheric lens. *Optical device.* Lens whose front surface is not curved as part of a sphere but is relatively flatter in the periphery. Aspheric spectacles are designed to provide better imagery with less aberrations; useful for correcting high refractive errors. See also SPHERICAL LENS, TORIC LENS.

aspheric lenticular spectacles. *Optical device.* Corrective eyeglasses worn after cataract extraction; each lens is composed of a 40 mm diameter nonspherical lens of high optical (plus) power set into a larger lens with no optical power. Provides better quality central image while minimizing lens thickness and weight. See also APHAKIC SPECTACLES, LENTICULAR LENS.

aspirate. 1. (ASS-pur-ayt). *Surgical procedure.* Withdrawing of fluid by suction, usually into a needle, as from a body cavity. 2. (ASS-pur-it). Fluid that has been aspirated.

aspiration-irrigation system. *Instrument.* Permits simultaneous removal of fluid and/or tissue from the eye and replacement with fluid or gas.

astereognosis (AY-steer-ee-ahg-NOH-sis). *Pathologic condition.* Inability to recognize objects or appreciate their form by touching them.

asteroid hyalosis (hi-uh-LOH-sis), **Benson's sign**. *Pathologic condition.* Degenerative process of having tiny, opaque, oval calcium deposits suspended in the vitreous; causes no decrease in vision. Occurs in the elderly, usually in one eye. See also SYNCHYSIS SCINTILLANS.

asthenopia (as-then-OH-pee-uh). *Symptom.* Vague eye discomfort arising from use of the eyes; may consist of eyestrain, headache, and/or browache. May be related to uncorrected refractive error or poor fusional amplitudes.

astigmatic axis (as-tig-MAT-ik). *Optics.* Meridional position of zero power in a cylindrical lens, perpendicular to the meridian containing maximum cylindrical power. Used for denoting proper lens orientation in correcting astigmatism.

astigmatic clock. See ASTIGMATIC DIAL.

astigmatic dial, astigmatic clock. *Test chart.* Radial (spoke-like) arrangement of lines used during refraction for subjectively determining the axis of an astigmatic refractive error. See also CLOCK DIAL, FAN DIAL, LANCASTER REGAN DIAL #2.

astigmatism (uh-STIG-muh-tiz-um). *Refractive error.* Optical defect in which refractive power is not uniform in all directions (meridians). Light rays entering the eye are bent unequally by different meridians, with maximum and minimum powers 90° to one another, which prevents formation of a sharp point focus on the retina. Instead, light rays form two focal lines separated by a focal zone. Usually results from corneal asphericity. Corrected by a cylindrical (toric) eyeglass or contact lens.

    "against-the-rule": optical power is greater in the horizontal meridian than in the vertical meridian. Can be corected by a plus-cylinder lens with its axis at 180°.

    compound: both focal lines lie in front of the retina (compound myopic astigmatism) or behind it (compound hyperopic astigmatism). Corrected by a sphero-cylindrical lens.

    corneal: variation in corneal curvature causes light rays to focus imperfectly on the retina.

    hyperopic: may be simple (one focal line lies on the retina, the other behind the retina) or compound (both focal lines behind the retina).

    irregular: distorted imagery caused by warped optical surfaces; warping is usually corneal and the result of scarring from trauma, inflammation, or developmental anomalies. May be corrected by contact lenses but not by standard eyeglasses.

    lenticular: caused by different curvature of one or both of the lens surfaces.

    mixed: one focal line lies in front of the retina; corrected by a minus cylinder lens. The other focal line lies behind the retina; corrected by a plus-cylinder lens.

    myopic: the two focal lines lie in front of the retina; corrected by a cylindrical (toric) lens. May be simple (one focal line on the retina and the other in the vitreous in front of the retina) or compound (both focal lines in front of the retina).

    radial: an image aberration created by light that hits a refractive surface obliquely; not a refractive error.

    residual: amount of astigmatism that remains after refractive error correction with contact lenses.

    simple: one focal line lies on the retina. In the meridian 90° away, light rays strike the retina before coming to another focal line (simple hyperopic), corrected by a plus cylinder lens; or they form another focal line in the vitreous before striking the retina (simple myopic), corrected by a minus-cylinder lens.

    "with the rule": optical power is greater in the vertical meridian of an eye than in the horizontal meridian. Corrected by a plus-cylinder lens with its axis at 90°.

astrocytoma. *Pathologic condition.* Non-malignant tumor in the central nervous system composed of astrocytes (supporting cells).

asymmetric surgery. *Surgical procedure.* Strabismus surgery performed on more than one muscle of the same eye, rather than on comparable muscles of both eyes. Used for correcting an inward or outward deviation.

asymptomatic. Having no symptoms of disease.

ataxia (ay-TAK-see-uh). *Functional defect.* Imprecise, uncoordinated movement of a voluntary muscle.

ataxia telangiectasia, Louis-Bar syndrome. *Pathologic condition.* Characterized by small, spidery blood vessels (telangiectasia) on the skin, conjunctiva, optic nerve and brain. Associated with immunoglobulin and lymphoproliferative abnormalities. Hereditary. See also PHAKOMATOSIS.

atenolol. *Drug.* Controls high blood pressure (hypertension) by its action as a beta blocker. Trade name: Tenormin. See also ACEBUTOLOL, LABETOLOL, METAPROLOL, NADOLOL, PINDOLOL, PROPANOLOL, TIMOLOL.

atheroma (ath-ur-OH-muh). *Pathologic condition.* Fatty deposit that thickens the inside wall of an artery. Can impede blood flow.

atherosclerosis (ath-ur-oh-skler-OH-sis). *Pathologic condition.* Form of arteriosclerosis in which fatty deposits form on the inner walls of medium-size arteries and interfere with smooth blood flow. Associated with heart attacks and strokes.

Athrombin K. *Drug.* Trade name of warfarin, a heart medication.

Atkinson facial nerve block. *Surgical technique.* Numbing the 7th (facial) cranial nerve with an anesthetic injected at the side of the eyelids near the top of the cheekbone, to decrease sensation in the lids and face. See also NABATH, O'BRIEN, AND VAN LINT FACIAL NERVE BLOCKS.

atopic conjunctivitis (ay-TAH-pik kun-junk-tih-VI-tis). *Pathologic condition.* Allergic reaction of the conunctiva (membrane covering white of eye and inner eyelids) to pollens, usually with hay fever. Characterized by tearing, swelling, and watery discharge containing eosinophils.

atresia (ay-TREE-zhuh). *Abnormal condition.* Absense or failure to open of a natural body passage, e.g., a tear duct.

Atromid S. *Drug.* Trade name of clofibrate; for lowering cholesterol levels.

atrophy (AT-roh-fee). *Anatomic defect.* Wasting away or loss of function of cells, tissue, or an organ.

atropine (AT-roh-peen). *Drug.* Eyedrop that blocks the parasympathetic nerves to the eye, paralyzing the iris sphincter and ciliary body and causing an enlarged pupil and blurred near vision. Used for cycloplegic refraction in children and for treating iritis. Effect is long-lasting (2–14 days). Trade names: Atropine-Care, Atropisol, Bufoptoatropine, Isopto Atropine.

attenuation (uh-ten-yu-AY-shun). 1. Dilution or weakening, as of the virulence of a disease-causing microorganism. 2. Narrowing of a hollow tube or blood vessel.

atypical monochromacy, cone monochromacy. *Congenital defect.* Rare inability to distinguish colors. Vision is relatively normal. Nonprogressive; hereditary. See also ROD MONOCHROMACY.

Aureomycin. *Drug.* Trade name of tetracycline, an antibiotic.

auscultation (ahs-kul-TAY-shun). *Procedure.* Listening to sounds arising within organs (e.g., lungs, heart) as an aid to diagnosis and treatment.

autofluorescence. *Characteristic.* Fluorescence (lighting up) of some tissues (e.g., disc drusen, lens) when stimulated by a cobalt blue (ultraviolet) light, even though no fluorescein dye is present.

autograft. *Surgical procedure.* Transfer of tissue to a new site on the same individual. See also HOMOGRAFT.

autoimmune disease. *Pathologic condition.* Attack by the body's immune system (immunologic reaction) to it's own tissues; occurs when antibodies lose the ability to distinguish between foreign antigens and body tissues. Examples: rheumatoid arthritis, sympathetic ophthalmia.

autokeratoplasty. *Surgical procedure.* Penetrating keratoplasty in which the full thickness of corneal tissue with a discrete opacity is excised, rotated, and resutured to shift the position of the opacity.

automated lamellar keratoplasty (ALK). *Surgical procedure.* Excision of the outer corneal layers (lamellae) with a computer-controlled keratome (knife), usually as a part of a refractive keratoplasty procedure (e.g., epikeratophakia, keratomileusis, LASIK).

automated perimeter. *Instrument.* Maps field of vision by presenting stationary (static) luminous stimuli in pre-arranged locations and plotted by computer. Trade names: Dicon, Humphrey Analyzer, Octopus, Squid. See also PERIMETRY.

automated refractor, auto refractor. *Instrument.* Electro-mechanical or computerized device used for determining an eye's refractive error.

autonomic drug. *Drug.* Acts upon autonomic (sympathetic and parasympathetic) nerve tissue to enhance or inhibit production of acetylcholine or epinephrine, chemicals in the body that transmit nerve impulses. Used for diagnostic eye tests and in treating eye disease. See also PARASYMPATHOLYTIC, PARASYMPATHOMIMETIC, SYMPATHOLYTIC AND SYMPATHOMIMETIC DRUGS.

autonomic nervous system (ANS). *Anatomy.* Group of involuntary nerves that monitor, process and control digestive and cardiovascular systems and functions that involve involuntary (smooth) muscles and the glands of internal organs. Eye functions under autonomic control include accommodation (focusing), miosis (pupil constriction), and mydriasis (pupil dilation). Comprised of sympathetic and parasympathetic systems.

Auto-Plot. *Instrument.* Trade name of screening device used for mapping central visual fields. Obsolete.

auto refractor. See AUTOMATED REFRACTOR.

a-wave. *Test.* Part of electroretinogram (ERG) action potential wave.

Axenfeld anomaly. *Congenital defect.* Eye malformation consisting of a white ring on the innermost surface of cornea (prominent Schwalbe's line). Associated with high intraocular pressure.

Axenfeld (loops of), intrascleral nerve loops. *Anatomy.* Condition in which a long ciliary nerve loops into the anterior sclera; gives rise to appearance of a minute dark spot of uveal tissue on the sclera near the limbus.

axes of Fick. Three imaginary reference lines in the eye, perpendicular to one another, intersecting at the center of rotation (x, y, and z axes of Fick).

axial hyperopia (AKS-ee-ul hi-pur-OH-pee-uh). *Refractive error.* Farsightedness caused by a short eyeball. See also AXIAL LENGTH.

axial length. *Anatomy.* Length of eyeball from center of cornea (anterior pole) to back of sclera (posterior pole); normally about 24 mm. See also A-SCAN.

axial myopia (mi-OH-pee-uh). *Refractive error.* Nearsightedness caused by a long eyeball. See also AXIAL LENGTH.

axis. *Optics.* Reference line. Plural: axes.

  astigmatic: meridional direction of minimum power in a cylindrical lens; perpendicular to the meridian of maximum cylindrical power. Used for denoting lens orientation for correcting astigmatism.

  optical: imaginary line in an eyeglass lens that passes through the optical centers of both surfaces. Also called lens axis, principal axis.

  visual: imaginary line connecting a viewed object with the fovea. See also FIXATION, PRIMARY LINE OF SIGHT.

axon. *Anatomy.* A nerve fiber; the part of a nerve cell that carries information away from the cell body.

axoplasmic flow. *Function.* Continuous pulsing movement of tissue metabolites and protoplasm between a neuron's cell body and its axon nerve fiber.

azathioprine. *Drug.* Anti-cancer drug. Used for immunosuppression in cases of lupus erythematosis, Behcet's disease, and Wegener's granulomatosis that do not respond to steroids.

B

Bacillus subtilis (buh-SIH-lus SUH-til-us). *Microorganism*. Large box-shaped rod bacteria found in soil and dust; can cause eye infection.

Baciquent. *Drug*. Trade name of bacitracin, an antibiotic.

bacitracin. *Drug*. Antibiotic used for treating external eye infections, such as bacterial blepharoconjunctivitis.

background diabetic retinopathy (BDR), nonproliferative retinopathy. *Pathologic condition*. Retinal changes associated with early stage of diabetic retinopathy. Common findings include microaneurysms, "dot and blot" hemorrhages, hard exudates, and dilation of the retinal veins. Excludes the presence of abnormal new blood vessels (neovascularization). See also PROLIFERATIVE RETINOPATHY.

back vertex power, effective *(or)* vertex power. *Measurement*. Power of a spectacle or contact lens, measured at the back surface (with a lensometer).

bacteremia (bak-tur-EE-mee-uh). *Pathologic condition*. Bacteria in the bloodstream.

bacterial conjunctivitis (kun-junk-tih-VI-tis). *Pathologic condition*. Infection of the conjunctiva (membrane covering white of eye and inner eyelids). Characterized by muco-pus discharge, redness, and a gritty feeling. Large numbers of polymorphonuclear cells are found in conjunctival discharge and scrapings.

bacteriophage. *Organism*. A virus that infects bacteria.

"bag," capsular bag. *Anatomy*. Bag-like lens capsule remnant remaining after cataract removal, that an intraocular lens is implanted into. Consists of the intact posterior capsule and the residual flap of anterior capsule.

Bagolini lenses (bag-oh-LEE-nee). *Test instrument*. Finely striated, clear lenses used for evaluating retinal correspondence in patients with eye deviations.

balanced salt solution. *Drug*. Sodium, potassium, calcium, and magnesium chloride in physiological concentration. Used during eye surgery to rinse or replace intraocular fluids. Trade name: BSS.

balancing. *Optics*. Refraction technique for relaxing accommodation equally in both eyes, to achieve an optimal correction.

Balint's syndrome. *Pathologic condition*. Paralysis of fixation resulting from bilateral brain lesions in the parieto-occipital area. Eyes move randomly with no voluntary control of fixation.

bandage lens. *Optical device*. Soft contact lens with no refractive power, used for protecting damaged or irregular corneal surfaces.

band keratopathy (kehr-uh-TAHP-uh-thee). *Pathologic condition*. Horizontal band of calcium deposits in superficial layers of the cornea; associated with chronic uveitis and other chronic ocular diseases.

bare sclera (SKLEH-ruh). *Surgical procedure*. Method of closing a conjunctival incision following extraocular muscle surgery or pterygium removal. The conjunctiva is attached directly to the sclera, allowing exposure of the sclera between the edge of the wound and the edge of the cornea.

baring of the blind spot. *Functional defect*. Visual field defect corresponding to a depression of retinal sensitivity just nasal to the physiologic blind spot, which enlarges beyond the normal temporal isopter. Associated with glaucoma.

Barkan's membrane. *Anatomy*. Thin membrane covering the trabeculum. May have etiologic significance in congenital glaucoma.

BARN (bilateral acute retinal necrosis). *Pathologic condition*. Severe retinal inflammation affecting both eyes; leads to patchy retinal thinning, hole formation, retinal detachment, and usually profound visual loss. Associated with herpes viruses, usually in healthy people. See also CMV RETINITIS, TOXOPLASMOSIS.

bar reader. *Instrument.* Separates a page into the parts seen by each eye, to aid eye coordination.

barrel distortion. *Optics.* Type of image distortion associated with high minus lenses; objects appear smaller at the edge of the lens than in the center (barrel-shaped).

basal cell carcinoma (BCC). *Pathologic condition.* Slow growing tumor; most common malignancy of the eyelids. Develops from the deepest (basal) layer of the skin, frequently near the medial canthus. Responds well to treatment. Does not metastasize.

basal iridectomy (BAY-zul ir-ih-DEK-tuh-mee). *Surgical procedure.* Peripheral iridectomy performed near the iris root, close to the angle.

basal lamina (LAM-ih-nuh). **Bruch's membrane, lamina vitrea**. *Anatomy.* Innermost layer of the choroid, lying directly under the retinal pigment epithelium. When damaged by disease or aging, responsible for many bleeding disorders of the macular area, e.g., macular degeneration.

basal tearing. *Function.* Tear secretion (mainly from tiny glands in the conjunctiva) that maintains normal moisture level in the tear film, to keep the conjunctiva and cornea moist. Reduced in dry eyes (keratoconjunctivitis sicca). See also REFLEX TEARING, SCHIRMER TEST.

base. In a prism, the thickest edge, opposite the apex.

baseball lens. *Optical device.* Type of vocational trifocal. Eyeglass lens that has semicircular segments of different plus powers at the bottom and top, giving the appearance of a baseball. See also ADD.

base curve. *Optics.* Usually refers to the curvature of the back surface of a spectacle or contact lens.

base-down prism (BD). *Optical device.* A prism whose thickest edge is downward. When placed in front of an eye, it moves the image upward and thus can be used to measure or treat an upward eye deviation (hypertropia, hyperphoria). Sometimes incorporated into eyeglasses.

Basedow's disease (BAZ-eh-dohz), **endocrine exophthalmos** *(or)* **ophthalmopathy, Graves'** *(or)* **thyroid eye disease, thyrotoxic** *(or)* **thyrotropic exophthalmos**. *Pathologic condition.* Eye signs that may occur in patients with excessive thyroid-related hormone concentration; includes eyelid retraction, lid lag on downward gaze, corneal drying, eye bulging (proptosis), fibrotic extraocular muscles, and optic nerve inflammation. See also DALRYMPLE'S SIGN, STELLWAG'S SIGN, VON GRAEFE SIGN.

base-in prism (BI). *Optical device.* A prism whose thickest edge is inward (toward the nose). When placed in front of an eye, it moves the image outward and thus can be used to measure or treat an outward eye deviation (exotropia, exophoria). Sometimes incorporated into eyeglasses.

basement membrane. *Anatomy.* Thin membranous layer of connective tissue at the base of every type of epithelial cell. Helps hold the cell in place.

base-out prism (BO). *Optical device.* A prism whose thickest edge is outward (toward the ear). When placed in front of an eye, it moves the image inward and thus can be used to measure or treat an inward eye deviation (esotropia, esophoria). Sometimes incorporated into eyeglasses.

base-up prism (BU). *Optical device.* A prism whose thickest edge is upward. When placed in front of an eye, it moves the image downward and thus can be used to measure or treat downward eye deviations (hypotropia, hypophoria). Sometimes incorporated into eyeglasses.

basic exotropia (eks-oh-TROH-pee-uh). See EXOTROPIA.

basic secretion test. Filter paper strips are placed in the anesthetized lower fornix for measuring the quantity of basic tear secretion when the eye in its resting state, without conjunctival irritation (which produces reflex tearing); part of Schirmer test.

basophil (BAY-soh-fil). *Anatomy.* Type of white blood cell.

basophilic adenoma (bay-soh-FIL-ik ad-ih-NOH-muh). *Pathologic condition.* Slow-growing pituitary tumor whose cells take up a basic dye. Rarely grows large, but may compress the chiasm from below and produce pressure on the optic nerves. Visual field defects appear in bitemporal inferior quadrants and expand slowly upward.

Bassen-Kornzweig syndrome (BAY-sen KORN-swige), **albetalipoprotein-emia**. *Pathologic condition.* Characterized by the body's inability to absorb fats (lipids), malformed red blood cells, progressive nervous system defects, and retinitis pigmentosa. Retinal changes resemble those in vitamin A deficiency (rod vision deteriorates before cone vision). Congenital; hereditary.

Batten-Mayou syndrome (MAY-oo), **Stock-Spielmeyer-Vogt** *(or)* **Vogt-Spiel-meyer syndrome**. *Pathologic condition.* Childhood form of amaurotic family idiocy, characterized by diffuse nervous system disease, macular lesions, and optic nerve degeneration.

Battle's sign. *Clinical sign.* A bruise (ecchymosis) over the mastoid area (behind the ear). Suggests a basal skull fracture.

Bayshet's disease. Incorrect spelling of BEHCET'S DISEASE.

B-cell. *Anatomy.* Type of white blood cell (lymphocyte) produced in the bone marrow; part of the body's immune system.

Bealshosky. Incorrect spelling of BIELSCHOWSKY.

Bear's disease. Incorrect spelling of BEHR'S DISEASE.

"bear tracks," congenital grouped pigmentation. *Anatomic variant.* Areas of excessively pigmented retinal pigment epithelium that resemble paw prints. Histopathology: hypertrophy of the pigment epithelium.

Beck's sarcoid Incorrect spelling of BOECK'S SARCOID.

bedewing (beh-DU-ing), **corneal bedewing, Sattler's veil**. *Pathological condition, clinical sign.* Swelling and clouding of superficial layers of the cornea, causing loss of surface smoothness, which reduces its image-forming properties. May be caused by prolonged increase in intraocular pressure or by contact lens overwear. See also OVERWEAR SYNDROME.

Behcet's disease (beh-SHETZ). *Pathologic condition.* Systemic disease, with chronic inflammation and vascular lesions in the mucous membranes of the mouth and genitalia. Eye findings include severe uveitis, optic neuritis, and iridocyclitis.

Behr's disease. *Pathologic condition.* Optic atrophy, with nystagmus, mental retardation, spasticity of limbs, and staggering gait. Occurs in childhood.

Beilshowsky. Incorrect spelling of BIELSCHOWSKY.

belladonna. Herb whose leaves and roots contain atropine and related anticholinergic alkaloids (chemicals).

Bell's palsy, facial palsy. *Pathologic condition.* Paralysis of muscles innervated by the 7th (facial) cranial nerve, which move facial structures surrounding the brow, eyelids and mouth. Eyelid on the affected side does not close properly, so corneal drying may become a problem.

Bell's phenomenon. *Function.* Upward and outward deviation of the eyes during sleep or with forcible closure of the eyelids.

Benadryl. *Drug.* Trade name of diphenhydramine; antihistamine for treating allergic and hypersensitivity reactions.

Benedikt's syndrome (BEN-uh-diktz). *Pathologic condition.* Paralysis of one eye accompanied by paralysis and tremor of the arm on other side of the body. Affected eye muscles are supplied by the 3rd (oculomotor) cranial nerve.

benign (buh-NINE). *Description.* Does not threaten health or life. Refers to a lesion or tumor that is non-cancerous (non-malignant).

benign essential blepharospasm (BEB) (BLEF-uh-roh-spaz-um), **essential blepharospasm**. *Functional defect.* Sudden, involuntary spasm of the orbicularis oculi muscle, producing uncontrolled blinking and lid squeezing. Involves both eyes and in advanced cases, muscles of the mouth or neck. Involuntary eyelid closure may result in temporary inability to see. See also BLEPHAROCLONUS, HEMIFACIAL SPASM, MEIGE SYNDROME.

benzalkonium chloride. *Chemical.* Preservative commonly used in ophthalmic solutions. Causes allergic reaction in some patients.

Benson's sign, asteroid hyalosis. *Pathologic condition.* Degenerative process of having tiny, opaque, oval calcium deposits suspended in the vitreous; causes no decrease in vision. Occurs in the elderly, usually in one eye. See also SYNCHYSIS SCINTILLANS.

Bergmeister's papilla (BURG-mi-sturz puh-PIL-uh). *Anatomy.* Cone-shaped mass of cells in the center of the optic disc during embryologic development; establishes depth of the optic cup. Usually degenerates before birth, but occasionally persists and obliterates the optic cup.

beriberi. *Pathologic condition.* Nervous system and gastrointestinal disturbances caused by vitamin B_1 (thiamine) deficiency. Associated with conjunctivitis and/or staphylococcal infection of the eyelids. If long-term, can lead to optic nerve damage and amblyopia.

birefringence. *Optics.* Characteristic of some crystalline materials to separate light into rays with two planes of polarization, 90° apart.

Berlin's edema, commotio retinae. *Pathologic condition.* Swollen, white, "bruised" retina that follows blunt trauma to the eye. Poor prognosis for vision recovery if it occurs in the macula (area of central vision).

Berman locator. *Instrument.* Magnetic device used for detecting and locating metallic foreign bodies in the eye, especially when visibility is hindered by bleeding or a cloudy cornea, lens or vitreous.

best-corrected visual acuity (BVA). *Measurement.* Vision obtained with best possible lens correction.

Best's disease, vitelliform degeneration. *Pathologic condition.* Retinal pigment epithelial degeneration that affects macular area primarily. Early lesion resembles an egg yolk; in later stages can look like scrambled egg. Hereditary.

beta adrenergic. *Drug.* Enhances action of sympathetic nerve fibers. Example: isoproterenol.

beta blocker, adrenergic blocking agent, sympatholytic drug. *Drug.* 1. Used topically for treating glaucoma. Blocks action of sympathetic nerve fibers by blocking beta adrenergic receptor sites for nerve impulse transmission; sometimes causes pupillary constriction. Betaxolol is a beta-one blocker; carteolol, levobunolol, metipranolol and timolol are beta-one and beta-two blockers. 2. Used systemically as heart medication to treat rapid arrhythmia and hypertension. Discontinuation may decrease intraocular pressure control.

Betagan. *Drug.* Trade name of levobunolol eyedrops, beta-one and beta-two blocking agent for treating glaucoma.

beta hemolytic (BAY-tuh hee-muh-LIT-ik). *Microorganism.* Type of streptococcal bacteria that fractures red blood cells and turns blood agar culture plate from red to clear. See also ALPHA HEMOLYTIC.

betaxolol (bay-TAKS-uh-lawl). *Drug.* Beta-one blocking agent that reduces aqueous secretion. Eyedrops used for treating glaucoma. Trade name: Betoptic. See also CARTEOLOL, LEVOBUNOLOL, METIPRANOLOL, TIMOLOL.

Betimol. *Drug.* Trade name of timolol; used for treating glaucoma.

Betoptic, Betoptic S (bay-TAHP-tik). *Drug.* Trade names for betaxolol eye-drops; used for treating glaucoma.

Bick procedure. *Surgical procedure.* Shortening technique for a lower eyelid that does not rest against the eyeball (ectropion). See also SENILE ECTROPION.

biconcave lens (bi-KAHN-kayv). *Optical device.* Minus-powered lens, thinner in the center and thicker at the edges, with inward curvature of both surfaces.

biconvex lens (bi-KAHN-veks). *Optical device.* Plus-powered lens, thicker in the center and thinner at the edges, with outward curvature of both surfaces.

Bielschowsky head tilt test (beel-SHAH/OW-skee). The head is tilted to one shoulder, then the other, to distinguish between a truly weak vertical muscle in one eye and an apparently weak vertical muscle in the other eye. See also INHIBITIONAL PALSY OF THE CONTRALATERAL ANTAGONIST.

Bielschowsky-Jansky disease. *Pathologic condition.* Characterized by diffuse nervous system disease, lesions in the macula, and optic nerve degeneration. See also AMAUROTIC FAMILIAL IDIOCY.

Bielschowsky-Lutz-Cogan syndrome, internuclear ophthalmoplegia. *Pathologic condition.* Eye movement abnormalities attributed to brainstem lesion. Eye on same side of body as the lesion has limited inward movement (adduction); other eye has jerky movements on outward gaze (abduction). Convergence is normal. Frequently accompanied by vertical oscillations (nystagmus), especially on up-gaze, and skew deviations. Associated with multiple sclerosis.

Bietti's marginal crystalline dystrophy (b/YEH-teez KRIS-tul-un DIS-troh-fee). *Pathologic condition.* Characterized by crystalline deposits in the corneal periphery associated with retinal pigmentation.

bifixation. See BIFOVEAL FIXATION.

bifocals. *Optical device.* Eyeglasses that incorporate two different powers in each lens, usually for near and distance corrections. See also ADD.

bifoveal. *Description.* The foveae of both eyes used together, as in bifoveal fixation.

bifoveal fixation (bi-FOH-vee-ul), **bifixation**. *Function.* Imaging an object on both foveae at the same time.

bifurcate (BI-fur-kayt). To divide into two branches, e.g., blood vessels.

bilateral. *Description.* Affecting or occurring on both sides.

bilateral acute retinal necrosis. See BARN.

Binkhorst equation. *Measurement.* One of several formulas used prior to cataract surgery for calculating the power for an intraocular lens.

binocular. *Description.* Referring to or affecting both eyes.

binocular depth perception, stereopsis, stereoscopic vision, 3rd grade fusion. *Function.* Visual blending of two similar images (one falling on each retina) into one, with visual perception of solidity and depth.

binocular field. Extent of the visual field seen by both eyes simultaneously. Consists of the overlapping part of each eye's monocular field.

binocular fixation pattern (BFP). *Test.* Used in conjunction with a cover test to determine if one eye is more often straight and preferred for fixation than the other.

binocularity. *Function.* Ability to use both eyes together.

binocular parallax. *Function.* As each eye views an object from a slightly different position, the two slightly different images are fused in the brain to create the perception of depth. See also PARALLAX.

binocular vision. *Function.* Blending of the separate images seen by each eye into one composite image. See also FUSION.

binocular visual acuity. *Function, test.* Quantitative assessment of vision with both eyes open.

biometry (ocular). *Test.* Measurement of the distance between various ocular structures, usually using A-scan and B-scan ultrasound instruments.

biomicroscope. See SLIT LAMP.

biomicroscopy (bi-oh-mi-KRAHS-cuh-pee. *Technique*. Microscopic examination of the cornea or lens with a slit lamp (biomicroscope).

bipolar cautery (bi-POH-lur), **bipolar coagulator**. *Surgical instrument*. Applies a tiny electric current to stop bleeding within a wet field, e.g., the vitreous.

bipolar cells. *Anatomy*. Retinal nerve cells that connect outer and inner layers of the sensory retina (connect rod and cone nuclei with ganglion cells).

bipolar coagulator. See BIPOLAR CAUTERY.

Bion Tears. *Drug*. Trade name of methylcellulose eyedrops; for treating dry eyes.

biprism (BI-prizm). *Instrument*. Two prisms placed base to base, for measuring relative tilt (cyclodeviations) between the two eyes.

bitemporal (bi-TEM-pur-ul). *Description*. Refers to the temporal visual field of each eye: the right eye's right half and the left eye's left half.

bitemporal hemianopsia (hem-ee-uh-NAHP-see-uh), **bitemporal hemianopia**. *Functional defect*. Visual field defect of the right half of the right eye's field and the left half of the left eye's field. Characteristic of lesions affecting the optic chiasm, e.g., pituitary tumors. See also SCOTOMA.

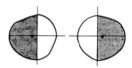

BITEMPORAL HEMIANOPSIA

bitoric contact lens (bi-TOR-ik). *Optical device*. Contact lens that has non-spheric (toric) curvatures on both front and back surfaces: on the front for astigmatic optical correction and on the back for stabilizing lens position to maintain its alignment on an astigmatic cornea.

Bitot's spot (BEE-tohz). *Clinical sign*. Pearly looking, foamy mass that forms superficially on a dry patch of bulbar conjunctiva near the cornea. Occurs with vitamin A difficiency.

Bjerrum scotoma (JEH-rum skuh-TOH-muh), **arcuate** *(or)* **comet** *(or)* **scimitar scotoma**. *Functional defect*. Arc-shaped blind area in the visual field; caused by damage to retinal nerve fiber bundles. Common in patients with glaucoma.

black sunburst. *Pathologic condition, clinical sign*. Melanin deposit on the retina caused by hemorrhage following small branch retinal artery blockage. Accompanies sickle cell disease.

bleb, filtering bleb. Bubble-like blister of conjunctiva. 1. *Surgical result*. Flap of tissue created for covering a sclero-corneal drainage channel, to enhance passage of fluid from the eye. Result of type of filtering procedure for treating some forms of glaucoma. 2. *Pathologic condition*. Follows inadvertent leak of aqueous fluid from a limbal wound, sometimes after surgery.

blef- Incorrect spelling of many words beginning BLEPH-.

blennorrhea (blen-uh-REE-uh). *Pathological condition*. Conjunctival inflammation producing mucous discharge. Obsolete term.

Blephamide (BLEF-uh-mide). *Drug*. Trade name of eyedrops containing prednisolone and sulfacetamide; for treating eyelid margin infections and some types of conjunctivitis.

blepharitis (blef-uh-RI-tus). *Pathologic condition*. Inflammation of the eyelids, usually with redness, swelling and itching. Many causes, e.g., infection, allergy.

    marginal: inflammation of the eyelid margin, with redness, swelling, itching and scaly skin.

    seborrheic (seb-ur-EE-ik): chronic dandruff-like inflammation of the eyelid margin, with redness, swelling, itching and scaly skin.

blepharo- (BLEF-uh-roh). Prefix: refers to the eyelids.

blepharochalasis (blef-uh-roh-kuh-LAY-sis), **dermatochalasis**. *Pathologic* *condition.* Excess eyelid skin, caused by atrophy of the elastic tissue. Usually a fold of tissue from the upper lid hangs over the eyelid margin. Associated with orbital septum defects or aging.

blepharoconjunctivitis (BLEF-uh-roh-kun-junk-tuh-VI-tis). *Pathologic condition.* Inflammation of the conjunctiva (membrane covering white of eye, undersurface of lids, and margins of upper and lower eyelids).

blepharophimosis (BLEF-uh-roh-fi-MOH-sis). *Congenital anomaly.* Narrower-than-normal opening between the upper and lower eyelids (palpebral fissure), with shorter-than-normal width of the opening. Often associated with excessive distance between the inner canthi and a drooping upper eyelid (blepharoptosis).

blepharopigmentation (blef-uh-roh-pig-men-TAY-shun), **microdermato-blepharopigmentation**. *Surgical procedure.* Application of tiny pigment granules under the skin between the lashes and/or eyebrows for cosmetic purposes. Results in "permanent eyeliner."

blepharoplasty (BLEF-uh-roh-plas-tee). *Surgical procedure.* Any plastic surgery of the eyelids.

blepharoptosis (blef-uh-rahp-TOH-sis), **ptosis**. *Functional defect.* Drooping of the upper eyelid. May be congenital or caused by paralysis or weakness (paresis) of the 3rd (oculomotor) cranial nerve or sympathetic nerves, or by excessive weight of the upper eyelids.

blepharospasm (BLEF-uh-roh-spaz-um). *Functional defect.* Sudden, involuntary spasm of the orbicularis oculi muscle, producing uncontrolled blinking and lid squeezing. See also BLEPHAROCLONUS.

    essential: involves both eyes and in advanced cases, muscles of the mouth or neck. Involuntary eyelid closure may result in temporary inability to see. Also called benign essential blepharospasm (BEB). See also HEMI-FACIAL SPASM.

blepharotomy (blef-uh-RAHT-uh-mee). *Surgical procedure.* Incision into an eyelid.

Bleph-10. *Drug.* Trade name of sulfacetamide antibiotic ointment; for treating external eye infections.

Blessig-Iwanoff cysts. *Pathologic condition.* Multiple, small, degenerative cystic (sac-like) spaces along the ora serrata in the peripheral retina. Common with aging.

"blind" goniotomy, direct goniotomy. *Surgical procedure.* Incision made in the trabecular meshwork without clear visualization of angle structures, e.g., when obscured by a cloudy cornea; used for treating congenital glaucoma.

blindness. *Functional defect.* Inability to see.

    cerebral: same as CORTICAL (below).

    color: see specific defects: CONE OR ROD MONOCHROMACY, DEUTERAN-OMALY, DEUTERANOPIA, PROTANOMALY, PROTANOPIA, TRITANOMALY, TRITANOPIA.

    cortical: caused by damage to the blood supply of the visual areas in the brain's occipital cortices. Retina appears normal; visually-evoked electrical response (VER) is markedly diminished. See also ANTON'S SYN-DROME, BRODMANN AREA 17.

    eclipse: macular damage caused by looking at the sun without protective filters, as during a solar eclipse. Intense radiant energy absorbed in the retina and pigment epithelium produces a dazzling light sensation that soon changes to a central blind spot (scotoma). Usually results in permanent reduction in central vision. Also called solar maculopathy.

    flash: caused by extremely bright light flash; usually temporary. Can be permanent if light is intense (e.g., from an atomic bomb blast).

    legal: best-corrected visual acuity of 20/200 or less, or reduction in visual field to 20° or less, in the better-seeing eye.

night: inefficient dark adaptation; markedly reduced vision in reduced illumination.

snow: inability to open the eyes due to severe, painful irritation of the cornea and conjunctiva; secondary to ultraviolet burns by sunlight rays reflected from snow, usually at high altitudes.

blind spot, scotoma. *Functional defect*. Non-seeing area within the visual field. May result from damage to the visual pathways or to the retina. A normal, physiological blind spot ("the blind spot" or blind spot of Mariotte) exists in all eyes and marks the site where the optic nerve enters the eye. Types listed under SCOTOMA.

blind spot mechanism, blind spot *(or)* Swan syndrome. *Functional defect*. Adaptive mechanism for avoiding double vision that may accompany an inward eye deviation (esotropia). Deviation increases until the image falls on the optic disc of the deviated eye, which eliminates double vision. Controversial concept; may not be clinically significant.

blink reflex. *Function*. Periodic contraction of orbicularis oculi muscle (5 second intervals), which spreads tears over eyeball surface and limits amount of light entering the eye. Additional blinking occurs with corneal or conjunctival irritation, bright lights, sudden loud noises, or sneezing.

Blocardren. *Drug*. Trade name of timolol; for controlling high blood pressure (hypertension).

Bloch-Stauffer syndrome, Rothmund *(or)* Thomson syndrome. *Pathologic condition*. Characterized by cataracts and skin pigmentation abnormalities. Congenital; hereditary.

Bloch-Sulzberger syndrome. *Pathologic condition*. Characterized by severe skin pigmentation defects and eye signs that include a white mass inside the eye and retinal malformation. Hereditary, X-linked.

blocked tear duct, nasolacrimal duct obstruction. *Pathologic condition*. Incomplete opening of a tear duct; causes continuous tearing. See also DACRYOCYSTORHINOSTOMY, LACRIMAL PROBE.

blood-aqueous barrier. *Function*. Physiological "filter" that keeps large molecules in the bloodstream (proteins, chemicals, drugs) from reaching the aqueous. Any disruption, e.g., from inflammation, trauma or surgery, allows leakage into the aqueous. Probably located in the ciliary body and iris at the tight cellular junctions between capillary cell walls and non-pigmented ciliary epithelial cells.

blood agar. *Lab medium*. Red-colored culture material that contains nutrients for growth of most oxygen-requiring bacteria and many fungi. See also CHOCOLATE AGAR.

blood urea nitrogen level. See BUN LEVEL.

blood pressure (BP). *Function*. Tension of blood within the arteries, measured in mm of mercury.

diastolic (di-uh-STAHL-ik): lowest pressure in cardiac cycle; occurs during heart relaxation phase.

systolic (sis-TAHL-ik): highest pressure in cardiac cycle; occurs when the heart contracts.

"blown pupil," fixed dilated pupil. *Anatomic defect*. Enlarged pupil that does not constrict in response to a light stimulus, a near object, or a light stimulus in the other eye.

blowout fracture. *Injury*. Break in the bony orbital floor or walls caused by blunt trauma to eye or orbit. Intraorbital contents are pushed into one or more of the paranasal sinuses. See also ORBITAL FLOOR FRACTURE.

blue sclera. *Clinical sign*. Thin sclera that has a translucent blue appearance from the underlying pigmented ciliary body and choroid. Hereditary. Sign of osteogenesis imperfecta (brittle bones).

blur and clear. *Eye exercise.* Orthoptic exercise for accommodative esotropia; patient practices keeping the eyes straight by relaxing accommodation and allowing image to blur.

blur circle. *Optics.* Refers to an unfocused image of an object point. Light rays focused by a lens system converge to form a small circle of light rather than a sharp point. The size of this circle on the retina (influenced by the degree of refractive error and diameter of the pupillary opening) determines how blurred an image looks.

blur point. *Measurement.* Point at which a change in prism or lens blurs vision (as gradually increasing amounts of prism or lenses are placed before the eyes); used for measuring range of single binocular vision. See also BREAK POINT, FUSIONAL AMPLITUDES.

bobbing. *Clinical sign.* Disordered, spontaneous, fast jerk of both eyes followed by a slow return to the straight-ahead (primary) position. Related to advanced disease of the brainstem, usually in a comatose patient.

> **ocular**: begins with a downward jerk.

> **reverse**: begins with an upward jerk.

Boeck's sarcoid (beks SAHR-koyd), **sarcoid, sarcoidosis**. *Pathologic condition.* Inflammatory disorder of unknown origin affecting almost all systems of the body; characterized by microscopic nodule formation. Most common eye findings are large mutton fat keratic precipitates, iritis with iris adhesions to the lens, and heavy vitreous deposits. See also "CANDLEWAX DRIPPINGS," MIKULICZ'S SYNDROME, "SNOW-BALLS," "STRING OF PEARLS."

bolus (BOH-lus). Small round mass, such as a concentrated lump of food or medication.

Boosacka nodules. Incorrect spelling of BUSACCA NODULES.

Botox. *Drug.* Trade name of freeze-dried form of botulinum toxin; injected into muscles for temporary paralysis.

botulinum toxin (bah-tchu-LI-num). *Chemical.* Poison derived from botulinum bacterium. Paralyzes muscle fibers temporarily. Used as an alternative or addition to surgery to correct eye misalignments or to paralyze a facial nerve causing uncontrollable lid spasms. Trade names: Botox, Oculinum. See also BLEPHAROSPASM.

botulism (BAH-tchu-lizm). *Pathologic condition.* Poisoning from food containing the bacterium *Clostridium botulinum.* Eye signs, possibly the first indicators of poisoning, include double vision (from extraocular muscle palsies), loss of clear near vision, dilated pupils, nystagmus and ptosis.

"bound down." *Description.* Refers to tissues that are adherent and not free to move normally.

> **muscle**: extraocular muscle scarred from trauma, disease or previous surgery, whose movement is restricted or prevented, usually in the direction opposite to its normal action.

bouquet of Rochon-Duvigneaud (roh-SHAHN du-vee-NOHD). *Anatomy.* 2,500 thin cones comprising the most central zone of the retinal foveal pit.

Bourneville's disease (BORN-vilz), **tuberous sclerosis**. *Pathologic condition.* Characterized by seizures, mental retardation, behavior disorders and skin tumors; eyes may show benign retinal tumors (resembling tapioca). Hereditary.

Bowen's disease (BOH-enz), **corneoconjunctival intraepithelial neoplasia, intraepithelial epithelioma**. *Pathologic condition.* Slow-growing, malignant tumor, commonly arising at multiple sites near the corneoscleral junction (limbus) but limited to the epithelial layer. May be caused by chronic sun exposure.

Bowman's membrane. *Anatomy.* Corneal layer just under the epithelium and above the corneal stroma.

boxcarring. *Anatomic defect.* Segmentation and sludging of blood in retinal blood vessels; associated with sluggish retinal blood flow.

box sarcoid. Incorrect spelling of BOECK'S SARCOID.

brachy- Prefix: flat

brachytherapy (BRAK-ee-ther-uh-pee). *Treatment.* Application of radioactive plaques to the sclera (outer layer of eye), for treating intraocular tumors.

bradycardia (bray-dih-KAHR-dee-uh). *Clinical sign.* Unusually slow heart rate. May be normal or pathological.

brain cortex. *Anatomy.* Outermost layers of the cerebrum and cerebellum.

brainstem, brain stem. *Anatomy.* The part of the central nervous system that connects the cerebral hemispheres and the spinal cord. Contains nerve centers that control eye movements.

branch artery occlusion (BAO), branch retinal artery occlusion. *Pathologic condition.* Blockage of blood flow through any of the branches of the central retinal artery, usually from an embolus. Produces retinal damage and a corresponding visual field defect. See also BRANCH VEIN OCCLUSION.

branch retinal artery occlusion (BRAO). See BRANCH ARTERY OCCLUSION.

branch retinal vein occlusion (BRVO). See BRANCH VEIN OCCLUSION.

branch vein occlusion (BVO), branch retinal vein occlusion. *Pathologic condition.* Blockage of blood flow through a branch of the central retinal vein (usually superior temporal), usually by an overlying hardened retinal artery. Associated findings include retinal vein engorgement, flame- shaped hemorrhages, macular edema, cotton-wool spots, and reduced vision. See also BRANCH ARTERY OCCLUSION.

break point. *Measurement.* Point at which a change in prism or lens induces double vision; occurs as gradually increasing amounts of prism or lenses are placed before the eyes to measure the range of single binocular vision. See also BLUR POINT, FUSIONAL AMPLITUDES.

breakup time (BUT). *Measurement.* Test for tear function. Time interval between a blink and the development of a dry spot in the pre-corneal tear film; less than 10 seconds is abnormal. Spot is visible after fluorescein staining, especially with the cobalt blue beam on the slit lamp.

brewey, brewy. Incorrect spelling of BRUIT.

bridle suture. *Surgical aid.* Loop of thread placed under a muscle (usually superior rectus) to help steady the eyeball. Often used in cataract surgery.

Brodmann area 8, frontal eye fields. *Anatomy.* Area in the frontal lobe of the brain; responsible for rapid, voluntary eye movements (saccades). See also BRODMANN AREA 19, FAST EYE MOVEMENTS.

Brodmann area 18, parastriate area. *Anatomy.* Visual association area in the occipital lobe of the brain, surrounding Brodmann area 17 (the primary visual cortex); helps to interpret visual messages from area 17. See also BRODMANN AREA 19, OCCIPITAL CORTEX.

Brodmann area 19, peristriate area. *Anatomy.* Visual association area in the brain surrounding the parastriate area (Brodmann area 18). Interprets images in area 17; begins the occipito-mesencephalic pathways for pursuit eye movements. See also OCCIPITAL CORTEX.

Brodmann area 17, primary visual cortex, striate area. *Anatomy.* Area in the occipital lobe of the brain (cerebral end of sensory visual pathways that begin at the retina), where initial conscious registration of visual information takes place. See also OCCIPITAL CORTEX.

bromocriptine. *Drug.* Anti-cancer drug; shrinks pituitary tumors by blocking prolactin secretion. Trade name: Parlodel.

brooks membrane. Incorrect spelling of BRUCH'S MEMBRANE.

Brookner test. Incorrect spelling of BRÜCKER (OR BRUECKNER) TEST.

browlift, browplasty. *Surgical procedure.* Removal of extra tissue above the eyebrow hairline, to repair drooping eyebrows.

Brown's syndrome, sheath *(or)* **superior oblique tendon sheath syndrome**. *Pathologic condition.* Sheath of superior oblique muscle that does not, or cannot, relax when the eye attempts to look upward and inward; mimics an inferior oblique palsy. Unilateral; may be congenital or acquired. See also RESTRICTIVE SYNDROMES.

browplasty. See BROWLIFT.

Bruch's membrane (brooks), **basal lamina, lamina vitrea**. *Anatomy.* Innermost layer of the choroid, lying directly under the retinal pigment epithelium. When damaged by disease or aging, responsible for many bleeding disorders of the macular area, e.g., macular degeneration.

Brückner test (BROOK-nur); also spelled Brueckner. For detecting eye misalignment (strabismus). When a bright light stimulus shining into both eyes elicits an equal brightness of the red reflex in each eye, there is no deviation; if different, the eye with the brighter reflex is deviating. See also RED REFLEX.

Brueckner test. See BRÜCKNER TEST.

bruit (BRU-ee). *Functional defect.* "Blowing" sound heard in any large artery when blood flow is turbulent; usually associated with blood vessel abnormalities or narrowing, as in atherosclerosis. In the carotid artery, can be a sign of carotid cavernous sinus fistulas, or orbital or intracranial tumors.

brunescent cataract. *Pathologic condition.* Cloudy crystalline lens that is brown, rather than gray or white. Occurs in the elderly as an advanced stage of nuclear sclerosis.

Brushfield spots. *Clinical sign.* Gray or brown spots on the iris, associated with mongolism (Down's syndrome). Also found in many normal children.

B-scan. *Instrument.* Ultrasound device that provides a cross-section view of tissues that cannot be seen directly. High frequency waves are reflected by eye tissues and orbital structures and converted into electrical pulses, which are displayed on the printout as bright spots on a black background. See also A-SCAN, ECHOGRAPHY, ULTRASONOGRAPHY.

BSS. *Drug.* Trade name of balanced salt solution; used for irrigating eyes during surgical procedures.

buckle. *Surgical procedure.* Used in retinal detachment surgery to help seal a tear or reduce vitreous traction. Material (usually silicone) is sutured onto the sclera to indent it and apply localized pressure over the retina.

bulbar. *Description.* 1. Refers to the eyeball. 2. Refers to globe-like expansion of a tubelike structure, such as the medulla oblongata of the brainstem.

bulbar conjunctiva. *Anatomy.* Mucus membrane covering the external eyeball (except the cornea). See also PALPEBRAL CONJUNCTIVA.

bullae (BU-lee). *Pathologic condition.* Small, fluid-filled blisters seen on the corneal surface when the cornea is swollen.

bullous (BULL-us). *Description.* Blister-like.

bullous keratopathy (kehr-uh-TAH-puh-thee). *Pathologic condition.* Degenerative process characterized by small blister-like pockets that form in the swollen corneal epithelial layer; markedly reduces vision. See also FUCHS' DYSTROPHY.

bull's-eye maculopathy (mak-yu-LAH-puh-thee). *Pathologic condition.* Alternating ring-like zones of pigmentation and depigmentation of the retinal pigment epithelium and choroid in the macular area. May result from long-term chloroquin use.

BUN (blood urea nitrogen) level. *Test.* Amount of urea in the blood, measured by the nitrogen content. Rough indicator of kidney function.

buphthalmos (boof-THAL-mus), **hydrophthalmos**. *Pathologic condition.* Abnormally large eyeball ("ox-eye") caused by glaucoma in a young, stretchable eye. See also CONGENITAL GLAUCOMA, MACROPHTHALMOS, MEGOPHTHALMOS.

bupivacaine. *Drug.* Long-acting anesthetic used for eye surgery. Trade name: Marcaine. See also LIDOCAINE, MEPIVACAINE, PROPARACAINE, XYLOCAINE.

Busacca nodules (bu-SAH-kuh). *Clinical sign.* Clumps of inflammatory cells on the front surface of the iris; associated with granulomatous uveitis. See also KOEPPE NODULES.

buttonhole. *Surgical complication.* Small tear or cut in a sheetlike tissue, e.g., the conjunctiva.

b-wave. *Test.* The part of the electroretinogram (ERG) wave (highest upward spike) thought to reflect Mueller cell function.

C

CAB (cellulose acetate butyrate). *Chemical.* Plastic used in making gas permeable hard contact lenses.

Calan. *Drug.* Trade name of verapamil, a heart medication.

calcarine fissure (KAL-kuh-rine). *Anatomy.* Midline groove in the occipital lobes of the brain that separate the upper and lower halves. Optic radiations end here, delivering visual information from the eyes.

Caldwell projection. Radiologic view useful in evaluating fractures of the orbit and face.

calipers. *Instrument.* Measuring device with two adjustable arms, for determining thickness, diameter, or distance between two surfaces.

caloric nystagmus (ni-STAG-mus), **labyrinthine *(or)* vestibular nystagmus.** *Abnormal function.* Involuntary, jerky eye movements caused by a disturbance in normal innervation from the labyrinths in the ears. Unrelated to visual stimuli. See also CALORIC TESTING.

caloric testing. Irrigation of an ear's auditory canal with warm or cold water, to test function of the vestibular system. See also COWS.

campimeter, tangent screen. *Test instrument.* Screen used for quantifying visual field defects within 30° of a fixation point. Testing is carried out at either 1 or 2 meters from the eye. See also PERIMETRY.

canaliculitis (kan-uh-lik-yu-LI-tus). *Pathologic condition.* Inflammation of the lacrimal canaliculusi, often caused by a fungus infection.

canaliculus (kan-uh-LIK-yu-lus), **lacrimal canaliculus.** *Anatomy.* Tiny channel in each eyelid that forms part of the tear drainage system. Begins at the lacrimal punctum in both upper and lower lids, joining to form the common canaliculus, which leads to the tear (lacrimal) sac and then through the nasolacrimal duct into the nose. Plural: canaliculi. See also PUNCTUM.

> **common c**: tiny channel under the skin formed by the junction of the upper and lower canaliculi; leads to the lacrimal sac.

canal of Schlemm. *Anatomy.* Circular channel deep in the corneo-scleral junction (limbus); conducts aqueous from the anterior chamber in the eye through aqueous veins into the bloodstream.

cancer, malignant lesion. *Pathologic condition.* Tissue of potentially unlimited growth that expands locally by invasion, and throughout the body by metastasis. See also CARCINOMA, SARCOMA.

candela (kan-DEH-luh). *Measurement.* Unit of luminous intensity of light based on a standard electric filament bulb.

candidiasis. *Pathologic condition.* Infection by the common fungus *Candida albicans.*

Candida albicans (KAN-dih-duh AL-bih-kanz). *Microorganism.* Yeast-like fungus. May infect eye structures, e.g., cornea, retina, vitreous. Drug addicts and immunocompromised patients are especially susceptible.

candle power. *Measurement.* Unit of luminous intensity of light based on a standard candle.

"candlewax drippings." *Clinical sign.* Clusters of waxy exudates in the vitreous and on the retinal surface; associated with ocular inflammation due to sarcoidosis. See also PERIVASCULITIS.

cannula (KAN-yu-luh). *Surgical instrument.* Small tube-like device for injecting or extracting fluids or air.

can-opener capsulotomy. *Surgical procedure.* Circular, jagged incision made in the anterior lens capsule for extracapsular cataract extraction. See also CAPSULE, CAPSULORHEXIS.

canthal resection. *Surgical procedure.* Removal of a section of inner or outer canthus (junction of upper and lower eyelids), e.g., during excision of an eyelid tumor.

cantholysis (kan-thoh-LI-sis). *Surgical procedure.* Loosening the attachment of the canthus (junction of upper and lower eyelids) to the tendon or bone, usually as part of eyelid plastic surgery.

canthoplasty (KAN-thoh-plas-tee). *Surgical procedure.* Reconstruction of the medial or lateral canthus (junction of upper and lower eyelids).

canthotomy (kan-THAH-tuh-mee). *Surgical procedure.* Horizontal incision at the canthus (junction of upper and lower eyelids) to temporarily enlarge lid separation, or as part of reconstructive lid plastic surgery.

canthus (KAN-thus). *Anatomy.* Angle formed by the inner or outer junction of the upper and lower eyelids. Plural: canthi.

> **medial**: canthus on the side near the nose.

> **lateral**: canthus on the side away from the nose.

(capillary) dropout. *Pathologic condition.* Loss of retinal capillaries. Occurs in various vascular diseases that affect the retina (e.g., diabetes, vein occlusions). Demonstrated by fluorescein angiography.

capillary hemangioma (hee-man-jee-OH-muh). *Pathologic condition.* Tumor composed of blood vessel cells; usually appears as grouping of bright red spots. Tends to be congenital, growing slowly for several years and then receding in size.

capsular bag, "bag." *Anatomy.* Bag-like lens capsule remnant remaining after cataract removal, that an intraocular lens is implanted into. Consists of the intact posterior capsule and the residual flap of anterior capsule.

capsular fixation. *Surgical technique.* One way an intraocular lens is held in place; a posterior chamber IOL is inserted completely within the capsular bag. See also SULCUS FIXATION.

capsule, lens capsule. *Anatomy.* Elastic bag enveloping the eye's crystalline lens. Helps control the shape of the lens for accommodation.

> **anterior c**: front of the capsule; lies in the posterior chamber just behind the iris.

> **posterior c**: rear of the capsule; lies against the anterior hyaloid membrane of the vitreous.

capsulectomy. *Surgical procedure.* Removal of part of the lens capsule. (Anterior capsulectomy is a routine part of extracapsular cataract extraction.)

capsulorhexis, capsulorrhexis (kap-suh-loh-REK-sis). *Surgical procedure.* Opening in the lens capsule (capsulotomy) made by a continuous tear to enable removal of opaque lens material during extracapsular cataract extraction. See also CAPSULOTOMY.

capsulotomy (kap-sul-AH-tuh-mee). *Surgical procedure.* Incision to open the lens capsule. See also CAPSULE, CAPSULORHEXIS.

> **anterior**: opening in the front lens capsule for extracapsular cataract extraction.

> **can-opener**: opening that has a circular jagged configuration; made in the anterior capsule as part of an extracapsular cataract extraction.

> **posterior**: opening in the rear lens capsule that has become opacified after previous cataract surgery; usually made with a YAG laser.

carbachol (KAHR-buh-kahl). *Drug.* Eyedrop that causes pupil constriction and increased aqueous outflow. Used for treating glaucoma. Trade names: Carcholin, Doryl, Isopto Carbachol.

carbenicillin. *Drug.* Antibiotic agent used for treating eye infections.

Carbocaine. *Drug.* Trade name of mepivacaine, an anesthetic used for eye surgery.

carbonic anhydrase inhibitor (kahr-BAHN-ik an-HI-drayz). *Drug.* Systemic or topical drugs that decrease aqueous production and secretion. For treating glaucoma. Examples: acetazolamide, dichlorophenamide, dorsolamide, ethoxamide, methazolamide.

Carcholin (KAHR-koh-lin). *Drug.* Trade name of carbachol; for treating glaucoma.

carcinoma. *Pathologic condition.* Cancer derived from epithelial cells, i.e., cells on the surface of a tissue or gland. See also SARCOMA.

    basal cell c: slow growing tumor; most common malignancy of the eyelids. Develops from the deepest (basal) layer of the skin, frequently near the medial canthus. Responds well to treatment. Does not metastasize.

    sebaceous gland c: malignant eyelid tumor arising from a meibomian or Zeiss gland. Often mistaken for a chalazion.

    squamous cell c. (SKWAY-mus): type of skin cancer. Malignant tumor arising from epithelial surface cells. May occur on any skin surface including the eyelids; can metastasize.

cardinal fields. *Test.* See DIAGNOSTIC FIELDS OF GAZE, the preferred term.

cardinal points. *Optics.* Six points (2 principal, 2 nodal, 2 focal) on the principal axis of any optical system that describe the focusing action of that system.

cardinal movements. *Function.* Four directions (right, left, up, down) that the eyes move in reaching the secondary positions. See also DIAGNOSTIC POSITIONS OF GAZE, YOKE MUSCLES.

cardinal positions of gaze. Six positions (right, left, up + right, down + right, up + left, down + left) used for testing the six pairs of muscles involved in eye movement coordination.

Cardrase (KAHR-drayz). *Drug.* Trade name of ethoxzolamide; for treating glaucoma.

carotid artery (kuh-RAH-tid). *Anatomy.* Major vessel carrying blood to the head (including both eyes) from the aorta; refers also to the internal and external branches of the carotid artery.

carotid cavernous fistula (CCF). See CAVERNOUS SINUS FISTULA.

carteolol. *Drug.* Beta-one and beta-two blocking agent that reduces aqueous secretion. Used as eyedrops for treating glaucoma. Trade name: Ocupress. See also BETAXOLOL, LEVOBUNOLOL, METIPRANOLOL, TIMOLOL.

caruncle (KEHR-un-kul). *Anatomy.* Pink, fleshy conjunctival tissue in the nasal corner of each eye over the semilunar fold.

caruncle epicanthus (ep-ee-KAN-thus), **epicanthal fold**. *Anatomy.* Vertical skin fold on either side of the nose, hiding the caruncle. Present in all infants (before bridge of nose is formed) and most Oriental adults. Often makes normal eyes appear crossed. See also PSEUDOSTRABISMUS.

catabolic. *Description.* Aspect of metabolism relating to processes that break down chemical bonds. See also ANABOLIC.

cataract. *Pathologic condition.* Opacity or cloudiness of the crystalline lens, which may prevent a clear image from forming on the retina. Surgical removal of lens may be necessary if visual loss becomes significant, with lost optical power replaced with an intraocular lens, contact lens or aphakic spectacles. May be congenital or caused by trauma, disease, or age. See also NUCLEAR SCLEROSIS.

    brunescent: brown in appearance (rather than gray or white); occurs in elderly as an advanced stage of nuclear sclerosis.

    congenital: present at birth. Many causes, often hereditary.

    cortical: radially arranged opacities in lens cortex following lens fiber swelling and fragmentation. Form of senile cataract; also called cortical spokes.

    cupuliform (kuh-PUH-lih-form): same as POSTERIOR SUBCAPSULAR (below).

    hypermature: totally opaque lens that has begun to shrink and liquify; the remaining hard nucleus floats in the lens capsule. Degraded lens protein molecules may leak into the aqueous through the capsule. See also PHACOLYTIC GLAUCOMA.

immature: cloudy lens that has some clear zones remaining; vision loss depends on extent of clouding.

incipient: cataract in its early stages, or one that has sectors of opacity with clear spaces intervening; little impact on visual acuity.

intumescent (in-tu-MEH-sent): lens that has swollen and enlarged as it became cloudy. May lead to secondary acute angle closure glaucoma.

lamellar (luh-MEH-lur): concentric thin layers (lamellae) of opacities surrounded by zones of clear lens; vision may be good.

mature: opaque lens having no clear zones remaining, but not yet shrunken. Causes marked vision decrease. Used to be called "ripe."

Morgagnian: same as HYPERMATURE (above).

posterior subcapsular: located within the rear surface of the lens. Occurs in elderly as a type of "senile cataract" or at any age after chronic intraocular inflammations or prolonged steroid drug use.

senile: lens opacity occurring in the elderly. Various forms, depending on the position of the opacity: cortical, nuclear.

traumatic: may develop within hours after injury to the eyeball.

zonular: same as LAMELLAR (above)

cataract extraction (cat. ext.). *Surgical procedure.* Removal of a cloudy lens from the eye.

extracapsular: method that leaves the rear lens capsule intact.

intracapsular: complete removal of lens with its capsule, usually by cryoextraction. See also PHACOEMULSIFICATION.

cataract glasses, aphakic spectacles. *Optical device.* Thick, plus-powered eyeglasses that replace optical power lost after cataract extraction, when no intraocular lens has been inserted. See also ASPHERIC LENTICULAR SPECTACLES.

cataractogenic. *Description.* Refers to anything that causes, or makes more likely, the formation of a cataract.

Catarase (KAT-uh-rayz). *Drug.* Trade name of alpha-chymotrypsin.

cat cry syndrome, cri-du-chat syndrome. *Congenital anomaly.* Uncommon chromosome abnormality characterized by a mewing cry by the affected infant. Associated with larynx abnormalities, heart disease, mental retardation, small head, poorly formed ears, widely set eyes, epicanthus, anti-mongoloid slant, outward eye deviation, refractive errors, and tortuous retinal blood vessels.

catecholamines. *Chemical.* Group of natural substances in the body that stimulate the sympathetic nervous system (adrenergic stimulating agents). Example: epinephrine.

cat eye syndrome. *Congenital anomaly.* Chromosome abnormality characterized by developmental and mental retardation, ear tags, macula underdevelopment, optic nerve degeneration, and an incomplete iris that looks like a cat's eye.

cat scratch fever. *Pathologic condition.* Systemic infection following contact with cats; possibly of viral origin. A cause of Parinaud's oculoglandular syndrome.

cat's eye reflex. *Clinical sign.* Unusual whitish glint in the normally black pupil; resembles the reflection seen when a light shines into a cat's eye at night. See also CATARACT, LEUKOCORIA, PHPV, RETINOBLASTOMA.

cavernous atrophy, Schnabel's atrophy. *Pathologic condition.* Form of glaucomatous optic atrophy characterized histologically by lacunae (pods of liquefaction) in the nerve, posterior to the lamina cribosa.

cavernous hemangioma (hee-man-jee-OH-muh). *Congenital anomaly.* Benign blood vessel tumor composed of large vascular channels; sometimes located in the upper eyelid or in the orbit above and behind the eyelid.

cavernous sinus. *Anatomy.* Intracranial collector channel of venous blood (from superior and inferior ophthalmic veins of eye) located behind the orbit. The 3rd (oculomotor), 4th (trochlear), 5th (trigeminal), and 6th (abducens) cranial nerves, with sympathetic nerves, travel through it toward the eye. The ophthalmic branch of the internal carotid artery also courses through this network of vessels.

cavernous sinus fistula (FIS-tyu-luh), **carotid cavernous fistula**. *Pathologic condition*. Abnormal connection between an artery and the cavernous sinus (intracranial space behind orbit); blood is shunted directly from arterial into venous circulation. Produces a painful, protruding eye, dilated conjunctival blood vessels, and a "blowing" sound (bruit) in the carotid artery. Sometimes associated with extraocular muscle palsies, dilated retinal veins, and decreased vision.

cavernous sinus syndrome, parasellar syndrome. *Pathologic condition*. Characterized by restricted eye movement, venous blood congestion, and swelling and engorgement of the eyelids, conjunctiva and orbital tissues, making the eye bulge forward (proptosis). Caused by a blood clot, tumor, or infection in the cavernous sinus (intracranial space behind orbit), producing a weakness of the 3rd (oculomotor), 4th (trochlear), 5th (trigeminal), and 6th (abducens) cranial nerves. See also ORBITAL APEX SYNDROME, SUPERIOR ORBITAL FISSURE SYNDROME, TOLOSA-HUNT SYNDROME.

cavernous sinus thrombosis (thrahm-BOH-sis). *Pathologic condition*. Clotting of blood in the cavernous sinus (intracranial space behind the orbit), causing a protruding eye, pain, swelling, extraocular muscle weakness or paralysis, and optic nerve swelling with decreased vision. May be fatal.

CBC (complete blood count). *Lab test*. Routine set of blood tests performed as part of a diagnostic evaluation of a patient. Usually consists of white and red blood cell count, differential count, hemoglobin, hematocrit.

cc (cubic centimeter). *Unit of measure*. Equivalent to 1 milliliter (1/1000 of a liter).

cc (with [cum] correction). Indicates that vision was tested with patient wearing refraction correction (eyeglasses or contact lenses).

cecal (SEE-kul). *Description*. Refers to the optic disc.

Cechlor. *Drug*. Trade name of cefachlor, an antibiotic.

cefazolin. *Drug*. Broad spectrum antibiotic; injected intramuscularly or intravenously. Trade name: Kefsol.

cefotaxime. *Drug*. Broad spectrum antibiotic. Trade name: Claforan.

"cell and flare." *Clinical sign*. Accumulation of white blood cells and increased protein in the aqueous, visible on slit-lamp examination of the anterior chamber. Associated with inflammation of the iris and/or ciliary body. See also AQUEOUS FLARE.

cellophane maculopathy (mak-yu-LAHP-uh-thee). See CELLOPHANE RETINOPATHY.

cellophane retinopathy (reh-tin-AH-puh-thee), **cellophane maculopathy, epiretinal membrane, epiretinal proliferation, macular pucker**. *Pathologic condition*. Retinal wrinkling in the macular area caused by contraction of the transparent membrane lying on the retinal surface; distorts vision.

cellulitis (sel-yu-LI-tis). *Pathologic condition*. Infection or inflammation of tissues.
  orbital: infection of orbital contents, often caused by streptococci or staphylococci. Produces swelling and redness of lids, bulging eye (proptosis), limitation of eye movement, and swelling of orbital tissues. Usually spreads from infected ethmoid, spheroid, maxillary or frontal sinuses.
  pre-septal: swelling or infection of eyelid tissue in front of the orbital septum. Does not affect the eyeball.

cellulose acetate butyrate. See CAB.

Celluvisc. *Drug*. Trade name of methylcellulose eyedrops; for treating dry eyes.

Celoxin. Incorrect spelling of CILOXAN.

center of rotation. Imaginary point near the center of the eyeball, 13 mm behind the cornea, around which the eye appears to revolve.

centrad. *Unit of measure.* Rarely used unit of prism strength. One centrad deviates light 1 cm of arc at a distance of 1 meter. See also PRISM DIOPTER.

central areolar choroidal atrophy, choroidal sclerosis. *Pathologic condition.* Patchy age-related degeneration of the choroid and pigment epithelium. One of the many forms of macular degeneration (with reduced vision) if the macular area is involved.

central fixation, fixation. *Function.* Coordinated accommodation and ocular movements that achieve and maintain an image of objects on the fovea.

central fusion. *Function.* Blending (in the brain) of similar macular images from the two eyes into one composite image; under appropriate conditions stereopsis results. See also BINOCULAR VISION, MONOFIXATION SYNDROME, PERIPHERAL FUSION.

centrally fixing eye, fixing eye. *Function.* Eye that looks directly at an object so that its image is focused on the fovea. Normally functioning eyes fixate together; if one eye is deviated, only the straight eye is a fixing eye.

central nervous system (CNS). *Anatomy.* Brain and spinal cord.

central posterior curve (CPC). *Optics.* Curvature of the inside surface (base curve) of a contact lens.

central retinal artery (CRA). *Anatomy.* First branch of the ophthalmic artery; supplies nutrition to the inner two-thirds of the retina. Enters the optic nerve behind the eye, extends forward to the optic disc, then divides into superior and inferior branches.

> **occlusion (CRAO)**: blockage of blood flow through the CRA (usually in one eye); causes sudden, permanent loss of vision. Retinal changes include opaque inner layers, cherry red macular spot (disappears after about 2 weeks), and markedly thin arteries.

central retinal vein (CRV). *Anatomy.* Blood vessel that collects retinal venous blood drainage; exits the eye through the optic nerve.

> **occlusion (CRVO)**: blockage of blood flow through the CRV; causes markedly decreased vision, which may improve over many months. Retinal findings include dilated and engorged veins, intraretinal and nerve fiber layer hemorrhages, swollen optic disc margins, and retinal thickening. Also called retinal apoplexy. See also HEMORRHAGIC RETINOPATHY.

central scotoma (skuh-TOH-muh). *Functional defect.* Loss of the central 5° of visual field, which can markedly decrease visual acuity.

central secal. Incorrrect spelling of CENTROCECAL.

central serous chorioretinopathy (SIH-rus KOR-ee-oh-ret-ih-NAH-puh-thee), **serous chorioretinopathy**. *Pathologic condition.* Blister-like elevation of sensory retina in the macula (area of central vision), with localized detachment from the pigment epithelium. Results in reduction and/or distortion of vision that usually recovers within a few months.

central suppression. *Functional defect.* In a misaligned eye, blocking (in the brain) of the retinal image when it is incompatible with the image from the fixing eye; occurs in deviations under 8$^\Delta$. See also FOUR-PRISM-DIOPTER TEST.

central threshold stimulus. *Test technique.* In visual field testing, the weakest light intensity detected outside the central visual area.

central vision. *Function.* An eye's best vision. Results from stimulation of the fovea and the macular area.

centrally fixing eye. See FIXING EYE.

centrocecal scotoma (sen-troh-SEE-kul skuh-TOH-muh. *Functional defect.* Non-seeing area (scotoma) that encompasses central vision and includes both the fixation point and the physiologic blind spot. Characteristic of toxic damage to the optic nerve. See also TOBACCO-ALCOHOL AMBLYOPIA.

cephalexin. *Drug.* Broad spectrum antibiotic. Trade name: Keflex.

cerclage (sur-CLAHJ). *Surgical procedure.* For retinal detachment repair, an encircling band of silastic rubber, suture material or piece of fascia lata muscle is anchored around the sclera near the eyeball's equator.

cerebellopontine angle tumor (seh-ruh-BEL-oh-PAHN-teen). *Pathologic condition.* Brain tumor between the pons and cerebellum. Characterized by impaired hearing, oscillating eye movements, spasms of eyelid muscles, and loss of corneal sensation. Damages the 5th (trigeminal), 6th (abducens), 7th (facial), and 8th (vestibular) cranial nerves.

cerebellum (sehr-uh-BEL-um). *Anatomy.* Part of the brainstem responsible for coordinating and smoothing out body movements. Lies behind the pons and the medulla, and under the back of the cerebrum.

cerebral blindness (suh-REE-brul). See CORTICAL BLINDNESS.

cerebral dyschromatopsia (dis-kroh-muh-TAHP-see-uh). *Functional defect.* Inability to recognize colors following bilateral occipital lobe disease.

cerebral hemispheres, cerebrum. *Anatomy.* Two large half-spheres that make up most of the brain. Responsible for the five senses (hearing, smell, taste, touch, vision) and voluntary movements.

cerebrospinal fluid (CSF). *Anatomy.* Fluid (produced in the ventricles of the brain) that circulates in the sub-arachnoid space surrounding the brain, spinal cord and optic nerves. Helps cushion the brain and supplies some nutrients to its surface.

cerebrovascular accident (CVA), stroke. *Pathologic condition.* Sudden loss of specific brain functions (speech, specific movements), resulting from interrupted blood supply, as by an embolism, thrombosis or hemorrhage. Usually from cerebral blood vessel disease (atherosclerosis).

cerebrum. See CEREBRAL HEMISPHERES.

cervical ganglion (SUR-vih-kul GANG-lee-un). *Anatomy.* Series of paired clumps of nerve junctions in the neck alongside the spine and internal carotid arteries. Plural: ganglia, ganglions.

    superior: one (of a pair) of ganglia in the neck alongside the spine and internal carotid artery. Contains sympathetic nerve fibers from the cervical and thoracic spinal nerves that supply the eye and orbit.

cervico-oculo-acoustic malformation, Wildervanck syndrome. *Congenital anomaly.* Consists of neck and cervical spine deformity, Duane's syndrome, and hearing loss. See also GOLDENHAR'S SYNDROME, KLIPPEL-FEIL SYNDROME.

Cestan-Chenais syndrome (ses-TAN sheh-NAY). See CESTAN'S SYNDROME.

Cestan's syndrome, Cestan-Chenais syndrome. *Pathologic condition.* Vertebral artery clot in the medulla area of the brainstem. Characterized by involuntary eye oscillations (nystagmus) and Horner's syndrome.

chalazion (kuh-LAY-zee-un). *Pathologic condition.* Inflammed lump in a meibomian gland (in the eyelid). Inflammation usually subsides, but may need surgical removal. Sometimes called an internal hordeolum. Plural: chalazia.

chalcosis (kal-KOH-sis). *Pathologic condition.* Deposit of copper in eye tissues; may follow penetration by a copper foreign body.

chalcosis lentis. *Pathologic condition.* "Sunflower" cataract produced by the toxic effect of a copper foreign body that has penetrated the eye.

Chandler's syndrome, essential iris atrophy. *Pathologic condition.* Progressive loss of iris stroma, with hole formation and pupil distortion, accompanied by severe glaucoma. Rare; tends to affect females ages 20–40. See also ICE SYNDROME.

Charcot triad (shahr-KOH TRI-ad). *Clinical sign.* Nystagmus, intention tremor, slurred speech. Late sign in demyelinating disease, e.g., multiple sclerosis.

check ligament. *Anatomy.* Fibrous tissue that attaches extraocular muscle sheaths to orbital walls, to limit the eye's rotations.

Chediak-Higashi syndrome (CHEH-dee-ak hih-GAH-shee). *Pathologic condition.* Characterized by albinism, neurologic deficits, and predisposition to infections; fatal. Rare, hereditary.

cheiroscope (KI-ruh-skohp). *Instrument.* Provides anti-suppression exercises for encouraging simultaneous use of both eyes; one eye views a picture while it is traced on paper placed in front of the other eye.

chemical burns. *Injury.* Alkali and acid burns; cause irreversible vision loss if neglected. Requires immediate, copious water irrigation for 30 minutes.

chemosis (kee-MOH-sis). *Pathologic condition.* Swelling of the conjunctiva.

cherry-red spot. *Clinical sign.* Apparent color change in the fovea (retinal area of sharpest vision). Results from opacification of the inner retinal layers around it, allowing red color of choroidal circulation to stand out. Occurs in central retinal artery occlusion and Tay-Sachs disease.

chiasm (KI-az-um), **optic chiasm.** *Anatomy.* X-shaped part of the retina-to-brain nerve chain, where retinal nerve fibers from the nasal side of both eyes cross to the opposite side and optic nerves from the two eyes join and form the optic tracts. Located at the base of the brain just above the pituitary gland. See also OPTIC TRACT.

chiasmal compression syndrome (ki-AZ-mul). *Pathologic condition.* Pressure exerted on the chiasm from above and below produces outer (temporal) visual field defects in both eyes. Rare.

chiasmal syndrome. *Pathologic condition.* Blind areas in the outer half of the visual field in both eyes, from damage to nasal optic nerve fibers at the chiasm. May be caused by various lesions. See also BITEMPORAL HEMIANOPSIA.

chiasmatic arachnoiditis. *Pathologic condition.* Inflammatory process involving a lining of the brain (arachnoid) in the region of the optic chiasm. May lead to unpredictable visual field defects.

Chibroxin. *Drug.* Trade name of norfloxacin antibiotic eyedrops.

Chievitz (fiber layer of) (sheh-VITZ). *Embryology.* Unusual arrangement of macular tissue existing from the 5th month of fetal development until shortly after birth. Significance not known.

chiroscope. Incorrect spelling of CHEIROSCOPE.

Chlamydia trachomatis (kluh-MID-ee-uh truh-KOH-muh-tus). *Microorganism.* Infectious agent, somewhat larger than bacteria, that causes trachoma, leading cause of blindness in world. See also TRIC.

chlorambucil (klor-AM-byu-sil). *Drug.* Anti-cancer drug also used for treating Behcet's disease, sympathetic ophthalmia, and ocular inflammation associated with juvenile rheumatoid arthritis.

chloramphenicol (klor-am-FEN-ih-kahl). *Drug.* Broad spectrum antibiotic. Trade names: AK-Chlor, Chloromycetin, Chloroptic, Echonochlor, Ophthocort.

chlorolabe (KLOR-oh-layb). *Anatomy.* Green-sensitive pigment found in retinal cones. See also CYANOLABE, ERYTHROLABE, TRITANOMALY.

Chloromycetin (klor-oh-mi-SEE-tin). *Drug.* Trade name of chloramphenicol (eyedrop or ointment), a broad sprectrum antibiotic.

Chloroptic (klor-AHP-tik). *Drug.* Trade name of chloramphenicol (eyedrops), a broad spectrum antibiotic.

chlorothiazide. *Drug.* Heart medication; increases urination to remove excess body fluid. Trade name: Diuril. See also FUROSEMIDE, HYDROCHLOROTHIAZIDE.

chloroquine (KLOR-oh-kwin). *Drug.* For treating autoimmune diseases such as arthritis and lupus. May cause retinal damage.

> **c. retinopathy.** *Pathologic condition.* Drug-induced bull's-eye maculopathy, frequently with impaired vision; may be reversible by stopping drug in early stages.

chocolate agar. *Lab medium.* Brown-color culture material consisting of heated blood cells in agar. Used for growing bacteria *(Hemophilus, Neisseria)* and fungi that thrive best in reduced oxygen. See also BLOOD AGAR.

choked disc, papilledema. *Clinical sign.* Swelling of the optic disc with engorged blood vessels, associated with elevated pressure within the skull. Characterized by blurred optic disc edges, flame-shaped nerve fiber layer hemorrhages next to the disc, and enlarged physiologic blind spot. Vision is normal.

cholinergic blocking agent (koh-lin-UR-jik), **parasympatholytic drug.** *Drug.* Blocks parasympathetic nerve fibers by inhibiting action of acetylcholine in nerve transmission, causing enlarged pupils (mydriasis) and ciliary muscle paralysis (cycloplegia), which results in loss of focusing ability at near (accommodation). Used for cycloplegic refraction and for treating uveitis. Examples: atropine, cyclopentolate, tropicamide.

cholinergic stimulating agent, parasympathomimetic drug. *Drug.* Mimics action of parasympathetic nerve fibers, causing small pupils (miosis), dilating blood vessels and increasing accommodation. Works by (1) simulating acetylcholine chemically (miotics), whiclh increases aqueous outflow and opens the trabecular meshwork to treat glaucoma; examples: carbachol, pilocarpine; (2) inactivating cholinesterase (anti-cholinesterase), for treating accommodative esotropia and myasthenia gravis; examples: diisopropyl fluorophosphate, echothiophate iodide, edrophonium chloride, pyridostigmine bromide.

cholinesterase (koh-lin-ES-tur-ayz). Natural body enzyme that breaks down acetylcholine at nerve junctions, preventing accumulation.

cholystyramine (koh-lee-STI-ruh-meen). *Drug.* Heart medication; for decreasing cholesterol levels. Trade names: Cuemid, Questran. See also CLOFIBRATE, LOVASTATIN.

choriocapillaris (kor-ee-oh-kap-ih-LEHR-is). *Anatomy.* Layer of small blood vessels closely packed in the innermost choroid, attached to outer surface of Bruch's membrane. Provides nourishment and oxygen to the pigment epithelium and outer layers of retina, including visual cells.

chorioretinitis (KOR-ee-oh-ret-ih-NI-tis). *Pathologic condition.* Inflammation of the choroid and retina.

choristoma (kor-is-TOH-muh). *Pathologic condition.* Tumor mass of normal tissue at an abnormal site; e.g., dermoid cyst. Congenital.

choroid (KOR-oyd). *Anatomy.* Vascular (major blood vessel) layer of the eye lying between the retina and sclera. Provides nourishment to outer layers of the retina. Forms part of the uvea, along with the ciliary body and iris. See also BRUCH'S MEMBRANE, CHORIOCAPILLARIS, HALLER'S LAYER, SATTLER'S LAYER, SUPRACHOROID.

choroidal detachment (kor-OY-dul). *Pathologic condition.* Separation of the choroid (blood vessel layer) from the sclera; caused by fluid leakage from the choroidal blood vessels. Usually related to excessively low intraocular pressure. May follow eye injury or eye surgery.

choroidal flush. *Clinical sign.* Filling of the choroidal blood vessels after intravenous fluorescein injection. First evidence of fluorescein dye reaching the eye during fluorescein angiography; occurs 8–20 seconds after injection.

choroidal folds. *Pathologic condition.* Lines, grooves or wrinkles in the choroid (blood vessel layer) at the posterior pole (back of eye). Usually signifies localized pressure on the eyeball or optic nerve, as by an orbital tumor. Made more visible by fluorescein angiography.

choroidal hemorrhage, expulsive hemorrhage. *Pathologic condition.* Bleeding from ruptured choroidal blood vesssels after a sudden decrease in intraocular pressure. Rare, serious complication of intraocular surgery that can result in the pushing out (extrusion) of intraocular contents through the surgical wound, with subsequent loss of vision.

choroidal hyperfluorescence (hi-pur-flor-ESS-enz). *Clinical sign.* Abnormally increased illumination of choroidal (blood vessel layer) areas following intravenous fluorescein injection (fluorescein angiography). Suggests choroidal fluid accumulation or defect in the pigment epithelium.

choroidal neovascular membrane (CNVM). *Pathologic condition.* Abnormal formation of new blood vessels in the choroid.

choroidal nevus (NEE-vus). *Anatomic defect.* Benign pigmented or non-pigmented lesion (freckle) in the choroid (blood vessel layer).

choroidal osteoma. *Pathologic condition.* Rare, yellow-white tumor with the density of bone. Hyperfluoresces on fluorescein angiography.

choroidals. *Anatomy.* Slang for choroidal detachment.

choroidal sclerosis. See CENTRAL AREOLAR CHOROIDAL ATROPHY.

choroideremia (kor-oy-dur-EE-mee-uh). *Pathologic condition.* Progressive loss of pigment epithelial and choroidal (blood vessel layer) tissue, advancing to degeneration of retinal visual cells and choroid. Initially characterized by night blindness; good vision may persist until late stages. Hereditary, X--linked (affects males predominantly).

choroiditis (kor-oy-DI-tis). *Pathologic condition.* Inflammation of the choroid.

choroidopathy (kor-oy-DAH-puh-thee). *Functional defect.* Degenerative abnormality that affects the choroid.

chromatic aberration (kroh-MAT-ik ab-ur-AY-shun). *Optics.* Distortion of an image into images with fuzzy and colored edges; caused by dispersion of light (by a lens or prism). Occurs because different wavelengths of light are refracted to different extents. See also CHROMATIC DISPERSION.

chromatic dispersion. *Optics.* Separation of white light (composed of many wavelengths) into a spectrum of colors, as by a prism. Basic cause of chromatic aberration.

chromatic perimetry (puh-RIM-uh-tree), **color perimetry.** *Test.* Visual field evaluation using red, blue or green targets instead of white.

chromophobe adenoma (KROH-muh-fohb). *Pathologic condition.* Common, slow growing tumor of the pituitary gland. Characterized by visual loss from pressure on the optic chiasm, and headache. May become large.

chromostereopsis (kroh-moh-steh-ree-AHP-sis). *Function.* Perception that different-colored objects or targets at the same distance from the eye are at different distances.

chronic (KRAH-nik). *Description.* Of long duration, or frequent recurrence over a long time, often by a slow progressive course of indefinite duration. See also ACUTE.

chronic angle closure glaucoma (glaw-KOH-muh). *Pathologic condition.* Form of narrow angle glaucoma. Repeated attacks of angle obstruction over a long period (months to years) eventually block the normal drainage channels permanently.

chronic open angle glaucoma (COAG) (glaw-KOH-muh), **open angle** *(or)* **primary open angle glaucoma.** *Pathologic condition.* Most common type of glaucoma. Caused by gradual blockage of aqueous outflow from the eye despite an apparently open anterior chamber angle. If untreated, results in gradual, painless, irreversible loss of vision. Usually affects both eyes.

chronic progressive external ophthalmoplegia (CPEO) (ahf-thal-muh-PLEE-juh), **progressive external ophthalmoplegia.** *Pathologic condition.* Degenerative disease, usually in elderly, characterized by droopy eyelids (ptosis), gradual paralysis of all extraocular muscles, and eventual loss of all eye movement. May be associated with paralysis of other muscle groups. See also EXTERNAL OPHTHALMOPLEGIA.

chronic spastic entropion. *Pathologic condition.* Inward turning of an eyelid against the eyeball from loss of elasticity of eyelid structures, with overactivity of the marginal muscle of Riolan.

chrysiasis (krih-SI-uh-sis). *Pathologic condition.* Gold deposits in the eye, especially in the corneal and conjunctival epithelium. See also ARGYROSIS.

cicatricial ectropion (sik-uh-TRISH-ul ek-TROH-pee-un). *Anatomic defect.* Eyelid that is pulled and held away from normal contact with the eyeball by a scar. May result from previous surgery, eyelid trauma, burns, infection, or inflammation.

cicatricial strabismus (struh-BIZ-mus), **adhesive syndrome.** *Pathologic condition.* Limitation of eye movement with damage and scarring of the muscle cone or supportive tissue (e.g., Tenon's capsule and fat); found after orbital trauma or surgery. See also RESTRICTIVE SYNDROME.

cicatrix. *Anatomic defect.* Scar.

C.I.E. Abbreviation for Commission Internationale de l'Eclairage, established in 1931 to standardize measurement of colors.

cilia (SIL-ee-uh). *Anatomy.* Eyelashes. Singular: cilium.

ciliary arteries (SIL-ee-eh-ree). *Anatomy.* Branches of the ophthalmic artery that supply nourishment to all structures within the eye but the inner retina. Enter the eyeball around the optic disc and rectus muscle insertions.

> **anterior:** seven blood vessels (forward extensions of the muscular arteries) that form the greater arterial circle and supply blood to the limbus, iris, ciliary body and ciliary processes (after joining the long posterior ciliary arteries).

> **posterior:** six to 20 *short* ciliary arteries that supply blood to the optic nerve head, choroid and choriocapillaris, and two *long* ciliary arteries that join the anterior ciliary arteries to form the major arterial circle of the iris.

ciliary block glaucoma (glaw-KOH-muh), **aqueous mis-direction syndrome, malignant glaucoma.** *Pathologic condition.* Increase in intraocular pressure accompanied by a shallow anterior chamber and forward displacement of the iris and lens. Complication following surgery for acute angle closure glaucoma; may be caused by aqueous trapped behind the vitreous.

ciliary body. *Anatomy.* Circumferential tissue inside the eye composed of the ciliary muscle (involved in lens accommodation and control of intraocular pressure) and 70 ciliary processes that produce aqueous.

ciliary flush, ciliary hyperemia *(or)* **injection.** *Clinical sign.* External eye redness caused by congestion of blood vessels surrounding the corneoscleral junction (limbus). Associated with corneal inflammation, iritis, or acute angle closure glaucoma. See also CONJUNCTIVAL INJECTION.

ciliary ganglion (GANG-lee-un). *Anatomy.* Small junction of nerves within the muscle cone behind the eyeball. Contains sympathetic nerve fibers that supply uveal blood vessels, parasympathetic nerve fibers that supply the iris sphincter and ciliary body, and fibers (or a branch) from the nasociliary nerve that supply sensation to the cornea, iris, and ciliary body.

ciliary hyperemia (hi-pur-EE-mee-uh). See CILIARY FLUSH.

ciliary injection. See CILIARY FLUSH.

ciliary muscle. *Anatomy.* Smooth muscle portion of the ciliary body. Responsible for relaxation of zonules, to allow the crystalline lens to focus for near (accommodate).

ciliary nerves. *Anatomy.* Motor and sensory nerves in the eye that innervate the iris, choroid and ciliary body. Three to six *short* ciliary nerves originate in the ciliary ganglion; two *long* ciliary nerves originate from the nasociliary division of the 5th (trigeminal) cranial nerve and provide sensory fibers from the dilator of the iris and choriocapillaris. See also NASOCILIARY NERVE.

ciliary processes. *Anatomy.* Innermost, epithelial portion of the ciliary body. Secretes aqueous fluid and serves as the attachment site for suspensory ligaments of the lens (zonules). See also PARS PLICATA.

ciliary spasm. *Functional defect.* Prolonged, painful contraction of the ciliary muscle, usually in response to corneal or iris inflammation.

ciliary sulcus (SUHL-kus). *Anatomy.* Groove in the posterior chamber between the ciliary body and the iris root. Sometimes used to help position an intraocular lens.

cilioretinal artery (SIL-ee-oh-RET-ih-nul). *Anatomic variant.* Blood vessel (present in about 15% of individuals) that nourishes an area of central retina, usually including or near the macula. Derived from ciliary and choroidal arteries at the disc margin instead of from the central retinal artery.

ciliospinal reflex (SIL-ee-oh-SPI-nul). *Function.* Pupil dilation in response to painful pinching of the skin at the back of the neck.

Ciloxan. *Drug.* Trade name of ciprofloxacin, a broad spectrum antibiotic.

cinch. *Surgical procedure.* Folding and overlapping an extraocular muscle onto itself, to strengthen it. Obsolete.

ciprofloxacin. *Drug.* Broad spectrum antibiotic eyedrops; used for treating corneal infections. Trade name: Ciloxan.

circadian heterotropia (sur-KAY-dee-un het-ur-oh-TROH-pee-uh), **alternate day *(or)* clock-mechanism esotropia, cyclic strabismus**. *Functional defect.* Eye deviation that follows 48-hour cycle, alternating 24 hours of normal binocularity with 24 hours of one eye turning inward (toward nose).

circinate exudate (SUR-sin-ayt EKS-yu-dayt). See CIRCINATE RETINOPATHY.

circinate retinitis. Incorrect term for CIRCINATE RETINOPATHY.

circinate retinopathy (ret-in-AHP-uh-thee), **circinate exudate**. *Pathologic condition.* Ring-shaped deposit of exudates within the retina from retinal vascular leakage; usually around the macular area (area of central vision). Many causes, especially diabetes.

circle of least confusion. *Optics.* Area within an astigmatic image (conoid of Sturm) where defocused vertical and horizontal meridians produce the smallest, clearest image.

Claforan. *Drug.* Trade name of cefotaxime, an antibiotic.

Claude's syndrome. *Pathologic condition.* Paralysis of cranial nerves III and IV on one side, with anesthesia and occasional taxia on the opposite side. Resembles Benedikt's syndrome.

Clear Eyes. *Drug.* Trade name of naphazoline decongestant eyedrops; for "whitening" the eyes.

climatic droplet keratopathy. See LABRADOR KERATOPATHY.

clindamycin (klin-duh-MI-sin). *Drug.* Broad spectrum antibiotic that is injected intramuscularly or intravenously.

clock dial, Lancaster Regan dial #1, "sunburst" dial. *Test chart.* Radial (spoke-like) arrangement of black lines used in refraction to subjectively refine the axis of an astigmatic refractive error. See also ASTIGMATIC CLOCK, FAN DIAL, LANCASTER REGAN DIAL.

clock-mechanism esotropia. See CIRCADIAN HETEROTROPIA.

clofibrate. *Drug.* Heart medication; for decreasing cholesterol levels. Trade name: Atromid S. See also CHOLYSTYRAMINE, LOVASTATIN.

Cloquet's canal (kloh-KAYZ), **hyaloid canal**. *Anatomy.* Pathway within the vitreous that extends from the optic disc to the lens. In the fetus, contains the hyaloid artery, which disappears before birth, though the canal remains. See also PHPV.

closed-angle glaucoma (glaw-KOH-muh), **angle closure *(or)* acute angle closure *(or)* narrow angle glaucoma**. *Pathologic condition.* Sudden rise in intraocular pressure. Aqueous behind the iris cannot pass through the pupil and pushes the iris forward, preventing drainage through the angle (pupillary block mechanism). Occurs in patients with narrow anterior chamber angles. See also OPEN-ANGLE GLAUCOMA.

Clostridium (klaws-TRIH-dee-um). *Microorganism.* Anaerobic, gram-positive, rod-shaped bacteria that causes tetanus (from a perforating wound with contaminated metal foreign body) and botulism.

clotrimazole (kloh-TRI-muh-zol). *Drug.* Topical agent used for treating ocular *Acanthomoeba* infections. Also injected intravenously to treat fungal eye endophthalmitis. See also AMPHOTERICIN B, FLUCYTOSINE, KETOCONAZOLE, MICONAZOLE, NATAMYCIN.

CMV retinitis, cytomegalic inclusion disease. *Pathologic condition.* Virus infection causing retinitis and vasculitis, with lesions that produce widespread destruction of retinal and choroidal structures. Occurs in infants and immunosuppressed adults, as in AIDS. See also ACUTE RETINAL NECROSIS, TOXOPLASMOSIS.

CN, N. Abbreviation for cranial nerve; used with nerve number (e.g., CN II, N II). Those involved with visual function:

    CN II (2nd cranial, optic): largest sensory nerve of eye. Carries impulses for sight from retina to brain. Composed of retinal nerve fibers that exit the eyeball through the optic disc and from the bony orbit through the optic foramen.

    CN III (3rd cranial, oculomotor): primary motor nerve to the eye. Originates in front of the cerebral aqueduct in the mid-brain area of the brainstem; runs through cavernous sinus to enter the orbit through the superior orbital fissure, where it divides into the superior division, which sends branches to superior rectus and levator muscles, and the inferior division, which sends branches to the medial and inferior rectus and inferior oblique muscles, and carries parasympathetic fibers to the pupil sphincter and ciliary body muscles.

    CN IV (4th cranial, trochlear): motor nerve that innervates the superior oblique muscle. Originates in the lower midbrain; travels forward into the orbit through the superior orbital fissure.

    CN V (5th cranial, trigeminal): large, three-branched sensory nerve originating in the pons area of the brainstem. The 1st branch (ophthalmic division) supplies sensation to the eyeballs, conjunctiva, eyelids, brows, forehead, and front half of scalp.

    CN VI (6th cranial, abducens): motor nerve that innervates the lateral rectus muscle, enabling the eye to move outward (away from nose). Originates in the lower pons area of the brainstem; enters the orbit through the superior orbital fissure.

    CN VII (7th cranial, facial): supplies motor impulses to the muscles of the scalp and face, including the orbicularis oculi surrounding the eye and tear (lacrimal) glands; also supplies taste sensation for front two-thirds of the tongue.

CNS (central nervous system). *Anatomy.* Brain and spinal cord.

coagulation (koh-ag-yu-LAY-shun). 1. *Function.* Process of blood clotting. 2. *Surgical procedure.* Destruction of tissue by heat or cold to form a scar, e.g., to seal a retinal tear. See also CRYOPEXY, DIATHERMY, PHOTOCOAGULATION.

Coats' disease, exudative retinitis. *Pathologic condition.* Chronic, progressive retinal disorder characterized by massive white exudates into and under the retina, with eventual detachment. Associated with malformed, tortuous retinal blood vessels with aneurysmal dilatations. Affects one eye; tends to occur in males. See also RETINITIS PROLIFERANS.

Coats' white ring. *Pathologic condition.* Small, inconsequential corneal opacity containing iron, located at the site of previous foreign body injury.

coaxial viewing (koh-AK-see-uhl). *Optics.* Feature of an optical instrument (e.g., a surgical microscope) to allow two or more individuals to view the operative field.

cobblestone degeneration, paving stone *(or)* **peripheral chorioretinal degeneration.** *Degenerative change.* Flat yellowish round areas of retinal thinning and loss of pigment near the ora serrata, through which the underlying choroid can be seen. Occurs with advancing age. No affect on vision.

"cobblestones." *Pathologic condition.* Flat-topped crusts on the conjunctiva (inner surface membrane) of the upper eyelid. Formed from hard, flat papillae that develop with vernal conjunctivitis or giant papillary conjunctivitis. Resemble a mosaic.

cocaine. *Drug.* Stimulates sympathetic nervous system; also causes mild pupillary dilation and constriction of conjunctival blood vessels. Used as a surface anesthetic (e.g., eyedrops) for the cornea and inner eyelids. Repeated doses are toxic to the corneal epithelium.

Cockayne's syndrome. *Congenital disorder.* Characterized by profound deafness and blindness (Usher's syndrome), dwarfism (long trunk, short legs), aged appearance, and mental retardation.

cocktail. *Drug.* Slang for drugs given in combination (orally or parenterally) for diagnosis or treatment.

co-contraction syndrome (Duane's), retraction syndrome, Duane's *(or)* **Stilling-Turk-Duane retraction syndrome.** *Congenital defect.* Eye muscle abnormality often accompanied by inward an eye deviation (esotropia). Characterized by inability to move one eye outward past the midline (abduction) and retraction of that eye into the orbit, with narrowing of the eyelid fissure on attempted movement of that eye toward nose (adduction).

Cogan's congenital oculomotor apraxia (KOH-ganz, ay-PRAKS-ee-uh). *Congenital abnormality.* Inability to make voluntary eye movements. Results in head-thrusting to bring the eyes into desired gaze positions. Usually improves with age.

Cogan's lid twitch. *Clinical sign.* Involuntary upper eyelid twitch that occurs when a patient with a droop (ptosis) of that eyelid shifts gaze from downward to straight ahead.

Cogan's microcystic dystrophy, corneal epithelial basement membrane disease, map-dot-fingerprint dystrophy. *Pathologic condition.* Common corneal epithelial basement membrane disease characterized by cysts, dots, or lines that may change in pattern and distribution over time and resemble a map. Bilateral; may be asymptomatic or may lead to recurrent corneal erosions. Hereditary, degenerative.

Cogan's syndrome. *Pathologic condition.* Corneal disorder characterized by abnormal growth of blood vessels into mid-corneal layers (interstitial keratitis), severe inflammation of iris and ciliary body (iridocyclitis), and deafness. Rare; affects young adults. See also ICE SYNDROME.

"cogwheeling." *Functional defect.* Fast, jerky, refixation eye movements that intermittently interrupt slow, smooth, following eye movements.

coherent light. *Optics.* Wavelengths of the same frequency (monochromatic) traveling in the same direction, with the waves in phase (identical peaks and troughs).

colchicine. *Drug.* Anti-cancer drug, also used for treating Behcet's disease and gout.

collagen (KAH-luh-jun). *Anatomy.* Connective tissue protein that is the primary structural component of sclera, cornea, fibrous tissue, tendons, ligaments and fascia.

collagen disease. *Pathologic condition.* Group of diseases that cause widespread pathologic changes in connective tissue, often in blood vessels; may cause inflammation. Example: lupus erythematosis.

collagen shield. *Protective device.* Contact lens used as a bandage to reduce wound leaks or help corneal ulcers heal. Made from pig sclera.

collarette. *Anatomy.* Zigzag circular line that divides the front surface of the iris into ciliary and pupillary zones.

collateral circulation. *Anatomy.* Alternate blood supply system that takes over when the primary blood vessel system becomes blocked; established through enlargement of minor vessels.

collicular plate, corpora quadrigemina. *Anatomy.* Area on the roof of the midbrain that contains both of the superior colliculi and inferior colliculi.

colliculi. *Anatomy.* Two pairs of mounds on the roof of the midbrain that contain nerve centers. Singular: colliculus. See also COLLICULAR PLATE, CORPORA QUADRAGEMINA.

    inferior: contain centers for responses to sound.

    superior: contain centers for coordination of eye movements.

Collier's sign. *Clinical sign.* Eyelid retraction that exposes excessive amount of the white of the eye above and below the iris. Bilateral; makes the eyes appear to be staring. Associated with midbrain lesions. See also DALRYMPLE'S SIGN.

collimated. *Optics.* Describes light rays that have been bundled and made parallel by an optical system.

collyrium (kuh-LIR-ee-um). Eyewash.

coloboma (kah-luh-BOH-muh). *Congenital anomaly.* Cleft or defect in normal continuity of a part of the eye, e.g., absence of lower segment of optic nerve head, choroid, ciliary body, iris, lens or eyelid. Caused by improper fusion of fetal fissure during gestation. May be associated with other abnormalities, including a small eye (microphthalmia). Plural: colobomata.

color blindness. See specific defects: DEUTERANOMALY, PROTANOMALY, TRITANOMALY; DEUTERANOPIA, PROTANOPIA, TRITANOPIA.

color perimetry (puh-RIM-uh-tree), **chromatic perimetry**. *Test.* Visual field evaluation using red, blue or green targets instead of white.

color vision. *Function.* Perception of color. Results from stimulation of red, green and blue cone receptors in the retina. See also CHLOROLABE, CYANOLABE, DEUTERANOMALY, ERYTHROLABE, FARNSWORTH D15, ISHIHARA TEST, PROTANOMALY, TRITANOMALY.

coma aberration (KOH-muh). *Optics.* Image distortion of points that lie off the optical axis; appear comma-shaped instead of dot-like.

Comberg lens. *Instrument.* Diagnostic contact lens that creates radio-opaque reference marks on x-rays of the orbit. For localizing an ocular foreign body.

comet scotoma (skuh-TOH-muh), **arcuate** *(or)* **Bjerrum** *(or)* **scimitar scotoma**. *Functional defect.* Arc-shaped blind area in visual field. Caused by damage to retinal nerve fiber bundles. Common in patients with glaucoma.

comitant strabismus (KAH-muh-tunt struh-BIZ-mus), **concomitant strabismus**. *Functional defect.* Eye misalignment in which the amount of deviation remains the same in every direction of gaze.

common canaliculus (kan-uh-LIK-yu-luhs). *Anatomy.* Tiny channel under the skin (between the eyelids and the nose) formed by the junction of the upper and lower canaliculi. Carries tears into the tear (lacrimal) sac, from which they drain into the nose.

commotio retinae (kuh-MOH-shee-oh RET-in-ee), **Berlin's edema**. *Pathologic condition.* Swollen, white, "bruised" retina that may follow blunt trauma to the eye. Prognosis for recovery of vision is poor if it occurs in the area of central vision (macula).

Compazine. *Drug.* Trade name of type of phenothiazine, a tranquilizing agent that also prevents vomiting.

complementary after-image. *Function.* After-image in the color that is complementary to the original stimulus. See also COMPLEMENTARY COLORS.

complementary chromaticities (kroh-muh-TIS-ih-tees). See COMPLEMENTARY COLORS.

complementary colors, complementary chromaticities. Paired samples of light that produce a colorless (achromatic) stimulus when combined in approriate proportions.

complete blood count (CBC). *Lab test*. Routine set of blood tests performed as part of a diagnostic evaluation of a patient. Usually consists of white and red blood cell count, differential count, hemoglobin and hematocrit.

compound astigmatism (uh-STIG-muh-tizm). *Refractive error*. Optical defect in which refractive power is not uniform in all directions (meridians). Light rays entering the eye are bent unequally by different meridians, preventing formation of a sharp point focus on the retina. Instead, light rays form two focal lines, both lying in front of or behind the retina. Corrected by a sphero-cylindrical lens.

>**hyperopic** (hi-pur-AHP-ik): the two focal lines form behind the retina; corrected by a plus sphero-cylindrical lens.

>**myopic** (mi-AHP-ik): the two focal lines form in front of retina; corrected by a minus sphero-cylindrical lens.

computerized perimeter, automated perimeter. *Instrument*. Field of vision is plotted by computer from luminous stimuli presented in pre-arranged locations. Examples: Dicon, Humphrey Analyzer. See also PERIMETRY.

computerized tomography, CT scan. *Clinical test*. Low dosage x-rays coupled with a computer to generate a film showing tissue detail.

concave cylinder, minus cylinder. *Optical device*. Toric lens that has maximum minus power in one meridian and no optical power in the meridian perpendicular to it. See also ASTIGMATISM.

concave lens, diverging *(or)* **minus lens**. *Optical device*. Lens that is thicker at the edges than in the center, increasing the divergence of incoming light rays. Corrects nearsightedness (myopia).

concavo-convex lens (kahn-CAY-voh), **meniscus lens**. *Optical device*. Lens that has an outward curving (convex) front surface and an inward curving (concave) back surface.

concomitant strabismus. See COMITANT STRABISMUS.

cone. 1. *Anatomy*. Light-sensitive retinal receptor cell that provides sharp visual acuity and color discrimination. See also PHOTOPIC VISION, ROD. 2. *Pathologic condition*. Conical-shaped portion of cornea, central or eccentric, that disturbs the normal image-forming properties, e.g., in keratoconus.

cone degeneration, cone dystrophy. *Functional defect*. Degeneration of retinal receptors (primarily cones); results in progressive, marked decrease in vision and loss of color discrimination. Hereditary. No known treatment. See also ROD DEGENERATION.

cone dystrophy (DIS-truh-fee). See CONE DEGENERATION.

cone monochromacy, atypical monochromacy. *Congenital defect*. Rare inability to distinguish colors. Vision is relatively normal. Nonprogressive; hereditary. See also ROD MONOCHROMACY.

conformer. Plastic shell sometimes used as a temporary "false eye" after removal of an eye (enucleation); placed under eyelids (over buried implant) to preserve their shape. Will later be replaced by a permanent prosthesis.

confrontation fields. *Test*. Screening method for gross visual field defects, using the examiner's eye as a fixation point and his moving fingers as peripheral targets.

confusion. *Functional defect*. Simultaneous perception of two objects in the same location in space. Occurs at the onset of an eye deviation, when the fovea of each eye is stimulated by a different object.

conge. Incorrect spelling of CONJ.

congenital amaurosis (am-uh-ROH-sis), **Leber's congenital amaurosis**. *Congenital defect*. Blindness or near-blindness in both eyes; may be accompanied by nystagmus, sensitivity to light, and sunken eyes. Marked reduction in retinal function, seen on an electroretinogram.

congenital bulbar paralysis, congenital facial diplegia, Moebius *(or)* **von**

Graefe's syndrome. *Congenital anomaly.* Bilateral malformation in the nuclei of the 6th (abducens) and 7th (facial) cranial nerves, resulting in inability to move either eye outward past the midline, inability to close the eyelids, large inward eye deviation (esotropia), and a droopy, expressionless facial appearance.

congenital cataract. *Pathologic condition.* Cloudy or opaque crystalline lens that is present at birth. Many causes; often hereditary.

congenital dystrophic ptosis (dis-TROH-fik TOH-sis). *Congenital anomaly.* Drooping eyelid(s) associated with a non-functioning levator muscle. Usually hereditary.

congenital esotropia (ee-soh-TROH-pee-uh), **infantile esotropia**. *Functional defect.* Inward (toward nose) eye deviation found at birth or within first 6 months; misalignment is usually large, and unaffected by eyeglasses. Requires surgery to straighten the eyes. See also CROSS-FIXATION.

congenital facial diplegia (di-PLEE-juh). See CONGENITAL BULBAR PARALYSIS.

congenital fibrosis syndrome. *Pathologic condition.* Inability of the eyes to look upward or to either side. Characterized by eyes fixed in downward direction, drooping eyelids (ptosis), and chin-up head position. Usually hereditary.

congenital glaucoma (glaw-KOH-muh), **infantile glaucoma**. *Congenital defect.* High intraocular pressure accompanied by hazy corneas and large eyes (buphthalmos) in newborn or within first 6 months. Developmental abnormalities in the anterior chamber angle obstruct normal fluid drainage mechanism. Characteristic symptoms are tearing, light sensitivity (photophobia) and uncontrolled blinking (blepharospasm). Requires early surgical correction. See also BUPHTHALMOS, CYCLO-CRYO, GONIOTOMY, TRABECULECTOMY AB EXTERNO.

congenital grouped pigmentation, "bear tracks." *Anatomic variant.* Areas of excessively pigmented retinal pigment epithelium that resemble paw prints. Histopathology: hypertrophy of the pigment epithelium.

congenital hypertrophy of the retinal pigment epithelium (CHRPE). *Pathologic condition.* Excessive black pigment on the fundus. Seen as a flat, round lesion with a thin, poorly pigmented border; depigmented holes may be found within the lesion. No visual significance unless large.

congenital nystagmus (ni-stag-mus). *Congenital defect.* Involuntary, rhythmic eye movements noted within first 6 months of life. There is usually one position of gaze in which the spontaneous movements are minimized or absent (null point). May be hereditary or result from decreased vision from corneal opacities, cataracts, albinism, chorioretinitis, aniridia, macular disease, or optic atrophy. See also NYSTAGMUS.

congenital oculomotor apraxia (COMA) (ay-PRAK-see-uh), **Cogan's congenital oculomotor apraxia**. *Congenital abnormality.* Inability to make voluntary eye movements; results in head-thrusting to bring the eyes into desired gaze positions. Usually improves with age.

congenital retinoschisis (ret-in-oh-SKEE-sis), **juvenile retinoschisis**. *Congenital anomaly.* Splitting of the retina into inner and outer layers; usually involves the macular area. Hereditary, X-linked. See also RETINOSCHISIS.

congenital stationary night blindness (CSNB). *Pathologic condition.* Nonprogressive retinal disorder characterized by poor night vision; rod function is abnormal. Retina appears normal. Hereditary. See also PARADOXIC PUPIL.

congested. *Description.* Refers to blood vessels that are engorged with blood.

congestive heart failure (CHF). *Pathologic condition.* The heart loses efficiency in pumping venous blood returned by the circulation, becoming unable to maintain adequate circulation to body tissues and thus incapable of supplying the oxygen demands of the tissues and organs.

congruous (KAHN-gru-us). *Description.* Refers to visual field defects that are similar (in extent and intensity) in both eyes. Typical of brain lesions in the occipital lobe.

conical cornea, keratoconus. *Pathologic condition.* Degenerative corneal disease characterized by generalized thinning and cone-shaped protrusion of the central cornea. Usually affects vision in both eyes and occurs during the second decade of life. Hereditary.

conj. *Anatomy.* Slang for conjunctiva.

conjugate foci (FOH-si). Optical relationship between the position of an object and its image by an optical system.

conjugate movement (KAHN-juh-gut), **conjunctive *(or)* gaze movement, version.** *Function.* Parallel movements of both eyes. See also PURSUIT MECHANISM, SACCADES.

conjunctiva (kahn-junk-TI-vuh). *Anatomy.* Transparent mucous membrane covering the outer surface of the eyeball except the cornea, and lining the inner surfaces of the eyelids. Plural: conjunctivae.

> **bulbar**: portion that covers the external eyeball.
>
> **palpebral**: portion that lines the eyelids.

conjunctival flap (kahn-junk-TI-vul). *Surgical procedure.* Tongue-shaped section of conjunctiva that is dissected on two or three sides. Used for exposing the sclera below, protecting a wound, covering a corneal defect, or covering a filtration site for aqueous humor, producing a filtering bleb. See also FORNIX-BASED FLAP, LIMBUS-BASED FLAP.

conjunctival hyperemia (hi-pur-EE-mee-uh). See CONJUNCTIVAL INJECTION.

conjunctival injection, conjunctival hyperemia. *Clinical sign.* Eye redness caused by congestion of blood vessels in the conjunctiva (membrane covering white of eye and inner eyelids); most prominent near the fornix and decreasing toward the corneo-scleral junction (limbus). Associated with all types of conjunctivitis. See also CILIARY INJECTION.

conjunctival sac, cul-de-sac, fornix. *Anatomy.* Loose pocket of conjunctiva between the upper eyelid and the eyeball, and the lower eyelid and the eyeball; permits the eye to rotate freely.

conjunctival scraping. *Surgical procedure.* Specimen obtained by scraping the conjunctiva at the site of a lesion or maximum disease involvement. Used for identifying cell types by means of smears, stains, and cultures. See also BLOOD AGAR, GIEMSA STAIN, GRAM STAIN, SABOURAUD'S DEXTROSE AGAR.

conjunctive movement. See CONJUGATE MOVEMENT.

conjunctivitis (kun-junk-tih-VI-tis), **"pink eye."** *Pathologic condition.* Inflammation of the conjunctiva (mucus membrane that covers white of eye and inner eyelid surfaces). Characterized by discharge, grittiness, redness and swelling. Usually viral in origin; may be contagious.

> **acute**: having sudden onset.
>
> **allergic**: hypersensitivity to foreign substances.
>
> **atopic**: allergic reaction to pollens; usually accompanies hay fever.
>
> **bacterial**: caused by infection; characterized by muco-pus discharge, redness, and a gritty feeling.
>
> **chronic**: persistent or intermittent.
>
> **contact**: caused by allergy or by irritation from eye medications or cosmetics used near the eye.
>
> **dermato-** involves bulbar and palpebral conjunctiva as well as the skin near the eyelid margins.
>
> **follicular**: characterized by hundreds of tiny, glistening, translucent elevations (follicles) composed of lymphoid tissue on undersurfaces of lids.
>
> **Parinaud's oculo-glandular**: characterized by conjunctival lesions surrounded by follicles, with fever and malaise. Rare; usually affects only one eye.

vernal: allergic reaction (itching, mucous); numerous small lumps (papillae) form on palpebral conjunctiva. Affects children; recurs in warm summer months.

viral: caused by a virus; characterized by discharge, grittiness, redness and swelling. Usually contagious.

conjunctivo-dacryocystorhinostomy (kun-junk-TI-voh-DAK-ree-oh-SIS-toh-ri-NAHS-toh-mee). *Surgical procedure.* Method of constructing a new tear drainage channel from the lacrimal sac to the nose, through the conjunctiva. See also JONES TUBE.

connective tissue. *Anatomy.* Body tissue that binds and supports other tissues. Composed primarily of collagen and elastic tissue.

conoid of Sturm (KOH-noyd). *Optics.* Somewhat cone-shaped image of a point created by a cylindrical (astigmatic) lens. Lies between the two focal line images (interval of Sturm) and contains the circle of least confusion.

consecutive esotropia (ee-suh-TROH-pee-uh). *Functional defect.* Inward (toward nose) deviation of an eye following surgical correction for an outward deviation (exotropia).

consecutive exotropia (eks-uh-TROH-pee-uh). *Functional defect.* Outward (away from nose) deviation of an eye following surgical correction for an inward deviation (esotropia).

consensual light reflex, consensual light response. *Function.* Decrease in pupil size (constriction) in one eye resulting from light stimulation to the other eye. See also SWINGING FLASHLIGHT TEST.

consensual light response. See CONSENSUAL LIGHT REFLEX.

constricted pupil. *Function.* Reduced pupil size due to constriction of the iris sphincter or relaxation of the iris dilator muscle. Associated with bright illumination, drugs, or as a consequence of ocular inflammation, e.g., iritis. See also MIOTIC.

contact arc, arc of contact. *Anatomy.* Distance between an extraocular muscle's initial point of contact with the sclera and its true insertion on the eyeball.

contact conjunctivitis. See CONJUNCTIVITIS.

contact dermatitis (dur-muh-TI-tis). *Pathological condition.* Irritant skin disorder, usually caused by direct application of drugs, chemicals or cosmetics. May affect eyelids.

contact lens. *Optical device.* Small plastic disc containing optical correction, worn on the cornea or sclera as substitute for eyeglasses.

bandage: worn to protect an eye with corneal disease.

corneal: hard or soft lens that floats on tear film over the cornea.

gas permeable (GP): made of rigid plastic that allows much more oxygen and carbon dioxide penetration than other hard contacts.

hard: made of rigid plastic, usually polymethyl methacrylate (PMMA).

rigid gas permeable (RGP). Same as GAS PERMEABLE (above).

scleral: large, rigid lens that may be molded to fit patient's cornea and sclera; rarely used.

soft: water-absorbing (hydrophilic); often more comfortable than a hard contact lens.

contacto gauge, radiuscope. *Instrument.* Used for measuring back surface curvature (base curve) of a contact lens.

contactoscope. *Instrument.* Used for magnifying contact lenses, for quality control inspection.

continuous sutures, running sutures. *Surgical technique.* Stitches that are not tied separately. See also INTERRUPTED SUTURES.

contralateral. *Description.* Refers to the opposite eye or the opposite side of the body. See also IPSILATERAL.

contralateral antagonist. *Function.* Extraocular muscle whose action is opposite to that of another muscle in the opposite eye (e.g., right superior oblique, left superior rectus).

contralateral synergists (SIN-ur-jists), **yoke muscles**. *Function*. Six pairs of extraocular muscles (one from each eye, e.g., right medial rectus and left lateral rectus) that move the eyes in parallel. See also DIAGNOSTIC POSITIONS OF GAZE.

contrast sensitivity. *Function*. Ability to detect detail having subtle gradations in grayness between test target and background. Tested with specially designed targets or cards, e.g., AO Contrast Sensitivity system, Arden plates, Nicolet system, Pelli-Robson charts, Vistech system.

contusion. *Injury*. Blunt injury that does not break the surface of the skin or the eye. A bruise.

conus of optic disc. *Anatomic deviant*. Condition in which the choroid and retinal pigment epithelium do not extend to the optic disc, allowing the sclera to be observed with an ophthalmoscope at its margin.

converge. 1. *Optics*. Refers to the coming together of light rays toward a focus. 2. *Function*. To move both eyes inward (toward each other), usually in an effort to maintain single binocular vision as an object approaches.

convergence. *Function*. Inward movement of both eyes toward each other, usually in an effort to maintain single binocular vision as an object approaches.

  accommodative: occurs in response to an increase in optical power for focusing (accommodation) by the eyes' lenses.

  fusional: amount of convergence the eyes can undergo while maintaining single vision. Measured with graduated base-out prisms.

  proximal: portion of convergence brought about by awareness of an object's nearness.

  relative: amount of prism power that can be overcome while single clear binocular vision is maintained. May be positive or negative, depending on the direction of the prism.

  tonic: portion of convergence that results from changing from sleeping to the awake state.

  voluntary: amount the eyes can voluntarily converge without regard to clarity or single image.

convergence amplitudes. *Measurement*. Amount the eyes can turn inward (toward each other) before double vision occurs. Measured in prism diopters.

convergence insufficiency. *Functional defect*. Eye muscle problem in which the eyes cannot be pulled sufficiently inward (toward each other) to maintain single vision when attempting to fixate on a near object. Characterized by eye fatigue or double vision. See also ASTHENOPIA.

convergence spasm. *Functional defect*. Inward eye deviation (esotropia), usually accompanied by small pupils and by excessive accommodation (focusing power) that causes blurred distance vision (near vision remains clear). Usually related to an emotional problem or hysteria.

convergent deviation. See ESOTROPIA.

converging lens. See CONVEX LENS.

converging rays. *Optics*. Light rays in the process of coming together after being refracted by a lens or reflected from a curved mirror.

convex lens, converging *(or)* **plus lens**. *Optical device*. Lens that is thicker in the center than at the edges, adding optical power to incoming light rays. Corrects farsightedness (hyperopia).

convexo-concave lens. See CONCAVO-CONVEX LENS.

"copper wiring." *Clinical sign*. Refers to the color of opacified retinal arteriolar walls. Commonly associated with arteriosclerosis and hypertension. See also "SILVER WIRING."

corectopia (kor-ek-TOH-pee-uh). *Anatomic defect.* Displacement of the pupil from its normal position.

coreoplasty (KOR-ee-oh-plas-tee) *Surgical procedure.* Any procedure that changes the size or shape of the pupil, usually to obtain dilation (pupillo-mydriasis).

Corgard. *Drug.* Trade name of nadolol; controls high blood pressure (hypertension).

cornea (KOR-nee-uh). *Anatomy.* Transparent front part of the eye that covers the iris, pupil and anterior chamber and provides most of an eye's optical power. Five layers: epithelium, Bowman's membrane, stroma, Decemet's membrane, and endothelium.

corneal abrasion (KOR-nee-ul). *Injury.* Scraped area of corneal surface, accompanied by a loss of superficial tissue (epithelium).

corneal anesthesia. *Sign.* Loss of corneal sensitivity. Sign of diseased or denervated cornea.

corneal apex, apex, apical zone, corneal cap. *Anatomy.* Central 3–5 mm of cornea, where the surface has greatest curvature; yields highest K-readings (steepest meridian) by keratometry.

corneal astigmatism (uh-STIG-muh-tizm). *Refractive error.* Variation in corneal curvature, causing light rays to focus imperfectly on the retina. May be corrected with glasses or some contact lenses. See also ASTIGMATISM, IRREGULAR ASTIGMATISM.

corneal bedewing (beh-DU-ing), **Sattler's veil.** *Pathologic condition, clinical sign.* Swelling and clouding of superficial layers of the cornea, causing loss of surface smoothness, which reduces its image-forming properties. May be caused by prolonged increase in intraocular pressure or by contact lens overwear. See also OVERWEAR SYNDROME.

corneal "button." *Anatomy.* Slang for disc of corneal tissue, usually 5-10 mm diameter, removed from donor and recipient eyes for corneal transplant surgery.

corneal cap. See CORNEAL APEX.

corneal dellen (DEL-in). *Pathologic condition.* Localized zone of corneal thinning, usually at the edge (limbus), caused by excessive dehydration. Reversible.

corneal dystrophy (DIS-truh-fee). *Pathologic condition.* Accumulation of abnormal material or excess water in the cornea, leading to corneal cloudiness and reduced vision later in life. May affect epithelium, stroma and endothelium. Many types; often hereditary.

corneal ectasia, keratectasia. *Pathologic condition.* Abnormal bulging forward of thinned cornea, as with keratoconus.

corneal edema, steamy cornea. *Clinical sign.* A hazy, swollen cornea.

corneal endothelium. *Anatomy.* Innermost, single-celled layer of the cornea between Descemet's membrane and the anterior chamber. Acts as a pump to keep excess water out of the corneal stroma. See also FUCHS' DYSTROPHY.

corneal epithelial basement membrane disease (CEBMD), Cogan's microcystic *(or)* map-dot-fingerprint dystrophy. *Pathologic condition.* Common corneal epithelial basement membrane disease characterized by cysts, dots or lines that may change in pattern and distribution over time and resemble a map. Bilateral; may be asymptomatic or may lead to recurrent corneal erosions. Degenerative; hereditary.

corneal epithelium. *Anatomy.* Outermost layer of the cornea between Bowman's membrane and the tear film.

corneal erosion. See RECURRENT CORNEAL EROSION.

corneal graft. See CORNEAL TRANSPLANT.

corneal hydrops (HI-drahps). *Pathologic condition.* Sudden, abnormal fluid accumulation within corneal tissue, resulting in clouded vision. Seen in keratoconus.

corneal lens. *Optical device.* Hard or soft contact lens that floats on tear film over the cornea, providing refractive correction or protection for a damaged cornea. See also SCLERAL LENS.

corneal melt, keratolysis. *Pathologic condition.* Superficial corneal layers that "melt" away. May be associated with severe inflammatory disease of the sclera or peripheral cornea, dry eyes (keratitis sicca), or rheumatoid arthritis. See also FURROWS.

corneal reflex. *Clinical sign.* 1. *Optics.* Mirror-like reflection of a bright light from the corneal surface. See also PURKINJE IMAGES. 2. *Function.* Neurologic response: blink caused by touching the cornea.

corneal relaxing incisions. *Surgical procedure.* Technique for flattening a corneal meridian to decrease astigmatism, especially if caused by trauma or by scarring after corneal surgery.

corneal scraping. *Surgical procedure.* Specimen obtained by scraping a corneal lesion or ulcer. Used for identifying cell types by means of smears, stains and cultures. See also BLOOD AGAR, GIEMSA STAIN, GRAM STAIN, SABOURAUD'S DEXTROSE AGAR.

corneal transplant, corneal graft, keratoplasty. *Surgical procedure.* Replacement of a scarred or diseased cornea with clear corneal tissue from a donor. See also CORNEAL "BUTTON."

corneal topography. *Measurement.* Map of the variations in front surface curvature of the cornea, much like making a contour map of land. See also PHOTOKERATOSCOPY, PLACIDO DISK.

corneal trephination (treh-fin-AY-shun). *Surgical procedure.* Making a circular hole in eye tissue, e.g., a corneal "button" for a corneal transplant.

corneal ulcer. *Pathologic condition.* Area of epithelial tissue loss from the corneal surface. Associated with inflammatory cells in the cornea and anterior chamber. May be caused by bacterial, fungal, or viral infection.

corneoconjunctival intraepithelial neoplasia, Bowen's disease, intra-epithelial epithelioma. *Pathologic condition.* Slow-growing, malignant tumor, commonly arising at multiple sites near the corneo-scleral junction (limbus) but limited to the epithelial layer. Precursor to squamous cell carcinoma. Cause may be chronic sun exposure.

corneo-scleral junction, limbus. *Anatomy.* Transitional zone, about 1–2 mm wide, where the cornea joins the sclera and the bulbar conjunctiva attaches to the eyeball.

corneo-scleral trephination. *Surgical procedure.* Removing a small circular disc of cornea and sclera (corneo-scleral button) to make an opening into the anterior chamber angle, for permanent drainage of aqueous. Obsolete treatment for glaucoma.

coroid. Incorrect spelling of CHOROID.

"coronary" (coronary artery occlusion), heart attack, myocardial infarction. *Pathologic condition.* Sudden blockage of a blood vessel that supplies nutrients to the heart. Results in death (infarction) of some of the heart muscle.

corpora quadrigemina, collicular plate. *Anatomy.* Area on the roof of the midbrain that contains both the superior colliculi and inferior colliculi.

corresponding points. *Concept.* One point in each retina, which, when both are simultaneously stimulated, results in a perception of haplopia (single binocular vision). See also DISPARATE RETINAL POINTS.

cortex. *Anatomy.* 1. Jelly-like main part of the crystalline lens, composed of millions of thin lens fibers. Located between the denser inner nucleus and elastic outer capsule. 2. Outermost layers of the cerebrum and cerebellum in the brain. Plural: cortices.

cortical. *Description.* Refers to brain function.

cortical blindness, cerebral blindness. *Functional defect.* Absence of vision caused by damage to the blood supply of the visual areas in the occipital cortices of the brain. Retina appears normal; visually-evoked electrical response (VER) is markedly diminished. See also ANTON'S SYNDROME, BRODMANN AREA 17.

cortical cataract. See CORTICAL SPOKES.

cortical spokes, cortical cataract. *Pathologic condition.* Radially arranged opacities in the lens cortex following lens fiber swelling and fragmentation. Form of senile cataract.

Corticosporin. *Drug.* Trade name of suspension or ointment combining hydrocortisone, neomycin, bacitracin and polymyxin B; for treating ocular infections.

corticosteroid, steroid. *Drug.* Cortisone derivative. For treating inflammatory and allergic diseases. Long-term use can have serious side effects, e.g., osteoporosis, immunosuppression, cataracts, glaucoma. See also DEXAMETHASONE, METHYLPREDNISOLONE, PREDNISONE, PREDNISOLONE, RIMEXOLONE.

cortisone, hydrocortisone. *Drug.* Steroid medication used for treating inflammatory and allergic diseases.

Corynebacterium xerosis (kor-ih-nuh-bak-TIR-ee-um zeh-ROH-sis), **diphtheroid**. *Microorganism.* Club-shaped, gram-positive bacteria that exists normally on eyelid skin.

cotton-wool spots, soft exudates. *Clinical sign.* "Fluffy-looking" white deposits (resembling small tufts of cotton) within the retinal nerve fiber layer that represent small patches of retina that have lost their blood supply from vessel obstruction. May be associated with hypertensive and diabetic retinopathies and certain collagen vascular diseases. Gradually disappear without treatment, leaving some functional loss.

couching. *Surgical procedure.* Archaic method of using direct blunt trauma to "remove" a cataract by dislodging the lens downward from its normal position, out of the line of sight. Dates from pre-Christian era.

Coumadin. *Drug.* Trade name of warfarin; heart medication.

counts fingers (CF). *Test measurement.* Patient's ability to count number of fingers presented, usually at a distance of 1 or 2 ft. Administered when vision loss is profound (acuity less than 20/400). See also HAND MOVEMENT, LIGHT PERCEPTION.

cover test (CT). Detects eye misalignment (tropia) or tendency toward misalignment (phoria).

    alternate cover test: the cover is shifted from eye to eye and the direction of each eye's movement is noted.

    cover/uncover test: as the subject views a fixation target, one eye is covered and other eye is observed for movement; then the cover is removed and movement of both eyes is noted.

COWS. *Test result.* Mnemonic (Cold Opposite, Warm Same) for normal result of caloric test of the nerves that affect balance, located in the inner ear. Cold water placed in the ear causes rhythmic eye oscillations (nystagmus) toward the opposite side, warm water causes oscillations toward the same side.

cranial arteritis (ahr-tur-RI-tis). See TEMPORAL ARTERITIS.

cranial nerves (CN, N). *Anatomy.* Twelve pairs of nerves that transmit information to and from the brain. Those involved with the eyes are the 2nd (optic), 3rd (oculomotor), 4th (trochlear), 1st (ophthalmic) division of the 5th (trigeminal), and 6th (abducens).

craniofacial dysostosis (kray-nee-oh-FAY-shul dis-ahs-TOH-sis), **Crouzon's syndrome**. *Congenital anomaly.* Characterized by multiple abnormalities of skull and jaw, e.g., short head, broad hooked nose, high palate, large earlobes, widely separated eyes, shallow orbits, optic nerve damage, corneal exposure, nystagmus, and outward eye deviation (exotropia). See also APERT'S SYNDROME.

craniopharyngioma (KRAY-nee-oh-fahr-in-jee-OH-muh), **Rathke's pouch tumor**. *Pathologic condition.* Congenital tumor that grows, in cyst form, into the 3rd ventricle of the brain, compressing visual fibers at the back of the chiasm. Eye signs are vision loss, swollen optic nerve heads (papilledema), and inferior temporal visual field loss (bitemporal hemianopsia). Usually apparent by age 10.

craniosynostosis (KRAY-nee-oh-sin-ahs-TOH-sis). *Pathologic condition.* Premature fusion of cranial bone junctions. See also APERT'S SYNDROME, CROUZON'S SYNDROME.

Crawford tubes. *Surgical appliance.* Tubes passed from the lacrimal puncta through the canaliculi, nasolacrimal sac and duct into the nose to overcome nasolacrimal duct obstruction. May be kept in place for months.

creatinine serum (kree-AT-ih-neen). *Test.* To determine creatinine in the blood. Elevated level indicates kidney damage.

Crede's prophylaxis (kreh-DAYZ). Routine administration of 1% silver nitrate solution eyedrops to newborn to prevent spread of maternal gonorrhea infection to infant's eyes. Becoming obsolete. See also OPHTHALMIA NEONATORIUM.

crescent (myopic). *Anatomy.* Semilunar-shaped zone just temporal to the optic disc, in high myopes. See also MYOPIC DEGENERATION.

Creutzfeldt-Jakob disease (KROYTS-feld YAH-kohb). *Pathologic condition.* Rare, infectious, progressive neurological disease caused by a slow-acting virus. Can be transmitted by donor tissue, e.g., corneal transplant. Fatal.

cribiform ligament (KRIB-ih-form), **ligamentum pectinatum iridis, scleral trabeculae, trabecular meshwork**. *Anatomy.* Mesh-like structure inside the eye at the iris-scleral junction of the anterior chamber angle. Filters aqueous and controls its flow into the canal of Schlemm, prior to its leaving the eye.

cribiform plate, lamina cribrosa. *Anatomy.* Thin, sieve-like portion of sclera at the base of the optic disc through which retinal nerve fibers leave the eye to form the optic nerve. See also LAMINA DOTS.

cri-du-chat syndrome (kree-du-SHAH), **cat-cry syndrome**. *Congenital anomaly.* Uncommon chromosome abnormality characterized by a mewing cry by the affected infant. Associated with larnyx abnormalities, heart disease, mental retardation, small head, poorly formed ears, widely set eyes, epicanthus, anti-mongoloid slant, outward eye deviation (exotropia), refractive errors, and tortuous retinal blood vessels.

crocodile shagreen, mosaic degeneration. *Pathologic condition.* Polygonal, light gray corneal opacities centrally located at Decemet's (posterior) or Bowman's (anterior) level. Represents a mild age-related degenerative change with little or no affect on vision.

crocodile tears. *Functional defect.* Tears and excessive saliva produced while eating. Occurs with paralysis of the 7th (facial) cranial nerve after salivary gland nerve fibers regenerate abnormally and grow into the lacrimal gland. See also ABERRANT REGENERATION.

Crolom. *Drug.* Trade name of cromolyn solution; for treating allergic conjunctivitis.

cromolyn (KROH-muh-lin). *Drug.* Used for treating allergic conjunctivitis. Trade names: Crolom, Optichrom. See also KETOROLAC TROMETHAMINE, LODOXAMIDE.

cross cover test, alternate cover test. For determining inward, outward, upward or downward eye deviations. As a target is viewed, a cover is moved from eye to eye and direction of eye movement is noted. See also PRISM + ALTERNATE COVER TEST.

cross cylinder, Jackson cross cylinder. *Optical device*. Single lens composed of a plus cylinder and a minus cylinder of equal optical strength, placed perpendicular to one another. Used in a refraction to determine the axis and power of an astigmatic correction.

crossed diplopia, heteronymous diplopia. *Symptom*. Double vision in which the image seen by the right eye appears to be to the left of the image seen by the left eye. Associated with outward eye deviation (exotropia). See also UNCROSSED DIPLOPIA.

cross-eyes, convergent deviation, esotropia, internal strabismus. *Functional defect*. Misalignment in which one eye deviates inward (toward nose) while the other fixates normally. Deviation is present even when both eyes are uncovered. See also ESOPHORIA.

cross-fixation. *Functional defect*. Viewing an object in left gaze with the right eye, and an object in right gaze with the left eye. Frequently associated with a large infantile esotropia.

Crouzon's syndrome (KRU-zahnz), **craniofacial dysostosis**. *Congenital anomaly*. Characterized by multiple abnormalities of skull and jaw, e.g., short head, broad hooked nose, high palate, large earlobes, widely separated eyes, shallow orbits, optic nerve damage, corneal exposure, nystagmus, and an outward eye deviation (exotropia). See also APERT'S SYNDROME.

crowding phenomenon, separation difficulty. *Functional defect*. Inability to read an entire line of letters despite ability to read a single, isolated letter of the same size. Characteristic of functional amblyopia.

cryo (KRI-oh). 1. Slang for any surgical procedure that uses intense cold (cryosurgery). 2. Prefix: cold. Refers to use of intense cold for many surgical purposes. See also CRYOEXTRACTION, CRYOPEXY, CRYOPHAKE, CRYOPROBE, CYCLOCRYOTHERAPY.

cryoablation. *Surgical procedure*. Destruction of tissue by freezing. See also CYCLOABLATION.

cryoextraction. *Surgical procedure*. Removal of a cloudy lens (cataract) with its capsule by freezing the lens to the cold tip of the surgical instrument (cryophake) and pulling the lens out of the eye. See also INTRACAPSULAR CATARACT EXTRACTION.

cryoglobulinemia. *Pathologic condition*. Large protein globulin molecules in the blood that tend to clump in the presence of cold; may cause blockage of blood vessels because of increased blood viscosity. Sometimes related to hepatitis C.

cryolathe (KRI-oh-layth). *Surgical instrument*. Used for freezing and grinding human corneal tissue into different refractive powers. See also EPIKERATOPHAKIA, KERATOMILEUSIS.

cryopexy (KRI-oh-pek-see), **cryoretinopexy, retinocryopexy**. *Surgical procedure*. Use of intense cold to seal a retinal hole by creating a chorioretinal cold-burn and scar to close a retinal tear or tack down a detached retina.

cryophake (KRI-oh-fayk). *Surgical instrument*. Instrument whose tip generates intense cold; used for removal of a cloudy lens (cataract). See CRYOEXTRACTION.

cryoprobe (KRI-oh-prohb). *Surgical instrument*. Pencil-like device whose tip can be cooled with carbon dioxide, nitrous oxide or liquid nitrogen to freeze tissue. Used for removal of cloudy lens (cataract) or for cryotherapy. See also CRYOPEXY, CYCLOCRYOTHERAPY.

cryoretinopexy (kri-oh-RET-ih-noh-pek-see). See CRYOPEXY.

cryosurgery, cryo. *Surgical procedure*. Any surgical procedure that uses intense cold.

cryptogenic. *Description*. Of unknown origin.

cryptophthalmus (kript-ahf-THAL-mus). *Congenital anomaly*. Fusion of eyelids over the eyeball, resulting in an apparent absence of eyelids.

crypts of Fuchs (fyooks), **iris crypts**. *Anatomy.* Pit-like depressions in the front surface of the iris.

crystalline lens. *Anatomy.* The eye's natural lens. Transparent, biconvex intraocular tissue that helps bring rays of light to a focus on the retina. Suspended by fine ligaments (zonules) attached between ciliary processes.

C_3F_8, perfluoropropane. *Gas.* Injected into the eye to produce a nontoxic, expansive gas bubble to tamponade (push) dislocated parts into place. See also PNEUMATIC RETINOPEXY, SULPHUR HEXAFLUORIDE.

CT scan, computerized tomography. *Clinical test.* Low dosage x-rays coupled with a computer to generate a film showing tissue detail.

Cuemid. *Drug.* Trade name of cholystyramine; for lowering cholesterol levels.

cul-de-sac, conjunctival sac, fornix. *Anatomy.* Loose pocket of conjunctiva between upper eyelid and eyeball or lower eyelid and eyeball; permits the eyeball to rotate freely.

culture medium. *Lab compound.* Provides nutrients for growth of bacteria and fungi to aid in their identification. See also CHOCOLATE AGAR, SABOURAUD'S DEXTROSE AGAR, THIOGLYCOLATE BROTH.

cup, optic cup. 1. *Anatomy.* White depression in the center of the optic disc; usually normal and occupies less than one-third of the disc diameter. See also CUP-TO-DISC RATIO. 2. *Embryology.* Early stage in developing eye; an outpouching from the primitive brain.

cupped disc, cupping. *Pathologic condition.* Abnormal enlargement of the optic cup (depression in center of optic disc). Most commonly due to prolonged increase in intraocular pressure.

cupping. See CUPPED DISC.

cup-to-disc ratio. *Measurement.* Numerical expression indicating percentage of disc occupied by the optic cup. Used for evaluating the progression of glaucoma.

cupuliform cataract (kuh-PUH-lih-form), **posterior subcapsular cataract**. *Pathologic condition.* Common opacity of the rear surface of the lens. One type of "senile cataract" affecting the elderly; may occur at any age after chronic intraocular inflammations or after prolonged use of steroid drugs.

cutaneous horn. *Pathologic condition.* Small, cylindrical skin growth on the eyelid; a precancerous condition. Occurs in elderly people. See also ACTINIC KERATOSIS.

Cutler-Beard procedure. *Surgical procedure.* Two-step technique for reconstructing a large rectangular defect of the upper eyelid, such as after a lid tumor has been excised. Involves filling the area with a section from the lower lid, temporarily closing the lids, then after a few months to allow healing, the lids are separated. See also HUGHES PROCEDURE.

cyanolabe (si-AN-oh-layb). *Anatomy.* Blue-sensitive pigment found in retinal receptors (cones). See also CHLOROLABE, DEUTERANOMALY, ERYTHROLABE.

cyanopsia (si-an-AHP-see-uh). *Symptom.* Vision abnormality; objects appear to be tinted blue. Can be caused by aphakia, specific drug intoxications, carbon monoxide poisoning or hysteria. See also XANTHOPSIA, ERYTHROPSIA.

cyclectomy (si-KLEK-toh-mee). *Surgical procedure.* Removal of a portion of the ciliary body, with or without the iris, usually to excise a malignant lesion. See also IRIDOCYCLECTOMY.

cyclic strabismus (struh-BIZ-mus), **alternate day** *(or)* **clock-mechanism esotropia, circadian heterotropia**. *Functional defect.* Eye deviation that follows a 48-hour cycle, alternating 24 hours of normal binocularity with 24 hours of a large inward (toward nose) deviation.

cyclitic membrane (si-KLIH-tik). *Pathologic condition.* Membrane of fibrous tissue and inflammatory cells that grows across the front surface of the vitreous. Can cause decrease in vision or even massive shrinkage (phthisis) of the eye. Results from extensive intraocular inflammations.

cyclitis (si-KLI-tis). *Pathologic condition.* Inflammation of the ciliary body.

cycloablation, cyclodestruction. *Surgical procedure.* Destruction of the ciliary body to decrease aqueous production and thus decrease intraocular pressure. Frequently a last resort in advanced glaucoma when intraocular pressure remains uncontrolled despite maximum medical therapy. See also CYCLOCRYOTHERAPY, CYCLODIATHERMY, CYCLOPHOTOCOAGULATION.

cyclo-cryo. *Surgical procedure.* Slang for cyclocryopexy.

cyclocryopexy (CCT) (si-kloh-KRI-oh-pek-zee). See CYCLOCRYOTHERAPY.

cyclocryotherapy, cyclocryopexy. *Surgical procedure.* Destruction of part of the ciliary body by freezing, to reduce aqueous production; for control of elevated intraocular pressure in glaucoma. See also CYCLOABLATION.

cyclodamia (si-kloh-DAY-mee-uh). *Test.* Deliberate blurring of vision with lenses (fogging). Used in non-cycloplegic refraction to balance the correction in both eyes. See also BALANCING.

cyclodestruction. See CYCLOABLATION.

cyclodialysis (si-kloh-di-AL-ih-sis). *Pathologic change, surgical procedure.* Separation of the ciliary body from the sclera. May result from blunt trauma to the eye, or from surgery to control glaucoma (making a channel between the anterior chamber and suprachoroidal space).

cyclodiathermy (si-kloh-DI-uh-thur-mee). *Surgical procedure.* Destruction of part of the ciliary body with heat (diathermy), to reduce aqueous production in glaucoma. Rarely used; replaced by cyclocryotherapy.

cycloduction (si-kloh-DUK-shun). *Function.* Rotation (in either direction) of the eye around the front-to-back axis. See also TORSION, Y AXIS OF FICK.

Cyclogyl (SI-kloh-jil). *Drug.* Trade name of cyclopentolate, parasympatholytic eyedrops; dilates the pupil and paralyzes accommodation for a cycloplegic refraction.

cyclopentolate (si-kloh-PEN-tuh-layt). *Drug.* Eyedrop that blocks the parasympathetic nerve fibers to the eye, producing enlarged pupil and paralysis of accommodation. Effect lasts several hours. Trade name: Cyclogyl. See also TROPICAMIDE.

cyclophosphamide. *Drug.* Anti-cancer drug that interfers with the growth of malignant cells. In the eye, used for treating Behcet's disease, cicatricial pemphigoid, Mooren's ulcer, and Wegener's granulomatosis.

cyclophotocoagulation. *Surgical procedure.* Use of a laser beam to destroy the ciliary processes, to decrease aqueous production in poorly controlled advanced glaucoma. See also CYCLOABLATION.

cyclopia (si-KLOH-pee-uh). See CYCLOPS.

cycloplegia (si-kloh-PLEE-juh). *Functional defect.* Paralysis of the ciliary muscle, eliminating accommodation. Clinically accomplished with eyedrops that temporarily block the action of the parasympathetic nerves in the eye.

cycloplegic (si-kloh-PLEE-jik). *Drug.* Eyedrop that temporarily blocks the action of the parasympathetic nerves in the eye, relaxing the ciliary muscle (to paralyze accommodation) and iris sphincter (to enlarge the pupil). Used for cycloplegic refraction and treating iritis. Examples: Atropine, Cyclogyl, Mydriacyl.

cycloplegic refraction. *Test.* Assessment of an eye's refractive error after lens accommodation has been paralyzed with cycloplegic eyedrops (to eliminate variability in optical power caused by a contracting lens).

cyclops (SI-klahps), **cyclopia.** *Congenital anomaly.* Presence of one partially formed, abnormal eye in the center of the forehead. Condition is incompatible with life. See also SYNOPHTHALMIA.

cyclotropia (si-kloh-TROH-pee-uh). *Functional defect.* Extraocular muscle imbalance in which the vertical axis of the eye tilts inward (toward nose) or outward.

cycloversion (si-kloh-VUR-zhun). *Function.* Tilting of vertical axes of both eyes in the same (right or left) direction. See also TORSION.

cylinder, cylindrical lens. *Optical device.* Lens that produces a different refractive power in each meridian (minimal power in one meridian, maximal in the perpendicular meridian); used for correcting ocular astigmatism. See also ASTIGMATISM, PRINCIPAL MERIDIANS, TORIC LENS.

> **axis**: the meridian that has least optical power.

> **power**: difference (in diopters) between maximum and minimum powers.

cyst. *Anatomy.* Thin-walled sac, usually containing a liquid or semisolid. May be normal or abnormal.

cystic microphthalmia (SIS-tik mike-rahf-THAL-mee-uh). *Congenital defect.* Small, rudimentary non-functioning eyeball caused by failure of normal embryonic development.

cystinosis (sis-tin-OH-sis). *Pathologic condition.* Metabolic defect characterized by cystine crystal deposits throughout the body (including cornea and conjunctiva), dwarfism, and renal failure. There is also a less serious juvenile form and a benign, acquired adult form. Rare; hereditary.

cystoid macular edema (CME) (SIS-toyd MAK-yu-lur). *Pathologic condition.* Retinal swelling and cyst formation in the macular area; usually results in temporary decrease in vision, though may be permanent. Frequently occurs to some extent after cataract surgery. Specific cause is unknown. See also IRVINE-GASS SYNDROME.

cystotome (SIS-tuh-tohm). *Surgical instrument.* Used for opening the front capsule of the lens during extracapsular cataract extraction.

cyclosporine. *Drug.* Anti-cancer drug used for preventing the body's rejection of organ transplants. Also for treating non-infectious uveitis that does not respond to steroids.

cytomegalic inclusion disease (CMI) (si-toh-meh-GAL-ik). See CYTOMEGALO-VIRUS RETINITIS.

cytomegalovirus (CMV) (SI-toh-meg-al-oh-VI-rus). *Pathologic condition.* Large virus commonly present in the urinary tract. Rarely causes disease unless the individual is immunosuppressed (has poor immune response), e.g., in AIDS, in which case it can cause serious disease, e.g., CMV retinitis.

cytopenia. *Pathologic condition.* Below-normal blood cell count.

cytotoxic. *Description.* Refers to substances that are poisonous to certain cells of the body.

cytotoxic agent (si-toh-TAHK-sik). *Drug.* Destroys cells, e.g. cancer cells; also used for treating non-cancerous conditions, e.g., severe uveitis. See also ANTI-CANCER DRUGS.

Cytovene. *Drug.* Trade name of ganciclovir. For treating severe herpetic eye infections.

Cytoxan. *Drug.* Trade name of cyclophosphamide. For treating cancer.

D

D (diopter). *Optics.* Basic unit of lens refractive power; equal to the focal length (in meters) of a lens, e.g., a 2-diopter lens brings parallel rays of light to a focus at 1/2 meter. Also a measure of the degree that light converges or diverges, i.e., the reciprocal of the distance (in meters) between an object or image and any reference plane. See also PRISM DIOPTER.

dacryo- (DAK-ree-oh). Prefix: relating to tears.

dacryoadenitis (DAK-ree-oh-ad-ih-NI-tis). *Pathologic condition.* Inflammation of the lacrimal gland. Often chronic and caused by a granulomatous disease; acute form occurs with mumps and infectious mononucleosis.

dacryocystectomy (DAK-ree-oh-sis-TEK-toh-mee). *Surgical procedure.* Removal of the tear sac.

dacryocystitis (DAK-ree-oh-sis-TI-tis). *Pathologic condition.* Inflammation of the tear sac. Associated with faulty tear drainage.

dacryocystogram (DAK-ree-oh-SIS-toh-gram). *Test.* X-ray of tear drainage channels using radio-opaque dyes.

dacryocystography with radionuclide (dak-ree-oh-sys-TAW-gruh-fee ray-dee-oh-NU-clide). *Test.* Computerized x-ray study of tear drainage channels using a radioactive dye tracer.

dacryocystorhinostomy (DCR) (DAK-ree-oh-sis-toh-ri-NAHS-toh-mee). *Surgical procedure.* Construction of a new tear drainage channel from the lacrimal sac into the nose.

dacryoscintigraphy (dak-ree-oh-sin-TIG-ruh-fee), **scintigraphy**. *Test.* Photographing and measuring a radioactive tracer in the tear film as it travels through the tear drainage system.

dacryostenosis (dak-ree-oh-sten-OH-sis). *Anatomic defect.* Abnormally narrow opening of the tear sac.

Dalcaine. *Drug.* Trade name of lidocaine anesthetic; used for eye surgery.

Dalen-Fuchs nodules (DAY-lin fyooks). *Pathologic condition.* Microscopically visible inflammatory cell clusters lying beneath the retinal pigment epithelium. Associated with sympathetic ophthalmia.

Dalrymple's sign (DAL-rim-pulz). *Clinical sign.* Widened eyelid opening caused by upper eyelid retraction, resulting in a stare-like appearance. Associated with an overactive thyroid. See also COLLIER'S SIGN, STELLWAG'S SIGN, VON GRAEFE'S SIGN.

Dandy-Walker syndrome. *Congenital anomaly.* Malformation and narrowing (stenosis) of the normal openings in the 4th ventricle of the brain (foramina of Magendie and Luschka) with resulting hydrocephalus (water on the brain). Eye signs include ptosis, 6th nerve palsy, and papilledema.

dapsone. *Drug.* Anti-cancer drug used for immunosuppression. For treating cicatricial pemphigoid.

Daranide (DER-uh-nide). *Drug.* Trade name of dichlorophenamide; for treating glaucoma.

dark adaptation. *Function.* Process of an eye adjusting to decreased illumination and becoming more sensitive to light. See also SCOTOPIC VISION.

darkroom provocative test. For angle closure glaucoma in a glaucoma suspect. Intraocular pressure is checked after 1 hour in the dark; an increase to 8.5 mm is considered positive. See also MYDRIATIC PROVOCATIVE TEST.

debridement (deh-BREED-ment). *Surgical procedure.* Removal of dead or infected tissue and foreign material, to aid in healing.

Decadron (DEK-uh-dron). *Drug.* Trade name of dexamethasone, an anti-inflammatory steroid.

decentration. *Optics*. 1. Misalignment of the optical center of an eyeglass lens with the visual axis of the eye. 2. Re-positioning of the optical center of an eyeglass lens to align it with visual axis of a deviated eye. See also PRENTICE'S RULE.

decibel (dB). *Measurement*. 1. Unit of sound intensity. 2. In automated perimetry, the amount of light intensity an eye can detect, expressed in logarithmic units.

decompression (lateral orbital), Krönlein procedure. *Surgical procedure*. Partial removal of the bony orbital wall (zygoma) and/or floor (maxillary sinus roof) to relieve forward pressure on the eye when the orbital contents have increased in size (e.g., in Graves' disease). See also THYROID EYE DISEASE.

decongestant. *Drug*. Weak sympathomimetic eyedrops that constrict conjunctival blood vessels to "whiten" the eye and relieve minor eye irritation. Examples: ephedrine, phenyleprine, oxymetazoline, naphazoline, tetrahydrozoline.

decussation (deh-kuh-SAY-shun). Crossing, as of nerve fibers or light rays, to form an X.

degenerative myopia (mi-OH-pee-uh), **malignant myopia**. *Pathologic condition*. Uncommon form of myopia (nearsightedness) accompanied by progressive stretching changes and gradual damage to the retina, choroid, vitreous, sclera, and optic nerve.

Degest-2. *Drug*. Trade name of naphazoline eyedrops; contricts blood vessels to "whiten" the eye.

degree. *Unit of measure*. 1/360 of a circle. Used as an angular measure in visual field testing or (rarely) as a measure of eye misalignment: $1° = 1.7^\Delta$ (prism diopters).

dehiscence (dee-HISS-untz). *Pathologic condition*. Coming apart or breaking open of tissue, as a wound that has been previously repaired.

dellen (DEL-in), **corneal dellen**. *Pathologic condition*. Localized zone of corneal thinning, usually at the limbus, caused by excessive dehydration. Reversible.

demecarium bromide (dem-ek-EHR-ee-um). *Drug*. Anti-cholinesterase effect stimulates parasympathetic nerve fibers, increasing aqueous outflow. Powerful, long-acting. Used rarely for treating glaucoma. Trade name: Humorsol.

demyelination (dee-mi-uh-lin-AY-shun). *Pathologic condition*. Loss or destruction of the myelin covering of nerve fibers, such as in multiple sclerosis.

dendrite. *Anatomy*. Branch-like process of a nerve that conducts impulses toward the nerve cell body.

dendriform. *Description*. Branching; resembling a tree.

dendritic keratitis (den-DRIT-ik kehr-uh-TI-tus). *Pathologic condition*. Superficial corneal infection characterized by branch-shaped corneal ulcers. Characteristic of herpes simplex virus infection.See also KERATITIS.

denervation supersensitivity (dee-nur-VAY-shun). *Functional defect*. Marked increase in effect on eyes (usually pupil size) of chemicals that normally transmit nerve impulses. Follows structural damage to autonomic nerves. See also MECHOLYL TEST.

densitometry, reflection densitometry. Laboratory measurement technique to determine amounts of various retinal photopigments in visual cells.

deorsumvergence (dee-or-sum-VUR-junz). *Function*. Downward movement of one eye relative to the other, usually to maintain single binocular vision, e.g., when increasing amounts of base-up prism are placed in front of that eye.

deorsumversion (dee-or-sum-VUR-zhun). *Function*. Downward movement of both eyes from the straight-ahead position. See also DEPRESSION, INFRADUCTION.

Depo-Medrol (deh-poh-MEH-drawl). *Drug*. Trade name of methylprednisolone in a form that releases the drug slowly.

depression. *Function*. Downward movement of one or both eyes from the straight-ahead position. See also DEORSUMVERSION, INFRADUCTION.

depressors. *Anatomy*. Extraocular muscles (inferior rectus, superior oblique) that move the eye downward.

deprivation amblyopia (am-blee-OH-pee-uh). *Functional defect*. Type of functional amblyopia in which an eye loses visual acuity after central fixation disuse (due to cloudy cornea, cataract, droopy lid, etc.).

depth of field. *Optics*. Range (distances) in which an image created by an optical system is acceptably sharp.

depth perception. *Function*. Awareness of the relative spatial location of objects, some being closer to the observer than others.

    binocular: visual blending of two similar images (one falling on each retina) into one, with visual perception of solidity and depth. Also called stereopsis, 3rd grade fusion.

dermatochalasis (DUR-muh-toh-kal-AY-sis), **blepharochalasis**. *Pathologic condition*. Excess eyelid skin caused by atrophy of the elastic tissue. A fold of tissue from the upper lid usually hangs over the eyelid margin. Associated with orbital septum defects or aging.

dermatoconjunctivitis (DUR-muh-toh-kun-junk-tuh-VI-tis). *Pathologic condition*. Inflammation of the conjunctiva (membrane covering white of eye and inner lids) and skin near the eyelid margins.

dermatomyositis (DUR-muh-toh-mi-oh-SI-tis). *Pathologic condition*. Collagen disease characterized by inflammation of muscles, skin and blood vessels. Common eye signs are reddish-brown swollen eyelids, eye oscillations (nystagmus), eye movement restrictions, scleral inflammation, and retinal cotton-wool spots.

dermoid, dermoid cyst, epibulbar dermoid. *Congenital anomaly*. Tumor containing skin elements such as epithelium, fat, and hair; usually found at the corneo-scleral junction (limbus) or the lateral side of the upper eyelid. See also GOLDENHAR'S SYNDROME.

desaturated 15 hue test, Lanthony's desaturated 15 hue test. Sensitive color vision test for detecting congenital or acquired color deficiencies. See also MUNSELL SCALE.

descemetocele (dez-MET-oh-seel), **keratocele**. *Pathologic condition*. Protrusion of Descemet's membrane into the cornea to "plug" a defect after an ulcer has eroded the overlying stroma. Protects the eye from "blowing out."

Descemet's membrane (DES-uh-mayz). *Anatomy*. Thin, elastic layer deep in the cornea, formed by the endothelium and composed of collagen and elastic fibrils. See also DESCEMETOCELE.

detachment. *Pathologic condition*.

    choroidal (kor-OY-dul): separation of the blood vessel layer (choroid) from the sclera. Caused by fluid leakage from choroidal blood vessels; may follow eye injury or eye surgery. Related to excessively low intraocular pressure.

    retinal: separation of the sensory retina from the underlying pigment epithelium; almost always caused by a retinal tear. Disrupts visual cell structure, markedly disturbing vision. Often requires immediate surgical repair. See also CRYORETINOPEXY, DIALYSIS, GIANT TEAR, HORSESHOE TEAR, MORNING GLORY DETACHMENT, RHEGMATOGENOUS RETINAL DETACHMENT, SCLERAL BUCKLE, SEROUS DETACHMENT, TRACTION DETACHMENT.

    vitreous: separation of vitreous gel from retinal surface. Usually innocuous, but can cause retinal tears, which may lead to retinal detachment. Frequently occurs with aging as the vitreous liquifies, or in some disease states, e.g. diabetes and high myopia.

deuteranomaly (du-tur-uh-NAH-muh-lee). *Functional defect.* Most common type of color vision deficiency, mildly affecting red-green discrimination. Hereditary, X-linked (affects 5% of males). See also CHLOROLABE, PROTANOMALY, TRITANOMALY.

deuteranopia (du-tur-uh-NOH-pee-uh). *Functional defect.* Color vision deficiency, moderately affecting red-green discrimination. Form of dichromatism in which only two cone pigments are present. Hereditary; X-linked (affects 1% of males).

deviation, heterotropia, squint, strabismus, tropia. *Functional defect.* Eye misalignment caused by extraocular muscle imbalance: one fovea is not directed at the same object as the other. Present even when both eyes are uncovered. See also PHORIA.

    primary: (smaller) deviation caused by a paralyzed muscle when the uninvolved eye is fixating.

    secondary: (larger) deviation caused by a paralyzed muscle when the involved eye is fixating.

de Vick's disease. Incorrect spelling of DEVIC'S DISEASE.

Devic's disease (DEV-iks), **neuromyelitis optica**. *Pathologic condition.* Demyelinating central nervous system disorder characterized by paraplegia and inflammation of both optic nerves, causing marked vision loss. Similar to multiple sclerosis. Rare.

dexamethasone (deks-uh-METH-uh-zohn). *Drug.* Anti-inflammatory steroid ointment or suspension used for treating ocular infections. Trade names: Decadron, Maxidex, TobraDex.

dextroversion (deks-troh-VUR-zhun). *Function.* Parallel movement of both eyes to the right.

DFP (diisopropyl fluorophosphate). *Drug.* An anticholinesterase, parasympathomimetic drug that produces ciliary muscle contraction (accommodation), small pupils (miosis), and increased aqueous outflow. Used in diagnosis and treatment of accommodative esotropia and for treating glaucoma. Trade name: Floropryl.

DiaBeta. *Drug.* Trade name of glyburide medication; for controlling diabetes.

diabetic retinopathy (ret-in-AHP-uh-thee). *Pathologic condition.* Spectrum of retinal changes accompanying long-standing diabetes mellitus. Early stage is background retinopathy (non-proliferative). May advance to proliferative retinopathy, which includes the growth of abnormal new blood vessels (neovascularization) and accompanying fibrous tissue.

diagnostic positions of gaze, fields of gaze. *Test.* Nine positions (straight ahead, up, down, right, left, up + right, down + right, up + left, down + left) to which both eyes are moved as the head faces forward; for evaluation of extraocular muscles, versions and double vision. See also DIPLOPIA FIELDS, SECONDARY POSITIONS, TERTIARY POSITIONS, YOKE MUSCLES.

dialysis (di-AL-ih-sis). *Pathologic condition.* Break or tear of an ocular structure (retina, iris or ciliary body), usually at its peripheral edge. See also GIANT TEAR. 2. *Medical procedure.* For filtering abnormal components from body fluids.

diamond conjunctival resection, tarsalconjunctival spindle excision, tarsalconjunctival resection below the punctum. *Surgical procedure.* Removal of a spindle- or diamond-shaped section of conjunctival tissue from inside the lower lid parallel to the eyelid margin, to invert a malpositioned punctum and reposition the lower lid against the globe. See also ECTROPION.

Diamox (DI-uh-mahks). *Drug.* Trade name of acetazolamide, a carbonic anhydrous inhibitor; for treating glaucoma.

diaphoresis (di-uh-fur-EE-sis). *Clinical sign.* Profuse sweating.

diaphoretic. *Description.* Refers to an agent (drug or activity) that causes sweating.

diastolic blood pressure (di-uh-STAHL-ik). *Function.* Lowest pressure during the cardiac cycle (measured in mm of mercury); occurs during heart relaxation phase. See also SYSTOLIC BLOOD PRESSURE.

diathermy (DI-uh-thur-mee). *Surgical instrument.* Apparatus that generates focal heat. When applied to affected tissue, coagulates it. Can seal retinal tears, stop surface bleeding, or selectively destroy tissue.

dichlorophenamide (di-klor-oh-FEN-uh-mide). Oral medication that decreases aqueous fluid formation. For treating glaucoma. Trade names: Daranide, Oratol. See also CARBONIC ANHYDRASE INHIBITOR.

dichromatism (di-KROH-muh-tizm). *Functional defect.* Moderately severe color vision defect in which one of the three basic color mechanisms is absent or not functioning. Hereditary, X-linked (affects males predominantly). See also DEUTERANOPIA, PROTANOPIA, TRITANOPIA.

dictyoma. Incorrect spelling of DIKTYOMA.

differential (white blood cell count). *Lab test.* Percentage of each of the major types of white blood cells present in the circulating blood.

diffraction. *Optics.* Property of light that permits it to bend around sharp edges.

diffuse (dih-FYOOS). *Description.* Affecting a broad area, widespread. See also FOCAL.

diffuse angiokeratoma (an-jee-oh-ker-uh-TOH-muh), **angiokeratoma corporis diffusum universale, Fabry's disease.** *Pathologic condition.* Enzyme deficiency disease affecting fat (lipid) metabolism. Eye signs include whorl-like corneal opacities, star-shaped lens haze, and tortuous conjunctival and retinal veins. Hereditary, X-linked. See also SPHINGOLIPIDOSES.

diffuse unilateral subacute neuroretinitis (DUSN), "wipe-out" syndrome. *Pathologic condition.* Insidious, gradual loss of vision in one eye, usually in children. Thought to be caused by an intraocular *Toxocara* worm.

digitalis toxicity (dij-ih-TAL-is). *Pathologic condition.* Adverse reaction to digitalis (drug usually taken for heart problems). Eye signs include blurred vision, disturbed color vision, abnormal sensitivity to light (photophobia), light flashes, and fleeting blind spots.

digito-ocular reflex. *Sign.* Sensation of light in a blind eye, as a response to pressing or rubbing firmly on the eye, which mechanically stimulates photoreceptors.

diisopropyl fluorophosphate (di-I-soh-PROH-pil FLOR-oh-FAHS-fayt). See DFP.

diktyoma (dik-tee-OH-muh). *Pathologic condition.* Malignant ciliary body tumor. Occurs in children.

dilate (DI-layt). *Function, procedure.* To widen an opening, such as the pupil or lacrimal punctum.

dilated pinhole test (DI-lay-tid). For testing macular function in the presence of optical opacities, e.g., cataract, corneal scar. Vision is tested as the dilated eye looks through small hole(s) in an opaque disc. See also PINHOLE.

dilated pupil. *Anatomic change.* Enlarged pupil, resulting from contraction of the dilator muscle or relaxation of the iris sphincter. Occurs normally in dim illumination, or may be produced by certain drugs (mydriatics) or result from blunt trauma.

dilator muscle (DI-lay-tur), **dilator pupillae, iris *(or)* pupil dilator**. *Anatomy.* Smooth muscle of iris that contracts to enlarge the pupillary opening. Extends like wheel spokes from the pupillary margin to iris periphery. Innervated by sympathetic nerves.

dilator pupillae (pyu-PIL-ee). See DILATOR MUSCLE.

diopter (D) (di-AHP-tur). *Unit of measure.* Unit to designate the refractive power of a lens, or the degree of light convergence or divergence. Equal to the reciprocal of a lens' focal length (in meters), e.g., a 2-diopter lens brings parallel rays of light to a focus at 1/2 m. See also PRISM DIOPTER.

diphtheroid (DIF-thuh-royd), ***Corynebacterium xerosis***. *Microorganism.* Club-shaped, gram-positive bacteria; exists normally on eyelid skin.

dipivefrin (di-PIV-if-rin). *Drug.* Sympathomimetic eyedrop that converts to epinephrine inside the eye, decreasing aqueous secretion and increasing aqueous outflow. For treating glaucoma. Trade name: Propine.

diplopia, double vision. *Functional defect.* Perception of two images from one object; images may be horizontal, vertical or diagonal.

> **crossed**: image seen by the right eye appears to the left of that seen by the left eye. Associated with an outward eye deviation (exotropia).
>
> **heteronymous**: same as CROSSED (above).
>
> **homonymous**: same as UNCROSSED (below).
>
> **monocular**: multiple images seen with one eye. Commonly caused by an early cataract or irregular cornea.
>
> **paradoxic**: unexpected spacial location of images relative to actual eye position. Only found after strabismus surgery; usually temporary.
>
> **pathologic**: caused by misalignment of one eye. Temporary in children; permanent in adults.
>
> **physiologic**: doubling of distant objects when near object is viewed, and vice versa, for objects not directly fixated by both eyes. Normal.
>
> **uncrossed**: image seen by the right eye appears to the right of the left eye's image. Associated with an inturning eye (esotropia).

diplopia fields. *Test.* 1. Determination of the amount and direction of double vision in each of the nine diagnostic eye positions, evaluated with a fixation light, red filter, or Maddox rod and prisms. 2. Visual field analysis of both eyes simultaneously to distinguish areas of single vision from double vision.

dipping. *Sign.* Slow downward movement of both eyes followed by a delay, then a fast upward movement to primary position. Seen in comatose patients. See also BOBBING, REVERSE BOBBING.

direct antagonist, ipsilateral antagonist. *Anatomy.* Extraocular muscle whose action opposes that of another muscle in the same eye (e.g., medial rectus and lateral rectus).

direct goniotomy, "blind" goniotomy. *Surgical procedure.* Incision made in the trabecular meshwork without clear visualization of angle structures, e.g., when obscured by a cloudy cornea. Used for treating congenital glaucoma.

direct light response. *Function, test.* Decrease in pupil size (constriction) elicited when a light is directed toward that eye; tested in dim illumination with patient looking into the distance.

direct ophthalmoscope (ahf-THAL-muh-skohp), **direct scope**. *Instrument.* Hand-held device for visualizing interior of the eye (fundus). Provides a magnified (15x) upright image of the retina, with a small (8°) field of view. See also INDIRECT OPHTHALMOSCOPE.

direct scope. See DIRECT OPHTHALMOSCOPE.

disc, optic disc *(or)* nerve head. *Anatomy.* Ocular end of the optic nerve. Denotes the exit of retinal nerve fibers from the eye and entrance of blood vessels to the eye.

disc cupping. *Pathologic condition.* Enlarged and deepened optic cup, e.g., in glaucoma. See also CUP.

disc diameter. *Unit of measure.* Diameter of the optic nerve head (about 1.5 mm); used in describing location and size of fundus lesions.

disc drusen (DRU-sen), **hyaline masses**. *Pathologic condition.* Glistening nodules within the optic nerve head. May blur disc margins. Sometimes mistaken for chronic papilledema.

disciform degeneration of the macula (DIS-kih-form, MAK-yu-luh), **Kuhnt-**

Junius disease. *Pathologic condition.* Retinal degeneration leading to permanent loss of central vision (peripheral vision stays intact). Begins with a fluid leak under the retinal pigment epithelium in the macular area, usually followed by hemorrhage and scarring. Most common cause of blindness in persons over age 50. See also MACULAR DEGENERATION.

disciform keratitis (kehr-uh-TI-tus). *Pathologic condition.* Corneal stromal inflammation, probably related to an immune response. Appears as a disc-shaped, gray lesion. Usually related to herpes simplex virus infection. See also KERATITIS.

discission (dih-SIH-zhun). *Surgical procedure.* 1. Puncturing or cutting the opaque pupillary membrane or posterior lens capsule remnant to recreate a clear optical opening. 2. Puncturing a cataractous lens, allowing it to mix with aqueous, with resulting absorption of lens material.

disc neovascularization (nee-oh-vas-kyu-lur-ih-ZAY-shun). *Pathologic condition.* Abnormal formation of new blood vessels on or around the optic nerve head. May occur in diabetic retinopathy (proliferative phase) or after retinal vein occlusion.

disconjugate movement. See DISJUNCTIVE MOVEMENT.

disinsertion (dis-in-SUR-shun). *Surgical procedure.* Cutting an extraocular muscle free from its attachment on the eyeball. Used as a muscle weakening procedure to correct an eye deviation.

disjugate movement (DIS-juh-gut). See DISJUNCTIVE MOVEMENT.

disjunctive vergence, disconjugate *(or)* disjugate movement, vergence. *Function.* Movement of both eyes in opposite directions (toward or away from each other, up and down) to obtain or maintain single binocular vision.

dislocated lens. *Pathologic condition.* Partial or complete displacement of the crystalline lens from its normal position; caused by broken or absent zonules. See also ECTOPIA LENTIS, HOMOCYSTINURIA, LUXATION, MARCHESANI'S SYNDROME, MARFAN'S SYNDROME, SUBLUXATION.

disodium EDTA. 1. *Chemical.* Chelating (binding) agent used for removing abnormal calcium deposits from the corneal surface (e.g., for band keratopathy) and may help protect the cornea from ulceration after a chemical burn. 2. *Drug enhancer.* Enhances antibacterial activity of preservatives commonly used in topical eyedrops and increases drug penetration across the cornea. See also BENZALKONIUM CHLORIDE.

disparate retinal points (DIS-pur-it RET-in-ul). *Concept.* Points on each retina that, when stimulated by an object, give rise to perception that the object is in two different positions in visual space, i.e., seen double. See also CORRESPONDING POINTS.

dispensing optician. Professional who makes optical aids such as eyeglass lenses from refraction prescriptions supplied by an ophthalmologist or optometrist.

disposable lens. *Optical device.* Soft, hydrophilic contact lens designed to be discarded after wear (usually 1 week).

dissociated double hypertropia (hi-pur-TROH-pee-uh). See DISSOCIATED VERTICAL DEVIATION.

dissociated nystagmus (ni-STAG-mus). *Functional defect.* Involuntary, rhythmic, rapid side-to-side eye movements that differ in the two eyes as to speed, direction or amount. See also NYSTAGMUS.

dissociated position, fusion-free *(or)* heterophoric position, physiologic position of rest. *Function.* Position assumed by the eyes, relative to each other, when one eye is covered or its vision obstructed. See also PHORIA.

dissociated vertical deviation (DVD), alternating sursumduction, dissociated double hypertropia, double hypertropia. *Functional defect.* Eye deviation in which one eye drifts upward and rolls outward (extorts) whenever the two eyes are not working together.

distal. *Location*. Farther from a point of reference or away from the midline of the body. See also PROXIMAL.

distance and near (D + N). Reference points for measuring visual acuity: distance is usually 20 ft. (6 m); near is usually 16 in. (40 cm). See also DISTANCE VISION, NEAR VISION.

distance vision. *Measurement*. Visual acuity measured with target at 20 ft., the optical equivalent of "infinite distance." See also NEAR VISION.

distichiasis (dis-tih-KI-uh-sus). *Congenital anomaly*. Double row of eyelashes. Usually irritates the cornea.

distometer (dis-TAHM-ih-tur). *Instrument*. Caliper for measuring the distance between the back surface of an eyeglass lens and the front of the cornea. See also VERTEX DISTANCE.

distortion. *Optics*. 1. Imperfectly shaped image created by an optical system of lenses or mirrors. 2. Perception created by a wrinkled or irregular retina. See also METAMORPHOPSIA.

diuresis. *Clinical sign*. Increased urination.

diuretic. *Drug*. Substance that stimulates or permits the kidneys to excrete more urine.

Diuril. *Drug*. Trade name of chlorothiazide; for increasing urination and lowering blood pressure.

divergence. 1. *Optics*. Refers to the spreading apart of light rays as they leave an object or a minus-powered lens. 2. *Function*. Outward (away from each other) eye rotation, usually in an effort to maintain single binocular vision.
> **relative**: amount of base-in prism that can be overcome while maintaining clear binocular single vision. Also called relative fusional divergence.

divergence amplitudes. *Measurement*. Amount both eyes can rotate outward (away from each other) before double vision is induced. Measured in prism diopters.

divergence excess. *Functional defect*. Type of outward deviation (exotropia) that is greater when the target is at a distance (20 ft.) than at near (16 in.). See also BASIC EXOTROPIA, CONVERGENCE INSUFFICIENCY.

divergence insufficiency. *Functional defect*. Type of inward deviation (esotropia) that exists only for distances beyond about 5 ft.

divergent strabismus (struh-BIZ-mus), **exotropia, external strabismus, wall-eyes**. *Functional defect*. Eye misalignment in which one eye deviates outward (away from nose) while other fixates normally. See also EXOPHORIA.

diverging lens, concave lens, minus lens. *Optical device*. Lens that is thicker at the edges than in the center, increasing the divergence of incoming light rays. Corrects nearsightedness (myopia).

Dk level (Dk/L). *Measurement*. Amount of oxygen transmission per unit thickness of a contact lens.

doll's head phenomenon. *Function*. Eye movement in the direction opposite to head motion; keeps eyes on object of fixation when the head is passively moved side to side or up and down. See also VESTIBULO-OCULAR REFLEX.

dominant eye. *Function*. 1. Preferred eye for various visual tasks, e.g., sighting. 2. The eye that leads and controls the other during binocular eye movements. Usually on same side of body as dominant hand.

Donder's chart (DAHN-durz). *Measurement*. Standard table showing the relationship between advancing age and decrease in focusing ability (accommodation). Varies slightly from Duane's accommodation chart.

Donder's law. An eye moving from one position to another is always oriented identically in the new position no matter what path it took to arrive there.

Donder's line. *Measurement*. Graph showing the linear relationship between focusing ability (accommodation) and the amount of convergence required to maintain binocular fixation on an object as its distance from the eyes varies.

donor eye. Eye tissue (cornea and sclera) removed from a donor at death, for transplant. See also DONOR TISSUE.

donor tissue, graft. Eye tissue (cornea and sclera) removed upon a donor's death. Used for corneal transplant or for patching the sclera.

Dorello's canal (dor-EL-ohz). *Anatomy.* Opening in the brain where the 6th (abducens) cranial nerve enters the cavernous sinus.

dorsal. *Location.* Nearer to the back of the body. Often same as posterior.

dorsal midbrain syndrome, Parinaud's *(or)* **pretectal** *(or)* **Sylvian aque-duct** *(or)* **tectal midbrain syndrome**. *Pathologic condition.* Decreased ability to move the eyes up or down. Attributed to a brainstem lesion near the vertical gaze center. May be associated with inability to converge and poor pupil response to light. See also ARGYLL-ROBERTSON PUPILS.

dorsum sellae. *Anatomy.* Flat segment of the sphenoid bone (the quadri-lateral plate) that forms the posterior boundary of the sella turcica, which surrounds the pituitary gland.

Doryl (DOR-il). *Drug.* Trade name of carbachol eyedrops, for treating glaucoma.

dorzolamide. *Drug.* Carbonic anhydrase inhibitor in eyedrop form. For treat-ing glaucoma. Trade name: Trusopf.

"dot and blot" hemorrhages. *Pathologic condition.* Tiny round hemorrhages in the retina, usually in the outer plexiform later. Typically associated with diabetes.

dot dystrophy. Term sometimes used for MAP-DOT-FINGERPRINT DYSTROPHY.

double arcuate scotoma (AR-kyu-it skuh-TOH-muh). *Pathologic condition.* Two curved blind areas in the visual field, one up and one down, extend-ing from the physiologic blind spot in an arc around the fixation spot and ending at the horizontal raphe. Caused by damage to the retinal nerve fiber bundles. See SCOTOMA.

double dissociated hypertropia (DDH). See DISSOCIATED VERTICAL DEVIATION.

double elevator palsy. *Congenital anomaly.* Paralysis of extraocular muscles responsible for moving the eye upward (superior rectus, inferior oblique). May be associated with convergence, pupil and eyelid abnormalities.

double homonymous hemianopsia (hoh-MAH-nih-mus hem-ee-uh-NAHP-see-uh). *Pathologic condition.* Visual field loss of entire right and left sides with the exception of central vision (macular sparing). Caused by injury to the occipital lobes on both sides of the brain.

double hypertropia (hi-pur-TROH-pee-uh), **alternating sursumduction, dis-sociated double hypertropia, dissociated vertical deviation**. *Function-al defect.* Eye deviation in which one eye drifts upward and rolls outward (extorts) whenever the two eyes are not working together.

double ring. *Sign.* Small optic disc surrounded by a halo of decreased pig-ment and sometimes an additional halo of retinal pigment. Sign of optic nerve hypoplasia.

double vision, diplopia. *Functional defect.* Perception of two images from one object; images may be horizontal, vertical, or diagonal. Types listed under DIPLOPIA.

Douvas roto-extractor (DU-vahs). *Surgical instrument.* Device with a rotating cutting tip through which fluid can be injected and removed from the eye.

downbeat nystagmus (ni-STAG-mus). *Pathologic condition.* Involuntary, rapid, rhythmic vertical eye movements that have a faster downward movement. Occurs in patients with brainstem disease or drug intoxication.

down-gaze. Position of eye(s) following downward eye rotation (with the head in straight-ahead position). See also DEPRESSION, DEPRESSORS.

Down's syndrome, mongolism, trisomy 21. *Congenital defect.* Mental retardation associated with an extra chromosome (#21). Eye signs include lower eyelid margins that slant upward toward lateral canthi (mongoloid slant), Brushfield spots in iris, cataracts, inward deviation (esotropia), near-sightedness (myopia), blepharitis, and keratoconus.

Doyne's syndrome. *Pathologic condition.* Degenerative central retinal disorder characterized by white, hyaline deposits (drusen) under the pigment epithelium in the macular area. Hereditary.

Draeger tonometer (DRAY-ghur toh-NAH-muh-tur). *Instrument.* Hand-held device that measures intraocular pressure by flattening the cornea. See also APPLANATION TONOMETRY.

dragged disc. See DRAGGED RETINA.

dragged macula (MAK-yu-luh), **ectopic macula, foveal dystopia**. *Pathologic condition.* Displacement of the macular region of the retina by traction. Seen with retinopathy of prematurity, intraocular worm, previous inflammation and other forms of retinal scarring, and following retinal detachment surgery.

dragged retina, dragged disc. *Pathologic condition.* Retinal traction abnormality in which the retina and retinal vessels are pulled from their normal positions. Associated with retinopathy of prematurity, intraocular worm, or previous inflammation. Can affect one or both eyes.

dropout. *Pathologic condition.* Loss of retinal capillaries. Occurs in various vascular diseases that affect the retina (e.g., diabetes, vein occlusions). Demonstrated by fluorescein angiography.

Druault's bundle (DRU-ahltz). *Anatomy.* Group of vitreous fibrils that appear during embryologic development, and disappear when lens zonules form.

drug abuse retinopathy (ret-in-AHP-uh-thee). *Pathologic condition.* Retinal pathology caused by long-term intravenous drug abuse.

drusen (DRU-zin). *Anatomic defect.* Tiny, white hyaline deposits on Bruch's membrane (of the retinal pigment epithelium). Common after age 60; sometimes an early sign of macular degeneration.

drusen (disc), hyaline masses. *Pathologic condition.* Glistening nodules within the optic nerve head. May blur the disc margins. Sometimes mistaken for chronic papilledema.

dry eye syndrome, keratitis sicca, keratoconjunctivitis sicca. *Pathologic condition.* Corneal and conjunctival dryness due to deficient tear production, predominantly in menopausal and post-menopausal women. Can cause foreign body sensation, burning eyes, filamentary keratitis, and erosion of conjunctival and corneal epithelium. See also SJÖGREN'S SYNDROME.

D-seg, flat top. *Optical device.* Bifocal segment having a short horizontal upper line separating it from the main portion of the lens. Looks like a tipped over D. See also ROUND TOP.

D-SEG

D trisomy syndrome (TRI-soh-mee), **Patau's syndrome, trisomy 13 syndrome**. *Congenital anomaly.* Multiple defects in the brain, face and eyes caused by an extra chromosome.

Duane's accommodation chart. *Measurement.* Standard table showing relationship between age and decrease in focusing ability (accommodation). Varies slightly from Donders' chart.

Duane's syndrome, Duane's co-contraction *(or)* retraction syndrome, Stilling-Turk-Duane retraction syndrome. *Congenital defect.* Eye muscle abnormality characterized by inability to move one eye outward past the midline (abduction) and retraction of that eye into the orbit, with narrowing of the eyelid fissure on attempted movement of that eye toward the nose (adduction). Often accompanied by an inward eye deviation (esotropia).

duction (DUK-shun). *Function.* Movement of one eye; refers to movement ability measured independently from that of the other eye.

duochrome test (DU-oh-krohm). Method of refining a refraction by comparing the relative clarity of equal-size objects seen on red, then a green background. See also BALANCING, CYCLODAMIA.

Duolube. *Drug.* Trade name of polyvinyl alcohol eye ointment; for treating dry eyes.

Duratears. *Drug.* Trade name of polyvinyl alcohol eye ointment. For treating dry eyes.

dye dilution test, dye disappearance test. For detecting a blockage in the tear drainage (lacrimal) system. Involves instilling a few drops of fluorescein onto lower conjunctiva of both eyes and watching how long it remains.

dysarthria (dis-ARTH-ree-uh). *Clinical sign.* Inability to speak distinctly due to central nervous system disease.

dyscalculia. *Pathologic condition.* Impaired ability to do mathematical problems due to brain injury or lesion.

dyschromatopsia (dis-kroh-muh-TAHP-see-uh). *Functional defect.* Defective color vision (any type or degree).

dysconjugate. Incorrect spelling of DISCONJUGATE.

dyscoria (dis-KOR-ee-uh). *Anatomic defect.* Distorted shape of pupil.

dyscrasia (dis-KRAY-zhuh). *Pathologic condition.* Abnormal state of a part of the body, especially blood components.

dyslexia (dis-LEK-see-uh). *Functional defect.* Reading disability associated with problems in interpreting written symbols. Not related to visual acuity or intelligence, which are usually normal.

dysmetria (dis-MEE-tree-uh), **ocular dysmetria**. *Pathologic condition, clinical sign.* Uncoordinated eye movements, with "overshooting" of the eyes upon effort to view an object; small side-to-side eye movements occur until a stable end-point is reached. Sign of cerebellar system disease.

dysplasia (dis-PLAY-zhuh). *Pathologic condition.* Abnormal development or growth of cells, tissues or organs.

dysplastic coloboma (dis-PLAS-tik kohl-uh-BOH-muh). *Congenital anomaly.* Large, abnormal optic nerve head.

dysthyroidism (dis-THI-royd-iz-um). *Pathologic condition.* Disorder of the thyroid gland. Frequently associated with protruding eyes, eyelid retraction, and "stuck-down" and poorly moving extraocular muscles (especially the inferior recti). See also GRAVES' DISEASE.

dystichiasis. Incorrect spelling of DISTICHIASIS.

dystrophy (DIS-troh-fee). *Pathologic condition.* Progressive changes in a tissue or organ that may result from defective metabolism; usually genetically induced.

dystopia (foveal) (dis-TOH-pee-uh), **dragged** *(or)* **ectopic macula**. *Pathologic condition.* Displacement of the macular area of the retina by traction. Seen with retinopathy of prematurity, following retinal detachment surgery, intraocular worm, previous inflammation, and other forms of retinal scarring.

E

Eales' disease (eelz), **angiopathia retinae juvenilis, periphlebitis retinae, primary perivasculitis of the retina.** *Pathologic condition.* Characterized by inflammation and possible blockage of retinal blood vessels, abnormal growth of new blood vessels (neovascularization), and recurrent retinal and vitreal hemorrhages. Found in young men. Unknown cause.

Earl's fetal bovine serum. *Lab medium.* Used for growing viruses in the laboratory.

E carpine (KAHR-peen). *Drug.* Trade name of eyedrop containing epinephrine and pilocarpine; for treating glaucoma.

eccentric. *Description.* Off-center.

eccentric fixation. *Functional defect.* Visual abnormality in which a retinal area other than the fovea centralis is used for visual fixation. May occur as an adaptive mechanism with amblyopia or when the fovea has been destroyed.

ecchymosis (ek-ee-MOH-sus). *Pathologic condition.* Bleeding into the tissues, resulting in discoloration under the skin. A bruise.

echography (ek-AHG-ruh-fee), **ultrasonography, ultrasound**. *Test.* Transmission of high frequency sound waves into an eye, which are reflected by ocular tissues and displayed on a screen so that internal structures can be visualized. Aids in diagnosis of eye and orbital problems. See also A-SCAN, B-SCAN.

echothiophate iodide (ek-oh-THI-oh-fayt). *Drug.* Anticholinesterase eyedrop that stimulates parasympathetic nerve fibers, producing small pupils (miosis), ciliary muscle contractions (accommodation), and increased aqueous outflow. Used in treating open angle glaucoma and accommodative esotropia. Trade name: Phospholine Iodide.

eclipse blindness, solar maculopathy. *Pathologic condition.* Macular damage from staring at the sun without proper protective filters, usually during a solar eclipse. A dazzling light sensation soon changes to a central blind spot (scotoma), usually with some permanent reduction in central vision caused by intense radiant energy absorbed in the retina and pigment epithelium.

eclipse scotoma. *Pathologic condition.* Blind area in the central visual field caused by watching a solar eclipse. See also ECLIPSE BLINDNESS.

Econochlor (ee-KAHN-oh-klor). *Drug.* Trade name of chloramphenicol, a broad spectrum antibiotic.

Econopred (ee-KAHN-oh-pred). *Drug.* Trade name of prednisone acetate eyedrops, an anti-inflammatory steroid.

ectasia (ek-TAY-zhuh). *Pathologic condition.* Distention or expansion of a hollow organ or tube. In the eye, refers to a thin, stretched sclera or cornea, as can occur after congenital glaucoma or inflammation of the outer wall of an eye. If uveal tissue (iris, ciliary body, choroid) is included in the stretched area, the condition is called a staphyloma.

> **corneal**: abnormal bulging forward of thinned cornea, such as with keratoconus. Also called keratectasia.

ectopia, heterotopia (ek-TOH-pee-uh). *Pathologic condition.* Misplacement of parts. Commonly refers to dragged macula in ROP or other conditions that create retinal scars.

ectopia lentis. *Pathologic condition.* Partial displacement of the crystalline lens, caused by broken or absent zonules. May be hereditary. See also HOMOCYS-TINURIA, LUXATION, MARCHESANI'S SYNDROME, MARFAN'S SYNDROME, SUBLUXATION.

ectopic macula (ek-TAH-pik MAK-yu-luh), **dragged macula, foveal dystopia**. *Pathologic condition*. Displacement of the macular region of the retina by traction. Seen with retinopathy of prematurity, intraocular worm, previous inflammation and other forms of retinal scarring, and following retinal detachment surgery.

ectopic pupil, peaked *(or)* **up-drawn pupil**. *Abnormal condition*. Displacement of the pupil from its normal position. May result from a congenital defect, ocular surgery, or trauma.

ectropion (ek-TROH-pee-un). *Pathologic condition*. Outward turning of the upper or lower eyelid so that the lid margin does not rest against the eyeball, but falls or is pulled away. Can create corneal exposure with excessive drying, tearing, and irritation. Usually from aging. See also ENTROPION.

> **cicatricial** (sik-uh-TRISH-ul): caused by a scar (from previous surgery, eyelid trauma, burns, infection or inflammation).
>
> **involutional**: caused by horizontal weakening and stretching of the tarsal and conjunctival portions of an eyelid, usually in the elderly. Characterized by a loose lower eyelid, chronic eye irritation and excess tearing.
>
> **medial**: same as PUNCTAL (below).
>
> **punctal**: involves only the part of the lower lid closest to the nose.
>
> **senile**. Same as INVOLUTIONAL (above).

edema (eh-DEE-muh). *Clinical sign*. Swelling of tissue from excess fluid accumulation.

edetate disodium (ED-eh-tayt di-SOH-dee-um). *Chemical*. Preservative used in many contact lens wetting and cleaning solutions.

Edinger-Westphal (E-W) nucleus (EH-din-jur WEST-fahl). *Anatomy*. Portion of the 3rd (oculomotor) cranial nerve nucleus in the midbrain. Involved with parasympathetic nerve fibers for pupil constriction and accommodation.

EDMA (ethylene glyco-dy-methacrylate). *Chemical*. Plastic polymer used in making soft contact lenses. See also HYDROXYETHYL METHACRYLATE.

edrophonium chloride (eh-druh-FOH-nee-um). *Drug*. Short-acting anticholinesterase that aids nerve impulse transmission by stimulating parasympathetic nerve fibers. Used in testing for myasthenia gravis. Trade name: Tensilon.

EDTA (ethylene-diamine-tetra-acetic acid), disodium EDTA. 1. *Chemical*. Chelating (binding) agent used for removing abnormal calcium deposits from the corneal surface (e.g., for band keratopathy) and may help protect the cornea from ulceration after a chemical burn. 2. *Drug enhancer*. Enhances antibacterial activity of preservatives commonly used in topical eyedrops and increases drug penetration across the cornea. See also BENZALKONIUM CHLORIDE.

Edward's syndrome, E trisomy, 18 trisomy. *Congenital anomaly*. Chromosomal abnormality characterized by an inactive, poorly developed infant with multiple defects. Eye signs include small openings between eyelids, thick lower lids, epicanthus, incomplete choroid formation, small eyes (microphthalmia), congenital glaucoma, and corneal opacities. Fatal.

effective power, vertex *(or)* **back vertex power**. *Measurement*. Power of a spectacle or contact lens as measured at the back surface (with a lensometer).

efferent nerve (EF-ur-unt or EE-fur-unt), **motor nerve, output nerve**. *Anatomy*. Nerve that carries impulses away from central nervous system toward the surface of the body; e.g., the 3rd (oculomotor) cranial nerve. See also AFFERENT NERVE.

effusion (eh-FYU-zhun). *Clinical sign*. Escape of fluid into a body cavity or tissue. If excessive, can be drained by aspiration (sucking out through a needle).

efmoyd. Incorrect spelling of ETHMOID.

Egger's line, hyaloideo-capsular ligament, Weiger's ligament. *Anatomy.* A weak line of adherence between the anterior vitreous and the posterior surface of the lens, in the form of a ring 8–9 mm in diameter.

Ehlers-Danlos syndrome (AY-lurz). *Pathologic condition.* Congenital connective tissue disorder. Characterized by excessively flexible joints, stretchable skin ("India rubber man"), blood vessel disease, and defects of the heart, genitals, and respiratory and gastrointestinal tracts. Eye signs include epicanthus (skin folds near the nose), eyelids easily turned inside out, inward eye deviation (esotropia), blue scleras, glaucoma, dislocated lenses, and retinal hemorrhages.

eightball hyphema (hi-FEE-muh). *Pathologic condition.* Dark hemorrhage that fills the anterior chamber with blood. Usually follows trauma.

18 trisomy. See EDWARD'S SYNDROME.

eikonometer (i-kun-AHM-ih-tur). *Instrument.* Measures image size so that the difference between the two eyes can be compared. See also ANISEIKONIA.

electrocardiogram (ECG, EKG). *Test.* Graphic record of electrical waves produced from the contraction and electrical conduction of the heart.

electroencephalogram (EEG). *Test.* Graphic record of changes in electric signals produced by (cortical) activity in the brain. Detected by electric contact devices (electrodes) placed on the scalp.

electromagnetic spectrum. Range of radiant energy that has constant velocity but variable frequencies. Includes light, x-rays, radar and radio waves.

electro-oculogram (EOG). *Test.* Electrophysiologic test for function of the retinal pigment epithelium. Measures ratio of change in the corneo-retinal resting potential under conditions of light and dark adaptation.

electroperimetry (eh-LEK-troh-puh-RIM-uh-tree). *Test.* Computerized visual field testing; electrodes attached to the scalp record electrical impulses produced in response to visual stimuli.

electrophysiology. *Test.* Group of tests for evaluating various visual functions based on electrical phenomena associated with a physiological process, e.g., vision, brain activity, heart conduction. Examples: electro-oculogram, electroretinogram, visual evoked cortical potential, visual evoked response.

electroretinogram (ERG) (eh-LEK-troh-RET-in-oh-gram). *Test.* Electrophysiological measure of retinal function after light stimulation of retina. Consists of several wave forms, e.g., a-waves, which show rod and cone activity, and b-waves, which stem from Mueller and bipolar cells.

elevation. *Function.* Upward movement of one or both eyes. See also SUPRA-DUCTION, SURSUMVERSION.

elevators. *Anatomy.* Extraocular muscles (superior rectus, inferior oblique) that move the eye upward.

ELISA (enzyme-linked immunosorbent assay) (el-LI-zuh). *Test.* Blood test for determining presence of specific antibodies, e.g., for *Toxocara canis,* a worm that may migrate to the retina.

Elliot trephination. *Surgical procedure.* Removal of a full-thickness corneal button at the limbus under a conjunctival flap, using a trephine (instrument for cutting a small hole). Superceded by safer filtering procedures.

Elschnig pearls (EL-shnig). *Anatomic defect.* Cystic growth of lens epithelial remnants following an extracapsular cataract extraction. Cysts resemble single or clumped soap bubbles.

embolus (EM-boh-lus). *Pathologic condition.* Fragment of tissue (e.g., blood clot, tumor cell, air bubble, debris) that is free-floating in the bloodstream. Can obstruct a blood vessel and prevent normal blood flow. Especially dangerous in the brain or eye. Plural: emboli. See also THROMBUS.

embryotoxon (em-bree-oh-TAHK-sin). *Congenital defect.* Opacity of the innermost surface of the cornea at the periphery, resulting in an abnormally prominent Schwalbe's line.

emergent ray. *Optics*. Ray of light as it leaves a medium.

emesis (EM-uh-sus). *Clinical sign*. Vomiting.

emmetropia (em-uh-TROH-pee-uh). *Optics*. Refractive state of having no refractive error when accommodation is at rest. Images of distant objects are focused sharply on the retina without the need for either accommodation or corrective lenses.

emphysema (orbital). *Pathologic condition*. Presence of air in the orbit. Generally follows traumatic rupture of a nasal sinus, particularly the lamina papyracea of the ethmoid bone.

encephalofacial angiomatosis (en-SEF-uh-loh-FAY-shul an-jee-oh-muh-TOH-sis), **Sturge-Weber syndrome**. *Congenital anomaly*. Characterized by reddish pigmentation (port wine stain) usually on one side of the face, prominent in the area supplied by the 5th (trigeminal) cranial nerve. Associated with high intraocular pressure, large eye, and hemangiomas in the skin, choroid, and brain; if in the brain may result in seizures and mental retardation. Hereditary.

endocarditis (en-doh-kar-DI-tis). *Pathologic condition*. Inflammation or infection of the inside lining of the heart and its valves.

endocrine exophthalmos, endrocrine *(or)* Graves' ophthalmopathy, Basedow's disease, Graves' *(or)* thyroid eye disease, thyrotoxic *(or)* thyrotropic exophthalmos. *Pathologic condition*. Eye signs that may occur in patients with excessive thyroid-related hormone concentration. Includes eyelid retraction, lid lag on downward gaze, corneal drying, eye bulging (proptosis), fibrotic extraocular muscles, and optic nerve inflammation. See also DALRYMPLE'S SIGN, HYPERTHYROIDISM, STELLWAG'S SIGN, VON GRAEFE SIGN.

endocrine ophthalmopathy. See ENDOCRINE EXOPHTHALMOS.

endogenous (en-DAH-jun-us). Developing or originating from within the body. See also EXOGENOUS.

endoilluminator, fiberoptic light pipe. *Instrument*. Light source comprised of a flexible bundle of closely packed transparent fibers that conduct light; used for illuminating inside of eye during surgical procedures.

endolymph. *Anatomy*. Fluid present in the labyrinth of the inner ear.

endophthalmitis (en-dahf-thal-MI-tus). *Pathologic condition*. Inflammation of tissues inside the eyeball. Usually refers to purulent intraocular infection.

endophthalmos. See ENOPHTHALMOS.

entophytic. *Description*. Originating in the inner layers of the retina and growing into the vitreous. See also EXOPHYTIC.

endothelial (en-doh-THEE-lee-ul). *Description*. Relating to or produced from the endothelium.

endothelial camera, specular microscope. *Instrument*. Used for examining and photographing the size and regularity of the endothelial cells that line the undersurface of the cornea. Particularly useful in determining risk to the cornea from cataract extraction.

endothelial cell density (ECD). *Measurement*. Number of cells per square millimeter of corneal endothelium. Used for assessing the general health of the corneal endothelium and its potential for being damaged during eye surgery, such as keratoplasty.

endothelial dystrophy (DIS-truh-fee), **Fuchs' dystrophy**. *Pathologic condition*. Progressive corneal disorder characterized by hyaline endothelial outgrowths on Descemet's membrane, a cloudy waterlogged cornea, painful epithelial blisters and reduced vision. May require a corneal graft. Sometimes hereditary. See also BULLOUS KERATOPATHY, GUTTATA.

endothelium (en-doh-THEE-lee-um). *Anatomy*. Single-cell layer of tissue lining the innermost surfaces of many organs, glands, and blood vessels; also lines undersurface of the cornea, where it regulates corneal water content (hydration). Plural: endothelia.

corneal: innermost layer of the cornea between Descemet's membrane and the anterior chamber. Acts as a pump to keep excess water out of the corneal stroma. See also FUCHS' DYSTROPHY.

endpoint nystagmus (ni-STAG-mus). See NYSTAGMUS.

enophthalmos (en-ahf-THAL-mus), **endophthalmos**. *Anatomic defect.* Sinking of the eyeball into the orbit.

entoptic phenomenon (en-TAHP-tik). Visual sensation arising from unusual stimulation of the retina, such as by physical pressure on the side of the eyeball or by viewing a bright light (which produces an after-image and allows visualization of one's own retinal blood vessels). See also HAIDINGER BRUSH, PHOSPHENE, PHOTOPSIA.

entropion (en-TROH-pee-un). *Anatomic defect.* Inward turning of upper or lower eyelid so that the lid margin rests against and rubs the eyeball. See also ECTROPION.

cicatricial (sik-uh-TRISH-ul): caused by a scar. May result from previous surgery, eyelid trauma, burns, infection or inflammation.

involutional: same as SENILE (below).

senile: caused by anatomic changes associated with aging. Characterized by inturned lashes, foreign body sensation, and lower lid retraction on looking down.

spastic: *acute*: follows acute lid infections or long-term patching of the eye; *chronic*: caused by loss of elasticity of lid structures with overactivity of the marginal muscle of Riolan.

enucleation (ee-nu-klee-AY-shun). *Surgical procedure.* Removal of the eyeball, leaving eye muscles and remaining orbital contents intact. See also EVISCERATION, EXENTERATION.

enzymatic cleaner (en-zih-MAT-ik). *Chemical.* Tablets (dissolved in water) that remove protein and deposits from the surface of soft contact lenses. Used in addition to cleaning and sterilization.

enzyme. Chemical facilitator produced by the body that changes the speed of some specific chemical reaction in the body.

enzyme-linked immunosorbent assay. See ELISA.

eosinophil (ee-oh-SIN-uh-fil). *Anatomy.* Type of white blood cell. Found in abnormally high numbers in tissues affected by allergy, parasitic infection or toxin.

epiblepharon (ep-ee-BLEF-ur-ahn). *Congenital defect.* Abnormal skin fold across the upper or lower eyelid.

epibulbar dermoid, dermoid, dermoid cyst. *Congenital anomaly.* Tumor containing skin elements such as epithelium, fat or hair; usually found at the corneo-scleral junction (limbus) or lateral side of upper eyelid. See also GOLDENHAR'S SYNDROME.

epicanthal fold (ep-ee-KAN-thul), **epicanthus**. *Anatomy.* Vertical skin fold on either side of nose, hiding the caruncle. Present in all infants before bridge of nose is formed, and in most Oriental adults. May make normal eyes appear crossed.

epicanthus (ep-ee-KAN-thus). See EPICANTHAL FOLD.

epicanthus inversus (in-VUR-sus). *Congenital anomaly.* Vertical skin fold arising from the lower eyelid and inserting laterally into the upper lid.

epicapsular lens stars (ep-ee-KAP-suh-lur). *Congenital defect.* Small deposits of brown pigment on the front surface of the crystalline lens. Vision is rarely diminished.

epidemic keratoconjunctivitis (EKC) (KEHR-uh-toh-kun-junk-tih-VI-tis). *Path-*

ologic condition. Contagious infection of cornea and conjunctiva, caused by an adenovirus.

Epifrin (EP-ih-frin). *Drug.* Trade name of epinephrine eyedrops, for treating glaucoma.

epikeratophakia (EKF) (eh-pee-kehr-ih-toh-FAY-kee-uh). *Surgical procedure.* Onlay of a preserved lathe-cut corneal button onto the corneal surface. Used for correcting refractive errors.

epikeratoplasty (eh-pee-KEHR-ih-toh-plas-tee). *Surgical procedure.* Modified version of epikeratophakia.

epilation (eh-pih-LAY-shun). *Surgical procedure.* Removal of hair or lashes, sometimes by electrolysis. See also DISTICHIASIS, TRICHIASIS.

E-Pilo (ee-PI-loh). *Drug.* Trade name of eyedrops containing pilocarpine and epinephrine, for treating glaucoma.

epimacular proliferation (EMP), epiretinal membrane *(or)* proliferation, cellophane maculopathy *(or)* retinopathy, macular pucker. *Pathologic condition.* Retinal wrinkling in the macular area caused by contraction of the transparent membrane lying on retinal surface. Distorts vision.

Epinal (EP-ih-nahl). *Drug.* Trade name of epinephrine eyedrops, for treating glaucoma.

epinephrine (ep-ih-NEF-rin). 1. *Chemical.* Found normally in the body; stimulates the sympathetic nerves. 2. *Drug.* Eyedrop used for treating glaucoma. Causes mild pupillary enlargement (mydriasis), blood vessel constriction, and increased aqueous outflow. Side effects include stinging, allergic reactions, poor corneal penetration, black conjunctival pigmentation, and swelling of the central retina (macular edema) in aphakes. Trade names: Epinal, E-Pilo, Epifrin, Eppy, Glaucon. See also CATECHOLAMINES.

epiphora (ee-PIF-ur-uh). *Functional defect.* Overflow of tears down the cheek; caused by a defect in the tear drainage system or by an excessive amount of tears.

epiretinal membrane (ERM) (eh-pee-RET-ih-nul). See EPIMACULAR PROLIFERATION.

episclera (ep-ee-SKLEH-ruh). *Anatomy.* Outermost layer of sclera, composed of loose, fibrous, elastic tissue; attaches to Tenon's capsule.

episcleral explant, episcleral exoplant. *Surgical device.* Silicone or silicone sponge sewn onto the sclera to indent it (creating a scleral buckle) for repair of a retinal detachment.

episcleritis (ep-ee-skler-RI-tus). *Pathologic condition.* Inflammation of the episclera, outermost layer of the sclera. Affected eye is painful and light sensitive (photophobic). In chronic disease, purple nodules may develop surrounded by localized swelling and redness.

epistaxis (eh-pihs-TAK-sus). Nosebleed.

epithelial (ep-ih-THEE-lee-ul). Pertaining to the epithelium.

epithelial downgrowth. *Pathologic condition.* Abnormal growth of epithelium into the eye, covering internal structures. Associated with a penetrating corneal injury and poor healing of a corneal wound. Rare complication of cataract extraction.

epithelium (ep-ih-THEE-lee-um). *Anatomy.* Membranous multicellular layer covering the internal and external surfaces of the body and its organs. In the eye, covers the cornea, conjunctiva and eyelid. Plural: epithelia.

    corneal e: outermost layer of the cornea, between Bowman's membrane and the tear film.

Eppy. *Drug.* Trade name of epinephrine eyedrops, for treating glaucoma.

equator, equatorial meridian, geometric equator. Imaginary ring around the eye at the intersection of a plane dividing the eyeball into front and back halves.

equatorial degeneration, lattice retinal degeneration. *Degenerative change.*

Retinal thinning with dense vitreous traction in a degenerative zone near the retinal equator. May lead to retinal tears and detachment. Common.

equatorial meridian. See EQUATOR.

erosion (recurrent corneal). *Pathologic condition.* Episodic, periodic loss of outer layer of cornea (epithelium) due to its failure to adhere properly to Bowman's membrane. May follow minor scratch-type injury.

ervine gas syndrome. Incorrect spelling of IRVINE-GASS SYNDROME.

erysiphake (ih-RIS-ih-fayk). *Surgical instrument.* Uses mild suction to grasp the lens during cataract extraction. Obsolete.

erythema (eh-rih-THEE-muh). *Clinical sign.* Abnormal skin redness produced by congestion of capillaries under the skin. Occurs in patches of variable size and shape.

erythema multiforme (mul-tee-FOR-muh). *Pathologic condition.* Allergic response characterized by rash, scarring of mucous membranes of nose and mouth, and connective tissue inflammation. Eye involvement, called Stevens-Johnson syndrome, consists of severe conjunctival inflammation that may cause adhesion of eyelids and conjunctiva to the globe (symblepharon), eyelid scarring, and dry eyes due to closing of tear ducts. May be caused by hypersensitivity to drugs, infections, or food. Usually occurs in children and young adults.

erythroclast (uh-RITH-roh-klast, **ghost cell**. *Anatomic abnormality.* Abnormal red blood cell that can clog the trabecular meshwork and elevate intraocular pressure.

erythroclastic glaucoma (uh-rith-roh-KLAS-tic glaw-KOH-muh), **ghost cell glaucoma**. *Pathologic condition.* Secondary glaucoma caused by erythroclasts (abnormal red blood cells) clogging the trabecular meshwork.

erythrocyte. *Anatomy.* Red blood cell.

erythrocyte sedimentation rate (ESR), sed *(or)* sedimentation rate. *Lab test.* The rate (in mm per hour) at which red blood cells settle to the bottom of a tube of unclotted blood. Non-specific test used for measuring the progress of various systemic inflammatory diseases.

erythrolabe (eh-RITH-roh-layb). *Anatomy.* Red-sensitive pigment in cones. See also CHLOROLABE, CYANOLABE, PROTANOMALY, RHODOPSIN.

erythromycin (eh-rith-roh-MI-sin). *Drug.* Broad spectrum antibiotic used for treating various ocular infections. Trade names: AK-Mycin, Ilotysin.

erythropsia (eh-rith-RAHP-see-uh). *Symptom.* Vision abnormality in which all objects appear to be tinted red. See also CYANOPSIA, XANTHOPSIA.

eserine (EZ-ur-in), **physostigmine**. *Drug.* Early ophthalmic drug for treating glaucoma; indirectly stimulates parasympathetic nerves. Prolonged use causes conjunctival irritation. Rarely used today. See also MIOCEL.

eso deviation (EE-soh). *Functional defect.* Inward deviation of one eye. Refers to esotropia or esophoria.

esophoria (E) (ee-soh-FOR-ee-uh). *Functional defect.* Tendency toward inward (toward nose) deviation of one eye when a cover is placed over that eye. When cover is removed, eye straightens. See also ESOTROPIA.

esotropia (ET) (ee-soh-TROH-pee-uh), **convergent deviation, cross-eyes, internal strabismus**. *Functional defect.* Eye misalignment in which one eye deviates inward (toward nose) while the other fixates normally. Present even when both eyes are uncovered. See also ESOPHORIA.

LEFT ESOTROPIA

    accommodative: caused by overactive convergence response to the accommodative effort necessary to keep vision clear; especially likely in farsighted (hyperopic) children. Eyeglass correction for the hyperopia relaxes accommodation, allowing eyes to align. Sometimes bifocals can correct the excessive inturning at near.

   acquired: appears after age 6 months. Often helped by eyeglasses.

   alternating: continuous switching between an inturning right eye with straight left eye, and an inturning left eye with straight right eye.

   A-pattern: deviation is greater in up-gaze than in down-gaze.

   consecutive: follows surgical correction of exotropia (outward deviation).

   infantile: found at birth or within first 6 months; usually a large deviation that requires surgery (unaffected by eyeglasses).

   intermittent [E(T)]: occasional deviation; sometimes the eyes look straight ahead and work together normally, other times one eye deviates inward while the other fixates normally.

   non-accommodative: excessive turning is not influenced by correcting the hyperopia (farsightedness).

   sensory: follows loss of vision in the affected eye.

   V-pattern: deviation is greater in down-gaze than up-gaze.

essential blepharospasm (BLEF-uh-roh-spaz-um), **benign essential blepharospasm.** Sudden, involuntary spasm of the orbicularis oculi muscle, producing uncontrolled blinking and lid squeezing. Involves both eyes and in advanced cases, muscles of the mouth or neck. Involuntary lid closure may result in temporary inability to see. See also BLEPHAROCLONUS, HEMIFACIAL SPASM, MEIGE SYNDROME.

essential iris atrophy (AT-roh-fee), **Chandler's syndrome.** *Pathologic condition.* Progressive loss of iris stroma with hole formation and pupil distortion, accompanied by severe glaucoma. Rare; most common in females, age 20–40. See also ICE SYNDROME.

Ethamide (ETH-uh-mide). *Drug.* Trade name of ethoxzolamide tablets, for treating glaucoma.

ethmoid bone. *Anatomy.* Thin bone forming part of the medial orbital wall. One of seven bones lining the orbit (eye socket).

ethmoid sinus. *Anatomy.* Mucus-lined air cavity within the ethmoid bones; one of the nasal sinuses that drains into the nose. Others are frontal, maxillary, and sphenoid.

ethoxzolamide (eth-ahks-OH-luh-mide). *Drug.* Carbonic anhydrase inhibitor that lowers intraocular pressure by decreasing aqueous secretion. Used as oral medication for treating glaucoma. Trade names: Cardrase, Ethamide.

ethylene-diamine-tetra-acetic acid. See EDTA.

ethylene glyco-di-methacrylate. See EDMA.

etiology. Cause(s) of a disease or abnormal condition.

E trisomy (TRI-suh-mee), **Edward's syndrome, 18 trisomy.** *Congenital anomaly.* Chromosomal abnormality characterized by an inactive, poorly developed infant with multiple defects. Eye signs include small openings between eyelids, thick lower lids, epicanthus, incomplete choroid formation, small eyes (microphthalmia), congenital glaucoma, and corneal opacities. Fatal.

eucatropine (yu-KAT-roh-peen). *Drug.* Eyedrop that blocks parasympathetic nerves, producing enlarged pupils with only mild decrease in focusing ability (accommodation). Used in testing for angle closure glaucoma. Milder action than atropine.

euthyscope (YU-thih-skohp). *Instrument.* Modified ophthalmoscope used in treating eccentric fixation; helps re-educate the fovea to resume normal fixation by dazzling the area surrounding it with a bright light.

eversion (of the eyelid). 1. *Technique.* Turning the lid over to allow examination of the undersurface. 2. *Pathologic condition.* Lid held in a turned-over position, as by a scar.

evisceration (eh-vis-ur-AY-shun). *Surgical procedure.* Removal of contents of an eyeball, leaving the scleral shell and sometimes the cornea intact. Usually for reducing pain in a blind eye. See also ENUCLEATION, EXENTERATION.

exacerbation. Flare-up or worsening of a previously existing disease or condition. See also REMISSION.

excimer laser (EKS-ih-mur). *Surgical instrument.* Class of ultraviolet lasers (argon-fluoride type), wavelength 193 nm, which is almost universally used for photorefractive keratectomy (PRK). Excimer refers to the molecular reaction (photodisruption) that removes tissue accurately without heating it or the surrounding tissue, resulting in a smooth surface that heals rapidly with minimal scarring. Combined with other technologies, e.g., with automated lamellar keratoplasty (ALK) to produce LASIK (laser in situ keratomileusis). See also KERATOREFRACTIVE SURGERY, PARTIAL EXCIMER TRABECULECTOMY, PHOTOREFRACTIVE KERATECTOMY, PHOTOABLATION.

excimer trabeculectomy (partial). *Surgical procedure.* Unroofing Schlemm's canal with an excimer laser, then creating a conjunctival flap to cover the opening, forming a filtering bleb. Decreases outflow resistance for glaucoma control.

excise. *Surgical technique.* To remove tissue. See also INCISE.

excision. *Surgical procedure.* Cutting out; removal or resection. See also INCISION.

excoriation. Abrasion or wearing off of skin, as from severe scratching.

excycloduction (ek-si-kloh-DUK-shun), **extorsion.** *Function.* Outward rotation of the eye; the 12 o'clock meridian rolls away from the nose.

excyclovergence. *Function.* Outward rotation of both eyes (from the 12 o'clock meridian) while maintaining single binocular vision.

executive bifocals. *Optical device.* Eyeglass lenses made from one piece of glass with the reading segment across the entire lower part.

executive trifocals. *Optical device.* Eyeglass lenses made from one piece of glass with the reading and intermediate-distance segments across the entire lower part.

exenteration (orbital) (eks-en-tur-AY-shun). *Surgical procedure.* Removal of entire the orbital contents, including eyeball, extraocular muscles, fat and connective tissues. Usually for a malignant orbital tumor. See also ENUCLEATION, EVISCERATION.

exfoliation (true). *Pathologic condition.* Shedding of superficial layers of the lens capsule. Usually accompanies exposure to extreme heat, e.g., molten glass. See also PSEUDOEXFOLIATION.

eximer laser. Incorrect spelling of EXCIMER LASER.

exo deviation. *Functional defect.* Outward deviation of one eye. Refers to exotropia or exophoria.

exogenous (eks-AH-ghuh-nus). Developing or originating from a source outside the body. See also ENDOGENOUS.

exophoria (eks-uh-FOR-ee-uh). *Functional defect.* Tendency toward outward (away from nose) deviation of one eye when cover is placed over that eye. Eye straightens to align with uninvolved eye when cover is removed. See also EXOTROPIA.

exophthalmometer (eks-ahf-thal-MAH-mih-tur). *Instrument.* Measures how far an eye protrudes from its orbit.

exophthalmos (eks-ahf-THAL-mus), **proptosis.** *Anatomic defect.* Abnormal protrusion or bulging forward of the eyeball.

> **endocrine**: associated with abnormalities of the thyroid gland.
> **ophthalmoplegic** (ahf-thal-moh-PLEE-jik): inability to rotate the eye because it protrudes.
> **pulsating**: associated with a carotid-cavernous fistula.

exophytic. *Description.* Originating in the outer layers of the retina and growing outward toward the choroid. See also ENDOPHYTIC.

exotropia (XT) (eks-oh-TROH-pee-uh), **divergent (or) external strabismus, wall-eyes**. *Functional defect*. Eye misalignment in which one eye deviates outward (away from nose) while the other fixates normally. See also CONVERGENCE INSUFFICIENCY, DIVERGENCE EXCESS, EXOPHORIA.

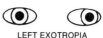

LEFT EXOTROPIA

> **A-pattern**: deviation is greater in down-gaze than in up-gaze.
> **basic**: measures the same at near (16 in.) as at distance (20 ft.).
> **consecutive**: follows surgical correction of inward deviation (esotropia).
> **intermittent [X(T)]**: sometimes eyes look straight ahead and work together; other times one eye deviates out while the other fixates normally.
> **secondary**: gradually develops in an esotropic (inturning) eye.
> **sensory**: follows loss of vision in the affected eye.
> **V-pattern**: deviation is greater in up-gaze than in down-gaze.

explant, episcleral explant (or) exoplant. *Surgical device*. Silicone or silicone rubber sponge attached onto the scleral surface to indent it (creating a scleral buckle), for retinal detachment repair.

> **circumferential**: encircles the eyeball.
> **radial**: attached in a front-to-back direction.

exposure keratitis (kehr-uh-TI-tus), **keratitis lagophthalmos**. *Pathologic condition*. Corneal irritation or inflammation caused by corneal drying, from incomplete eyelid closure.

expulsive hemorrhage, choroidal hemorrhage. *Pathologic condition*. Bleeding from ruptured choroidal blood vesssels after a sudden decrease in intraocular pressure. A rare, serious complication of intraocular surgery that can result in the pushing out (extrusion) of intraocular contents through the surgical wound, with subsequent loss of vision.

extended wear lens. *Optical device*. Soft hydrophilic contact lens designed to be worn for longer periods than daily-wear lenses before being removed for cleaning and sterilization.

external disease. *Pathologic condition*. Disease that affects the cornea, sclera, conjunctiva or eyelids.

external geniculate body (gen-IK-yu-lit), **lateral geniculate body**. *Anatomy*. Paired prominences at the sides of the midbrain (upper end of brainstem); neural way-station where optic tract fibers connect (synapse) to optic radiations and transmit visual information.

external hordeolum (hor-DEE-oh-lum), **stye**. *Pathologic condition*. Pustular infection of the oil glands of Zeis, located in the eyelash follicles at the eyelid margins. See also INTERNAL HORDEOLUM.

external levator resection (anterior approach) (luh-VAY-tur). *Surgical procedure*. Shortening of the levator muscle and reconstruction of the lid fold, to correct a moderate-to-severe drooping upper eyelid (ptosis). See also INTERNAL LEVATOR RESECTION.

external limiting membrane, outer limiting membrane. *Anatomy*. Layer of retina between the visual cells (rods and cones) and their nuclei.

external ophthalmoplegia (ahf-thal-moh-PLEE-juh). *Pathologic condition*. Acquired paralysis of the extraocular muscles, causing restriction of movement, and the levator muscle, causing a droopy eyelid (ptosis). May affect one or both eyes. See also CHRONIC PROGRESSIVE EXTERNAL OPHTHALMOPLEGIA.

external pterygoid-levator synkinesis (TEHR-ih-goyd, leh-VAY-tur, sin-kin-EE-sis), **Gunn (or) jaw winking (or) Marcus Gunn jaw winking syndrome**. *Congenital defect*. Droopy eyelid (ptosis) that opens widely when the patient chews, sucks or moves mouth to the opposite side. Caused by abnormal innervation of the levator muscle by the 5th (trigeminal) cranial nerve.

external strabismus. See EXOTROPIA.

extinction. *Functional defect*. Visual phenomenon in which a stimulus seen on one side of the visual field causes apparent disappearance of a stimulus on the opposite side; it will only be seen after the other stimulus is removed. Common following a stroke.

extorsion, excycloduction. *Function*. Outward rotation of one eye; the 12 o'clock meridian rolls away from the nose.

extracapsular cataract extraction (ECCE). *Surgical procedure*. Method of removing a cloudy lens (cataract) that leaves the rear lens capsule intact. See also INTRACAPSULAR CATARACT EXTRACTION.

extraocular muscles (EOM) (eks-truh-AHK-yu-lur), **extrinsic muscles**. *Anatomy*. Six muscles that move the eyeball (lateral rectus, medial rectus, superior oblique, inferior oblique, superior rectus, inferior rectus).

extraction. *Surgical procedure*. Removal of tissue, particularly the lens, e.g., cataract removal.

extremities. *Anatomy*. Arms and legs.

extrinsic muscles. See EXTRAOCULAR MUSCLES.

extrusion. Expulsion; pushing out.

exudate (EKS-yu-dayt). *Pathologic sign*. Blood cell-free fluid that leaks from blood vessels into the surrounding tissue or spaces. See also INFILTRATE.

exudates (retinal). *Pathologic condition*. Protein or fatty fluid that leaks from blood vessels into retinal tissue.

> **hard**: have less fluid content and higher density of fat and protein.

> **soft**: "fluffy looking" white deposits within retinal nerve fiber layer that represent small patches of retina that have lost their blood supply (ischemic infarcts) by vessel obstruction; not true exudates. May be associated with hypertensive and diabetic retinopathies and certain collagen vascular diseases. Gradually disappear without treatment, leaving some functional loss. Also called "cotton-wool" spots.

exudative retinitis (ret-ih-NI-tis), **Coats' disease**. *Pathologic condition*. Chronic, progressive retinal disorder characterized by massive white exudates into and under the retina with eventual detachment. Associated with malformed, tortuous, dilated retinal blood vessels. Affects one eye; tends to occur in males. See also RETINITIS PROLIFERANS.

eye, eyeball, globe. *Anatomy*. Sense organ for sight. Receives light imagery and transmits the visual information to the brain. Composed of three major structural layers (corneo-sclera, uvea and retina) and includes the lens, aqueous and vitreous.

eye examination. Evaluation that usually includes any or all of the following: visual acuity for distance and near (with and without correction), intraocular pressure, pupil functions, checks for external and internal infection, disease or defects, extraocular muscle function, inspection of lens and retina through a dilated pupil, plus others.

eyelids, lids. *Anatomy*. Structures covering the front of the eye, which protect it, limit the amount of light entering the pupil, and distribute tear film over the exposed corneal surface.

eye popping. 1. Self-inflicted finger pressure against upper and lower eyelid folds to push an eye partly out of its socket. May cause optic nerve compression. 2. *Test*. An infant's spontaneously opening the lids in response to dimming the room lights. Provides evidence of visual function.

eyestrain. *Symptom*. Discomfort while using the eyes for visual tasks. See also ASTHENOPIA.

F

Fabry's disease (fab-REEZ), **angiokeratoma corporis diffusum universale, diffuse angiakeratoma**. *Pathologic condition.* Enzyme deficiency disease affecting fat (lipid) metabolism. Eye signs include whorl-like corneal opacities, star-shaped lens haze, and tortuous conjunctival and retinal veins. Hereditary, X-linked. See also SPHINGOLIPIDOSES.

facial nerve. *Anatomy.* Seventh cranial nerve. Innervates muscles of the face and scalp, including the tear (lacrimal) glands; also carries taste sensation for the front two-thirds of the tongue.

facial palsy, Bell's palsy. *Pathologic condition.* Paralysis of muscles innervated by the 7th (facial) cranial nerve, which move facial structures surrounding the brow, eyelids and mouth. Eyelid on the affected side does not close properly so corneal drying may become a problem.

facility of outflow. *Measurement.* Rate at which aqueous fluid leaves the eye through the trabecular meshwork; measured by tonography. Abnormally low in glaucoma.

faco- Incorrect spelling of PHACO-.

facultative hyperopia (hi-pur-OH-pee-uh), **manifest hyperopia**. *Refractive error.* Farsighted defect in an eye's optical system. The amount is indicated by the strongest convex (plus) lens a patient will accept while retaining the best visual acuity.

facultative suppression. *Functional defect.* Non-perception of an image by a misaligned eye, with both eyes open. Image is seen when the straight eye is covered and the deviated eye is forced to fixate. Unconscious mechanism to avoid double vision (diplopia). See also OBLIGATORY SUPPRESSION.

Faden procedure (FAH-dun), **posterior fixation suture, retroequatorial myopexy**. *Surgical procedure.* Method of weakening a rectus muscle (medial, lateral, superior or inferior) by suturing it to the sclera 10–16 mm behind its insertion, thus restricting its action.

fakic. Incorrect spelling of PHAKIC.

fako-. Incorrect spelling of PHACO-.

falciform fold (FAL-sih-form). *Congenital anomaly.* Retinal fold extending from the optic disc toward the retinal periphery. Caused by traction from remnants of the primary vitreous and the hyaloid artery.

fallen eye syndrome. *Pathologic condition.* In a superior oblique palsy, refers to the lower, non-fixing, non-paretic eye that cannot elevate completely. Occurs years later, when the paretic eye is habitually used for fixation. See also INHIBITIONAL PALSY OF THE CONTRALATERAL ANTAGONIST, RISING EYE SYNDROME.

false image. In diplopia (double vision), image arising from the misaligned eye.

familial autonomic dysfunction, Riley-Day syndrome. *Pathologic condition.* Nervous system disorder characterized by reduced tear production (alacrima), decreased corneal sensation, outward eye deviation (exotropia), nearsightedness (myopia), excessive sweating, lack of pain sensitivity, excessive sensitivity to touch, incoordination, recurrent respiratory infections, absence of taste buds, and sudden, unexplained death. Hereditary; found only in Ashkenazic Jews.

familial exudative vitreal retinopathy (FEVR). *Pathologic condition.* Characterized by fluid leakage from the retina and vitreo-retinal membrane formation with new blood vessels. Affects both eyes. Resembles retinopathy of prematurity but lacks history of prematurity. Rare; hereditary.

familial lipoprotein deficiency (LI-poh-PROH-teen), **Tangier disease**. *Path-*

ologic condition. Congenital defect of fat (lipid) metabolism characterized by orange cholesterol deposits in the tonsils and tiny corneal deposits seen only by slit lamp. Does not affect vision.

fan dial. *Test chart.* Radial pattern of black lines used during refraction to subjectively determine the axis of an astigmatic error. See also ASTIGMATIC DIAL.

Farber's lipogranulomatosis (LI-poh-gran-yu-loh-muh-TOH- sus). *Congenital abnormality.* Fat (lipid) disorder characterized by the onset of a hoarse, weak cry soon after birth, cherry red spots in the macula, and glycolipid deposits in the retinal ganglion cell layer.

farinata (fehr-ih-NAH-tuh). *Anatomic defect.* Small, gray, dot-like opacities in the corneal stroma near Descemet's membrane. Visible on retroillumination. Incidental finding with no accompanying visual loss.

Farnsworth tests, Farnsworth-Munsell tests. For color vision; subject arranges 15 colored discs (D-15) or 86 discs (D-100) according to hue.

far-point of accommodation (fpa). Most distant point from the eye at which an object can be seen clearly.

farsightedness, hypermetropia, hyperopia. *Refractive error.* Focusing defect in which the eye is underpowered. Light rays coming from a distant object strike the retina before coming to sharp focus; true focus is said to be "behind the retina." Corrected with additional optical power supplied by a plus lens (spectacle or contact) or by excessive use of the eye's own focusing ability (accommodation).

Fasanella-Servat procedure (FAS-uh-NEL-uh SUR-vaht), **Fasanella procedure, internal tarsoconjunctival Müllerectomy.** *Surgical procedure.* Repair of a mildly drooping upper eyelid (ptosis) by removing a section of conjunctiva, Müller's muscle, and tarsus from the underside of the lid.

fascia (FASH-uh). *Anatomy.* Sheets of fibrous tissue that cover and connect organs, structures and muscles to help keep them in place.

fascia bulbi (BUL-bi), **Tenon's capsule.** *Anatomy.* Thin, fibrous, slightly elastic membrane that envelops the eyeball from the edge of the cornea (limbus) to the optic nerve. Attaches loosely to the sclera and to extraocular muscle tendons. See also INTERMUSCULAR MEMBRANE, MUSCLE SHEATHS.

fascia lata sling (LAH-tuh). *Surgical procedure.* Repair of a severely drooping upper eyelid (ptosis) by suspending the lid from the frontalis muscle with a sling of thin fibrous tissue transplanted from the thigh.

fascia (orbital). *Anatomy.* Protective and supportive tissue surrounding the eyeball; includes check ligaments, intermuscular membrane, muscle sheaths, orbital septum, periorbita, and Tenon's capsule.

fast eye movements (FEM), saccades. *Function.* Rapid simultaneous movements of both eyes in same direction; mechanism for fixation, refixation, and fast phase of optokinetic nystagmus. Initiated by frontal lobe of brain (Brodmann area 8). See also SLOW EYE MOVEMENTS.

febrile. *Clinical sign.* Having an elevated body temperature; feverish.

Fechner's law (FEK-nurz). *Optics.* The intensity of a visual sensation produced by a stimulus varies directly with the logarithm of the strength of the stimulus. See also WEBER'S LAW.

Feldstein suture plication, Snellen sutures. *Surgical procedure.* Repair of a senile entropion by tightening the inferior obicularis muscle in the lower eyelid.

Felty's syndrome. *Pathologic condition.* Rheumatoid arthritis, enlarged spleen, and lower-than-normal white count that develops gradually in middle age. Eye signs include dry eyes, keratoconjunctivitis and scleromalacia perforans.

Ferree-Rand perimeter. *Instrument.* Outdated visual field testing device.

Ferry's line. *Anatomic defect.* Linear abnormality that develops postoperatively in the corneal epithelium at the edge of a filtering bleb.

fetal alcohol syndrome. *Congenital abnormality.* Characterized by delayed growth, mental retardation, eyelid abnormalities, crossed eyes (esotropia), nearsightedness (myopia), and small (hypoplastic) optic nerves. Found in babies born to an alcoholic mother.

fetal fissure. *Anatomy.* Embryonic cleft along the bottom of the optic cup from front to back. Develops during the 4th week of embryonic life and closes by the 6th week.

fiber layer of Chevitz (sheh-VITZ). *Anatomy.* Structure of macular tissue that exists from the 5th month of fetal development until shortly after birth. Significance not known.

fiberoptic light pipe, endoilluminator. *Instrument.* Light source comprised of a flexible bundle of closely packed transparent fibers that conduct light; used for illuminating inside of eye during surgical procedures.

fibrin. *Chemical.* Protein in blood responsible for clot formation.

fibrosis (fi-BROH-sis). *Pathologic change.* Formation of fibrous connectve tissue, as in a scar. Often occurs after injury or degeneration.

fibrous dysplasia (dis-PLAY-zhuh). *Pathologic condition.* Characterized by enlarged orbital bones causing facial swelling, bulging of eye (proptosis), deformed orbits, and optic nerve degeneration. Occurs in children and young adults.

Fick's axes. Three imaginary reference lines in the eye (x, y, and z axes of Fick), perpendicular to one another, intersecting at the center of rotation.

field of vision, visual field. Full extent of the area visible to an eye that is fixating straight ahead. Measured in degrees from fixation.

fields of gaze, diagnostic positions of gaze. *Test.* Nine eye positions (straight ahead, up, down, right, left, up + right, down + right, up + left, down + left) to which both eyes are moved while the head faces forward; used for evaluation of extraocular muscles, versions, and double vision. See also DIPLOPIA FIELDS, SECONDARY POSITION, TERTIARY POSITION, YOKE MUSCLES.

fifth cranial nerve (N V), trigeminal nerve. *Anatomy.* Large three-branch cranial nerve originating in the pons area of the brainstem. First branch (ophthalmic nerve) conducts sensory impulses to the brain from the eyeballs, conjunctiva, eyelids, brow, forehead and front half of the scalp.

filamentary keratitis (kehr-uh-TI-tis). *Pathologic condition.* Strands of coiled, superficial corneal epithelium loosely attached to the cornea; when broken free, leave small, painful ulcers. Associated with keratoconjunctivitis sicca and trachoma.

filtering bleb. Bubble-like blister of conjunctiva. 1. *Surgical result.* Flap of tissue created to cover a sclero-corneal drainage channel, which enhances passage of fluid from the eye. Result of type of filtering procedure for the treatment of some forms of glaucoma. 2. *Pathologic condition.* Follows inadvertent leak of aqueous fluid from a limbal wound, sometimes after surgery.

filtering procedure. *Surgical procedure.* Creation of a drainage channel from the anterior chamber to the external surface of the eye under the conjunctiva, allowing aqueous to seep into a filtering bleb from which it is slowly absorbed. For controlling intraocular pressure in glaucoma.

fine needle aspiration (FNA). *Method.* Use of a fine (22 gauge), short (3.75 cm) needle to biopsy orbital masses behind the orbital septum.

finger counting, counts fingers. *Test measurement.* Patient's ability to count number of fingers presented, usually at a distance of 1 or 2 ft. Used when vision loss is profound (acuity less than 20/400). See also HAND MOVEMENT, LIGHT PERCEPTION.

fingerprint dystrophy. Term sometimes used for MAP-DOT-FINGERPRINT DYSTROPHY.

first grade fusion, superimposition. *Function.* Perceptual blending (superimposing) of two dissimilar images, one formed on each retina, into one composite image.

"fish mouth" tear. *Pathologic condition*. Retinal tear that opens wide when pressure is applied to the overlying sclera.

fissure height, fissure width, palpebral fissure height *(or)* **width**. *Measurement*. Distance from the center of the lower eyelid margin to the center of the upper eyelid margin, measured when the eye is open.

fissure length, palpebral fissure length. *Measurement*. Distance from the inner (nasal) to the outer (temporal) canthus of the eyelids.

fistula. *Pathologic condition*. Abnormal channel connecting an abscess or body organ to the body surface or to another internal structure.

5-fluorouracil (FLUH-roh-YUR-uh-sil). Anti-cancer drug; used in very low dose to prevent scar tissue from forming after filtering surgery for glaucoma.

fix. *Function*. Slang for fixate.

fixate. *Function*. To move an eye so that a viewed object is imaged on the fovea.

fixation, central fixation. *Function*. Coordinated accommodation and ocular movements that achieve and maintain the image of objects on the fovea.

fixation axis. Imaginary line connecting a viewed object with the eye's center of rotation. See also FIXATION.

fixation light. *Test object*. Small bright light used for controlling the patient's direction of attention, e.g., during eye muscle and pupil function evaluation.

fixation object. *Test object*. Item used for attracting and controlling the patient's direction of attention during certain diagnostic tests.

fixation preference (FP). *Test*. Use of a cover-uncover test to evaluate how well a misaligned eye maintains fixation. See also INDUCED TROPIA TEST.

fixation reflex. *Function*. Involuntary eye movement that positions the eye to image a viewed object on the fovea.

fixed dilated pupil, "blown pupil." *Anatomic defect*. Enlarged pupil that does not constrict in response to a light stimulus, a near object, or a light stimulus in the other eye.

fixing eye, centrally fixing eye. *Function*. Eye that looks directly at an object so that its image is focused on the fovea. Normally functioning eyes fixate together; if one eye is deviated, only the straight eye is a fixing eye.

flap. *Surgical procedure*. Tongue-shaped section of tissue (e.g., conjunctiva, sclera, skin) that is dissected on two or three sides and resutured.

    advancement: type of conjunctival or skin flap used for covering a defect or for reconstructing eyelids.

    conjunctival: used for exposing the sclera below, protecting a wound, covering a corneal defect, or covering a filtration site for aqueous humor, producing a filtering bleb.

    fornix-based: type of conjunctival flap. Opening the conjunctiva at the limbus (corneoscleral junction) and peeling up a flap toward the fornix, to cover a limbal incision site.

    limbal-based: type of conjunctival flap. Cutting the conjunctiva several millimeters behind the limbus (corneo-scleral junction) and making a flap toward the limbus, to cover a limbal incision site into the eye, e.g., during a cataract extraction.

    scleral: used for exposing the deeper sclera or inside of eye. Part of trabeculectomy procedure for glaucoma, iridocyclectomy for removal of a small intraocular tumor, and (seldom) for retinal detachment surgery.

    skin: cut to keep its blood supply intact. Often used for covering or filling a skin defect such as after removal of a tumor or scar.

    sliding: skin or conjunctiva dissected on three sides and stretched or slid over to cover an adjacent area. Common in reconstructive surgery.

flare, aqueous flare, Tyndall effect. *Clinical sign*. Scattering of a slit lamp light beam when it is directed into the anterior chamber;occurs when aqueous has increased protein content. Sign of iris and/or ciliary body inflammation (iritis).

Flarex. *Drug*. Trade name of fluorometholone, steroid used for treating external ocular inflammations.

flash blindness. *Pathologic condition*. Vision loss caused by viewing an extremely bright light flash. Usually temporary (can be permanent if light is especially intense, such as an atomic bomb blast).

flattest meridian, K. *Measurement*. Corneal surface direction (e.g., horizontal, vertical, oblique) having the flattest curvature or least optical power. Measured with a keratometer. See also K-READINGS, STEEPEST MERIDIAN.

flat top, D-seg. *Optical device*. Bifocal segment that has a short horizontal upper line separating it from the main portion of the lens. Looks like a tipped over D. See also ROUND TOP.

flavimacular retinopathy (flah-vee-MAK-you-lur ret-in-AHP-uh- thee), **fundus flavimaculatus**. *Pathologic condition*. Characterized by irregular, yellow flecked, deep retinal or pigment epithelial lesions. Often associated with a discrete macular abnormality. Vision may be affected. Rare; hereditary. See also STARGARDT'S DISEASE.

flecked retina syndromes. *Pathologic condition*. Several retinal diseases in which white or yellow flecks appear on the retina. See also BIETTI'S CRYSTALLINE DYSTROPHY, FUNDUS ALBIPUNCTATUS, FUNDUS FLAVIMACULATUS, STARGARDT'S DISEASE.

flecktenool. Incorrect spelling of PHLYCTENULE.

Fleischer ring (FLI-shur). *Pathologic change*. Ring-shaped brownish iron deposit at the base of an abnormal corneal zone. Occurs with keratoconus.

fleurette. *Pathologic condition*. Microscopic rose-petal-like arrangement of cells, sometimes seen in retinoblastoma.

Flexner-Wintersteiner rosettes. *Pathologic change*. Microscopic ring-like arrangement of retinoblastoma (malignant tumor) cells; when abundant and well-formed, believed to indicate a lower degree of malignancy.

flicker fusion frequency (FFF). *Test*. The number of flashes per second that is perceived as continuous rather than flickering. For assessment of rod and cone function.

flicktenular keratoconjunctivitis. Incorrect spelling of PHLYCTENULAR KERATOCONJUNCTIVITIS.

Flieringa ring (FLIR-ing-uh). *Surgical instrument*. Stainless steel ring sutured to the sclera during eye surgery to maintain the spherical shape of the eye; reduces the tendency of intraocular contents to be squeezed out when the globe is opened.

floaters, vitreous floaters. *Anatomic defect*. Particles that float in the vitreous and cast shadows on the retina; seen as spots, cobwebs, spiders, etc. Occurs normally with aging or with vitreous detachment, retinal tears, or inflammation.

floppy eyelid syndrome. *Pathologic condition*. The tarsus (eyelid framework) becomes loose and rubbery, allowing the eyelid to evert easily. Results in the eyelid losing contact with the eyeball during sleep.

Floropryl (FLOR-uh-pril). *Drug*. Trade name of diisopropylfluorophosphate.

flucytosine. *Drug*. Anti-fungal oral or topical drug used for serious eye infections. Related to fluorouracil. Trade name: Ancobon. See also AMPHOTERICIN B, CLOTRIMAZOLE, KETOCONAZOLE, MICONAZOLE, NATAMYCIN.

fluff balls. *Pathologic condition*. Slang description of white opacities found in the anterior vitreous in the presence of fungal endophthalmitis.

fluid gas exchange, air fluid gas exchange. *Surgical procedure*. Replacement of vitreal fluid with air or gas; sometimes used with vitrectomy surgery.

Liquid is drawn from the vitreous through one port (opening) of the vitrectomy instrument as air is injected into the vitreous through another port. See also PERFLUOROPROPANE, SULPHUR HEXAFLUORIDE.

fluorescein (FLOR-uh-seen), **fluorescein sodium**. *Chemical.* Yellow-green dye that fluoresces when illuminated with light of a specific wavelength, usually ultraviolet. Injected intravenously to study blood flow through the retina and choroid. Can also be applied directly to the cornea to detect abrasions or leakage from surgical wounds or to evaluate fit of hard and CAB contact lenses, or to the conjunctiva to evaluate tear drainage. See also FLUORESCEIN ANGIOGRAPHY.

fluorescein angiography (FA) (an-jee-AHG-ruh-fee), **intravenous fluorescein angiography**. *Test.* Used for evaluating retinal, choroidal, and iris blood vessels, as well as any eye problems affecting them. Fluorescein dye is injected into an arm vein, then rapid, sequential photographs are taken of the eye as the dye circulates. See also ARTERIAL PHASE, CHOROIDAL FLUSH, INDOCYANINE GREEN ANGIOGRAPHY.

fluorescein dye disappearance test. Evaluates the tear drainage system; dye dropped onto the conjunctiva of an eye with normal drainage should disappear within 5 minutes. See also JONES TEST.

fluorescein sodium. See FLUORESCEIN.

fluorescence (flor-ESS-enz). *Optics.* Capacity of a substance to absorb light of one wavelength and emit light converted to a longer wavelength.

fluorometholone. *Drug.* Steroid used for treating ocular inflammations. Trade names: Flarex, FML.

Fluor-Op. *Drug.* Trade name of fluorometholone, an anti-inflammatory steroid.

fluorophotometer (flur-oh-foh-TAHM-ih-tur). *Instrument.* Used for measuring the flow rate of fluids by dilution of fluorescein, e.g., for determining tear flow, or leakage from a retinal blood vessel.

fluorophotometry (flur-oh-for-TAHM-ih-tree). *Test.* Calculation of volume and rate of fluid flow.

flurbiprofen. *Drug.* Non-steroidal agent used for treating ocular inflammations and for inhibiting miosis during cataract surgery. Trade name: Ocufen.

flush (choroidal). *Clinical sign.* During fluorescein angiography, first evidence of fluorescein dye reaching the eye. Occurs 8 to 20 seconds after intravenous fluorescein injection.

flutter (ocular). *Clinical sign.* Brief, intermittent, spontaneous movements of both eyes. Occurs with cerebellar disease. See also ocular DYSMETRIA, OPSOCLONUS.

FML. *Drug.* Trade name of fluorometholone, an anti-inflammatory steroid.

focal. *Description.* 1. Localized area of a disease or chief site of a more generalized disease or infection. 2. Concerning a specific body area. See also DIFFUSE.

focal length, focal distance. *Optics.* Distance in meters from a lens (along its principal axis) to the position where that lens brings parallel light rays to a focus. Reciprocal of lens power; e.g., a 2-diopter lens has a focal length of 1/2 meter. See also FOCAL POINT.

focal point. *Optics.* Position on the principal axis of a lens system where parallel light rays are brought to a point focus. See also FOCAL LENGTH.

  primary: object point imaged at infinity, so light rays refracted from the lens emerge in parallel bundles.

  secondary: image point where parallel light rays from a distant object are brought to focus after refraction by the lens.

focus, image point. *Optics.* Point where light rays are brought to a sharp image point by a lens. Plural: foci.

Förster-Fuchs spot (FUR-ster fooks); also spelled Foerster. See FUCHS SPOT.

fogging. *Test*. Refraction refinement technique; plus-powered lens is placed before the eye to deliberately reduce visual acuity.

Folex. *Drug*. Trade name of methotrexate; for treating cancer.

follicles. *Pathologic condition*. Tiny, glistening, translucent (lymphoid) elevations on the undersurface of eyelids. Associated with viral conjunctival inflammation.

follicular conjunctivitis (kun-junk-tih-VI-tis) See CONJUNCTIVITIS.

foot-candle. *Measurement*. Unit of light intensity falling on a surface. One foot-candle of light falls upon 1 sq. ft. of surface located 1 ft. away from a light source of 1 international candle power.

foot-lambert. *Measurement*. Unit of luminance (light leaving a surface).

foramen (for-AY-min). *Anatomy*. A natural opening (hole) in bone through which nerves or blood vessels pass. Plural: foramina (for-AM-ih-nuh).

    optic f: opening in the sphenoid bone at the back of the orbit through which pass the ophthalmic artery, optic nerve, and sympathetic nerves.

forced duction test (DUK-shun)*,* **passive forced duction** *(or)* **traction test**. Forcibly moving the eyeball into different positions by grasping the anesthetized conjunctiva and episclera with forceps at the corneo-scleral junction (limbus). For determining if there are any mechanical restrictions to movement.

forced generation test. For determining function of a paralyzed extraocular muscle; patient attempts to move anesthetized eye held with forceps.

forced preferential looking (FPL). *Test*. Specific method of preferential looking technique. Vision is evaluated in preverbal children by noting whether they choose the blank side of a large rectangular card or the side with spatial frquency stripes. See also FIXATION PREFERENCE.

forceps. *Surgical instrument*. Used for grasping tissues or sutures.

forea. Incorrect spelling of PHORIA.

foreign body sensation (FBS). *Symptom*. Feeling of grittiness or having something in the eye. Frequently caused by a foreign body; other causes include corneal abrasion, corneal ulcer, inturned eyelash and conjunctivitis.

form fruste. *Pathologic condition*. Atypical or partial manifestation of signs and symptoms of a disease (that is often hereditary). Plural: formes frustes.

fornix (FOR-niks)*,* **conjunctival sac, cul-de-sac**. *Anatomy*. Loose pocket of conjunctiva between upper eyelid and eyeball, and lower eyelid and eyeball, that permits the eyeball to rotate freely. Plural: fornices.

fornix approach. *Surgical procedure*. Gaining access to eyeball, muscles, or orbital contents through the conjunctival fornix.

fornix-based flap. *Surgical procedure*. Type of conjunctival flap. Opening the conjunctiva at the limbus (corneo-scleral junction) and peeling up a flap toward the fornix, to cover a limbal incision site. See also LIMBAL-BASED FLAP.

foropter. Incorrect spelling of PHOROPTER.

fortified. Term applied to any standard eye medication to which additional active drug has been added to increase its concentration.

foscarnet. *Drug*. Injected intravenously for treating severe herpetic and cytomegalovirus eye infections. Trade name: Foscavir. See also ACUTE RETINAL NECROSIS, ACYCLOVIR, GANCICLOVIR.

Foscavir. Drug. Trade name of foscarnet. For treating CMV retinitis.

Foster-Kennedy syndrome, Kennedy syndrome. *Pathologic condition*. Characterized by optic nerve degeneration (atrophy) on same side as a frontal lobe brain tumor and optic nerve swelling on opposite side due to increased brain pressure.

fouropter. Incorrect spelling of PHOROPTER.

four-prism-diopter test (di-AHP-tur). For evaluating suppression in a minimally deviated eye. A 4$^\Delta$ prism is held base-out in front of the eye while the patient fixates on a light; absence of convergence movement indicates suppression. See also MONOFIXATION SYNDROME.

fourth cranial nerve (N IV), trochlear nerve. *Anatomy*. Motor nerve that innervates the superior oblique muscle of the eye. Originates in the lower midbrain; enters the orbit through the superior orbital fissure.

fourth nerve palsy, superior oblique palsy. *Pathologic condition*. Head tilt and upward eye deviation (hypertropia) caused by damage to the 4th (trochlear) cranial nerve; reduces the effectiveness of the superior oblique muscle.

fovea (FOH-vee-uh), **fovea centralis**. *Anatomy*. Central pit in the macula that produces sharpest vision. Contains a high concentration of cones and no retinal blood vessels. Plural: foveae.

foveal dystopia (FOH-vee-ul dis-TOHP-ee-uh), **dragged** *(or)* **ectopic macula**. *Pathologic condition*. Displacement of the macular region of the retina by traction. Seen with retinopathy of prematurity, intraocular worm, previous inflammation and other forms of retinal scarring, and following retinal detachment surgery.

foveal reflex. *Function*. Tiny optical reflection from the concave mirrorlike surface of the foveal depression in the retina. Visible with an ophthalmoscope.

foveola (foh-vee-OH-luh). *Anatomy*. Centermost, thinnest zone of the fovea.

Foville syndrome (foh-VEEL). *Pathologic condition*. Characterized by facial paralysis of one side of the face, and on the other side by inability to move the eye voluntarily toward the opposite side, and paralysis of body extremities. Pursuit movements and doll's head phenomenon are not affected. Caused by blood vessel disease in the pons.

Fox shield. *Protective device*. Pliable, oval metal disc that can be taped over a bandaged eye.

framing. *Exercise*. For increasing the ability to hold fusion while moving the eyes outward (divergence); as a pencil is held vertically in front of the nose (and seen double), a single distant object is moved closer until it appears "framed" between the two pencil images.

Franceschetti syndrome (fran-sus-KET-ee), **mandibulofacial dysostosis, Treacher-Collins syndrome**. *Congenital anomaly*. Bony deformity of skull and face; characterized by a bird-like appearance with small jaw and "parrot-beak" nose, indistinct orbital margins, notching of the lower eyelids (coloboma), and an anti-mongoloid slant of eyelids. Rare; hereditary.

Francois syndrome (fran-SWAH), **Hallermann-Streiff syndrome, oculomandibulodyscephaly**. *Congenital anomaly*. Bony deformity of skull and face. Characterized by a bird-like face with small jaw and "parrot-beak" nose, dwarfism, small eyes, congenital cataracts, and poor vision. Rare; hereditary.

free graft. *Surgical procedure*. Transplantation of tissue (e.g., skin, conjunctiva) with no attached blood supply, to cover a defect.

free tenotomy (ten-AHT-oh-mee). *Surgical procedure*. Cutting an extraocular eye muscle from its place of insertion on the eyeball, allowing it to retract. Rarely used. See also INTRASHEATH TENOTOMY.

Fresnel lens (freh-NEL), **Fresnel prism, "press-on."** *Optical device*. Flexible plastic lens or prism that has an adhesive side for adhering to an eyeglass lens. For correcting eye deviations or refractive errors. See also FRESNEL PRINCIPLE.

Fresnel principle. *Optics*. Ridged optical design that mimics the optical power of a standard lens or prism but greatly reduces its bulk and weight.

Fresnel prism. See FRESNEL LENS.

friable (FRI-uh-bul). *Description*. Fragile; easily crumbled or shredded.

frontal bone. *Anatomy*. Skull bone that forms forehead and orbital roof. One of seven bones forming the orbit.

frontal eye fields (FEF), Brodmann area 8. *Anatomy.* Area in the frontal lobe of the brain responsible for rapid, voluntary eye movements (saccades). See also BRODMANN AREA 19, FAST EYE MOVEMENTS.

frontal lobe. *Anatomy.* Large front part of each cerebral hemisphere in the brain. Contains centers for voluntary movements, including nerve fibers for fast voluntary eye movements (saccades). See also OCCIPITAL LOBE, PARIETAL LOBE, TEMPORAL LOBE.

frontal nerve. *Anatomy.* Largest branch of the ophthalmic nerve (1st division of the 5th [trigeminal] cranial nerve). Enters the orbit through the superior orbital fissure and divides into supratrochlear and supraorbital branches, providing sensation to the brow and forehead.

frontalis fixation, frontalis sling *(or)* **suspension.** *Surgical procedure.* Repair of a severely drooping upper eyelid (ptosis) by suspending the lid from the frontalis muscle by a sling of thin fibrous tissue transplanted from the thigh (fascia late sling), or by manmade absorbable or biologic nonabsorbable materials.

frontal sinus. *Anatomy.* Mucus-lined air cavity within the frontal bones; one of the nasal sinuses that drains into the nose. Others are the ethmoid, maxillary and sphenoid.

frosted branch angiitis (an-jee-I-tis). *Clinical sign.* Whitish sheathing around retinal blood vessels (usually veins); resembles frosted tree branches.

Frost suture. *Surgical procedure.* Method of temporarily closing the eyelids to protect the cornea following lid surgery, e.g., ptosis repair.

frozen globe. *Abnormal condition.* Eyeball that cannot move.

FTA-ABS. *Lab test.* Blood test: fluorescent treponema antibody absorption test for syphilis.

F_3T, TFT. See TRIFLUOROTHYMIDINE.

Fuchs (crypts of) (fyooks), **iris crypts.** *Anatomy.* Pit-like depressions in the front surface of the iris.

Fuchs' dystrophy (DIS-truh-fee), **endothelial dystrophy.** *Pathologic condition.* Progressive corneal disorder characterized by hyaline endothelial outgrowths on Descemet's membrane, a cloudy waterlogged cornea, painful epithelial blisters, and reduced vision. May require a corneal graft. Sometimes hereditary. See also BULLOUS KERATOPATHY, GUTTATA.

Fuchs' heterochromic cyclitis (HET-ur-oh-KROH-mik si-KLI-tus), **heterochromic uveitis.** *Pathologic condition.* Unilateral low-grade inflammation of the ciliary body and iris (which appears lighter in color than in the other eye). Secondary cataract and/or glaucoma may develop.

Fuchs' spot, Förster-Fuchs spot. *Pathologic change.* Pigmented, circular degenerative lesion that may develop in the macula of an extremely nearsighted eye, resulting in reduced vision. Thought to be caused by formation of new choroidal blood vessels (neovascularization). See also MYOPIC DEGENERATION.

fukes. Incorrect spelling of FUCHS.

fulminant. *Description.* Refers to a sudden, rapid, intense reaction.

functional amblyopia (am-blee-OH-pee-uh), **reversible amblyopia.** *Functional defect.* Vision deficiency in one eye with no detectable anatomic damage to visual pathways; vision usually recoverable in young patient. Four types: strabismic, deprivation, anisometropic, ametropic. See also AMBLYOPIA, NEUTRAL DENSITY FILTER.

functional defect. Abnormality attributed to patient's psychological state and not to any physical damage or disease process. See also HYSTERICAL AMBLYOPIA, SPIRAL FIELDS.

functional visual loss. *Symptom.* Decreased vision claimed by patient with no corroborating objective evidence of abnormality found on examination. See also HYSTERICAL AMBLYOPIA, MALINGERER.

fundoscopy (fun-DAHS-koh-pee). *Test.* Less preferred term for ophthalmoscopy (fundus examination with an ophthalmoscope).

fundus, fundus oculi. *Anatomy.* Interior posterior surface of the eyeball; includes retina, optic disc, macula, posterior pole. Can be seen with an ophthalmoscope.

fundus albipunctatus (al-bih-punk-TAH-tus). *Pathologic condition.* Characterized by night blindness and gray or whitish dot-like mottling of the fundus. Visual acuity, visual fields and color vision are not affected. Rare, hereditary.

fundus camera. *Instrument.* Camera used for taking pictures of the retina and inner lining of the eye, particularly the posterior pole. Based on the principle of monocular indirect ophthalmoscopy.

funduscope. *Instrument.* Less preferred term for ophthalmoscope.

fundus flavimaculatus (flah-vee-mak-yu-LAH-tis), **flavimacular retinopathy.** *Pathologic condition.* Characterized by irregular, yellow flecked, deep retinal or pigment epithelial lesions. Often associated with a discrete macular abnormality. Vision may be affected. Rare; hereditary. See also STARGARDT'S DISEASE.

fundus oculi. See FUNDUS.

fungal keratitis, keratomycosis. *Pathologic condition.* Gray, pus-producing corneal ulcer with irregular borders. Develops after eye injury from vegetable matter (tree branch, fingernail). See also CANDIDA ALBICANS, FUSARIUM.

Fungizone. *Drug.* Trade name of amphotericin; for treating fungal eye infections.

furosemide. *Drug.* Heart medication that increases urination so that excess body fluid is removed. Trade name: Lasex. See also CHLOROTHIAZIDE, HYDROCHLOROTHIAZIDE.

furrows. *Pathologic condition.* Peripheral corneal areas that have become thinner and produce gutter-like ulcers.

Fusarium (fyu-ZEHR-ee-um). *Microorganism.* Fungus that can cause corneal ulcers or endophthalmitis, especially in Florida.

fuscin (FYOOK-sin), **lipofuscin.** *Anatomy.* Fatty substance found in the retinal pigment epithelium. Excessive amounts are abnormal.

fused bifocal. *Optical device.* Eyeglass lens that has a plus-powered glass disc of high refractive index fused into its front surface, to provide added power for close work. See also ADD, D-SEG.

fusiform. *Description.* Shape of a structure that is tapered at both ends, resembling a spindle. Usually refers to bacteria.

fusion. *Function.* Perceptual blending of two similar images, one from each eye, into one image that is maintained as the eyes converge or diverge. See also CENTRAL FUSION, PERIPHERAL FUSION.

> **1st grade**: the superimposed images are dissimilar.
> **2nd grade**: vergence movements allow blending of the similar images into one as the images move off the fovea.
> **3rd grade**: binocular perception of depth (stereopsis) as slightly dissimilar images are blended.

fusional amplitudes, amplitudes, vergence ability. *Measurement.* Amount (in diopters) the eyes can move inward (converge) added to the amount they can move outward (diverge), while maintaining single vision.

fusional convergence. *Measurement.* Amount the eyes can converge while maintaining single vision. Measured with graduated base-out prisms.

fusion-free position, dissociated *(or)* heterophoric position, physiologic position of rest. *Function.* Position assumed by the eyes, relative to each other, when one eye is covered or its vision obstructed. See also PHORIA.

G

galactosemia (guh-lak-toh-SEE-mee-uh). *Pathologic condition.* Enzyme deficiency (galactokinase transferase) affecting children. Ingestion of milk, which contains galactose, causes cataracts, vomiting, dehydration, impaired liver function and mental retardation. Hereditary.

galactosyl ceramide lipidosis, Krabbe's disease. *Pathologic condition.* Hereditary defect of fat (lipid) metabolism caused by B-galactosidase enzyme deficiency. Onset in first 6 months of life, with irritability followed by progressive motor and mental deterioration, optic nerve degeneration, deafness, and death. See also SPHINGOLIPIDOSES.

gamma (angle). *Optics.* Angle formed at the center of rotation of an eye between the optic axis and the fixation axis.

ganciclovir (gan-SI-kloh-vir). *Drug.* Injected intravitreally to treat severe herpetic and cytomegalovirus eye infections. Trade name: Cytovene.

ganglion (GANG-lee-un). *Anatomy.* Group of nerve cell bodies located outside the central nervous system. Plural: ganglia, ganglions.

> **cervical** (SUR-vih-kul): series of paired clumps of nerve junctions in the neck alongside the spine and internal carotid arteries.

> > **superior cervical**: large clump (one of a pair) of neural interconnections in the neck, alongside the spine and internal carotid artery. Contains sympathetic nerve fibers from cervical and thoracic spinal nerves that supply the eye and orbit.

ganglion cell layer. *Anatomy.* Layer within the inner retina containing the nuclei of ganglion cells; gives rise to optic nerve fibers.

gangliosidosis (gang-lee-oh-si-DOH-sis). *Pathologic condition.* Hereditary defect in lipid (fat) metabolism caused by specific enzyme deficiencies; characterized by progressive motor and mental deterioration. Fatal. Includes juvenile Gm_1 and Gm_2 gangliosidosis; Pompe's, Sandhoff's and Tay-Sachs disease. See also SPHINGOLIPIDOSES.

Gantrisin (GAN-truh-sin). *Drug.* Trade name of sulfisoxazole, sulfa drug used for treating corneal and conjunctival infections.

ganzfeld. *Lab test.* Describes broad light stimulation of the full visual field. Used when recording electrical responses from the retina (ERG).

Garamycin (gar-uh-MI-sin). *Drug.* Trade name of gentamicin, an antibiotic.

gargoylism, Hurler's syndrome. *Pathologic condition.* Characterized by severe skeletal abnormalities, dwarfism, short spinal column, short fingers, depressed bridge of nose, joint stiffness, heart problems, severe mental retardation, retinal degeneration and corneal clouding. Form of mucopolysaccharidosis caused by enzyme alpha-L-iduronidase deficiency. Hereditary.

gas permeable lens (GP), rigid gas permeable lens. *Optical device.* Rigid plastic contact lens that allows oxygen and carbon dioxide penetration. See also HARD CONTACT LENS, SOFT CONTACT LENS.

Gasserian ganglion. *Anatomy.* Large group of nerve cell bodies that contain the ophthalmic, maxillary, and mandibular divisions of the 5th (trigeminal) cranial nerve, forming its sensory root.

Gaucher's disease (goh-SHAYZ). *Pathologic condition.* Genetic deficiency of enzyme B-glucosidase. Eye signs include yellowish-brown fleshy conjunctival deposits, corneal clouding, and macular degeneration. See also SPHINGOLIPIDOSES.

gaze movement, conjugate *(or)* subjunctive movement. *Function.* Parallel movements of both eyes. See also PURSUIT MECHANISM, SACCADES.

gaze palsy. *Functional defect*. Inability of the eyes to make parallel movements in a specific direction.

gaze paretic nystagmus (ni-STAG-mus). *Functional defect*. Involuntary eye oscillations that begin when the eyes attempt to look in a direction to which they cannot move easily. Associated with drugs, multiple sclerosis, tumors, and circulatory problems.

Geneva lens clock. *Instrument*. Device that measures surface curves and optical power of an eyeglass lens.

geniculate body (jen-IK-yu-lit), **external *(or)* lateral geniculate body**. *Anatomy*. Paired prominences at the sides of the mid-brain (upper end of brainstem); neural way-station where optic tract fibers connect (synapse) to the optic radiations and transmit visual information.

geniculo-calcarine tract (jen-IK-yu-loh-KAL-kuh-rine), **optic radiations**. *Anatomy*. Visual nerve pathway between the lateral geniculate body and the calcarine fissure of the occipital visual cortex in the brain. Consists of crossed nasal retinal fibers from one eye and uncrossed temporal retinal fibers from the other eye.

Genoptic. *Drug*. Trade name of gentamycin, an antibiotic.

Gentacidin. *Drug*. Trade name of gentamycin, an antibiotic.

gentamicin (jen-tuh-MI-sin). *Drug*. Antibiotic eyedrops or injection for treating external and internal eye infections caused by gram-negative bacteria. Trade names: Garamycin, Genoptic, Gentacidin.

geographic. *Description*. Refers to a condition whose shape resembles the irregular outline of a land mass, e.g., a corneal ulcer.

geographic choroidopathy, helicoid *(or)* serpiginous choroidopathy. *Pathologic condition*. Type of progressive, bilateral choroidal inflammation and degeneration that begins around the optic nerve head (peripapillary) and slowly, over months, extends in a creeping fashion.

geometric axis, optic axis. Imaginary line through the centers of curvature of the cornea and lens that passes through the nodal point of the eye.

geometric equator, equator, equatorial meridian. Imaginary ring around the eye at the intersection of a plane dividing the eyeball into front and back halves. See also ANATOMIC EQUATOR.

geometric perspective, linear perspective. *Psychophysics*. As parallel lines and planes recede into the distance, they appear to approach each other at the horizon. One of several monocular cues to depth perception. See also MONOCULAR DEPTH PERCEPTION.

German measles, rubella. *Pathologic condition*. Common viral disease. Mild in children; during the 1st trimester of pregnancy can generate fetal abnormalities such as mental retardation, heart disease, hearing defects, and eye defects, e.g., cataracts, glaucoma, retinal changes, eye deviations.

gerontoxon (JEH-run-TAHK-sin), **arcus senilis**. *Degenerative change*. Ring-shaped white deposit of fat near the peripheral edge of the cornea (limbus). Found typically in patients over age 60; also in young patients with abnormally high blood fat levels (arcus juvenilis).

Gerstmann's syndrome. *Pathologic condition*. Homonymous hemianopia, difficulty calculating numbers (dyscalculia), and right-left confusion resulting from a brain lesion in the area of the left angular gyrus on the dominant side.

ghost cell glaucoma, erythroclastic glaucoma. *Pathologic condition*. Secondary glaucoma produced by abnormal red blood cells (erythroclasts; also called ghost cells) clogging the trabecular meshwork.

ghost cells, erythroclasts. *Anatomic abnormality*. Abnormal red blood cells that can clog the trabecular meshwork and elevate intraocular pressure.

ghost vessels. *Pathologic condition*. Transparent, empty blood vessels that remain permanently in the cornea after regression of the inflammation that created them.

giant cell arteritis (ar-tur-I-tis), **cranial** *(or)* **temporal arteritis**. *Pathologic condition.* Inflammation of many of the arteries supplying the head and eyes. May be accompanied by severe headache, fever, weight loss, stroke and heart attack. Eye involvement includes sudden vision loss and optic nerve inflammation (caused by the closing off of the central retinal artery or a branch), double vision or droopy eyelids. Usually affects people over age 60.

giant papillary conjunctivitis (GPC) (kun-junk-tih-VI-tis). *Pathologic condition.* Allergic type of conjunctival inflammation often associated with continuous wearing of contact lenses. Hard, flat papillae form a cobblestone pattern on undersurface of the upper eyelid.

giant tear. *Pathologic condition.* Retinal tear of at least 1 quadrant (90°), usually located near the ora serrata or along an equatorial zone of lattice degeneration. Caused by trauma or hereditary predisposition. Likely to produce a retinal detachment that is difficult to repair. See also DIALYSIS.

Giemsa stain (GEEM-suh). *Test.* Stain applied to microscopic slides of corneal and conjunctival tear fluid or tissue samples. Helps to differentiate cell types, e.g., epithelial, neutrophil, eosinophil, lymphocyte, bacterial.

Gierke's disease (GIR-keez), **hepato-renal glycogenesis**. *Pathologic condition.* Characterized by inability of the body to store glycogen. Associated with cloudy corneal edges. Hereditary.

Girard procedure. *Surgical procedure.* Cataract extraction using ultrasonic vibrations (phacoemulsification) to help fragment and remove opaque lens material.

glabella (gluh-BEL-uh). *Anatomy.* Prominent area on the frontal bone between the eyebrows.

glabellar flap (guh-BEH-lur). *Surgical procedure.* V-shaped skin flap taken from between the eyebrows, for reconstructing an eyelid defect near the nose. See also MIDLINE FOREHEAD FLAP, V-TO-Y PLASTY.

glare. Undesirable sensation produced by brightness (within visual field) that is much greater than that to which the eyes are adapted. Causes annoyance, discomfort, or loss in visual performance.

glaucoma (glaw-KOH-muh). *Pathologic condition.* Group of diseases characterized by increased intraocular pressure resulting in damage to the optic nerve and retinal nerve fibers. Documented by typical visual field defects and increased size of optic cup. A common cause of preventable vision loss. May be treated by prescription drugs or surgery.

   absolute: end-stage, in which pressure remains elevated and vision is completely lost.

   acute angle closure: same as ANGLE CLOSURE (below).

   angle closure: sudden rise in intraocular pressure. Aqueous fluid behind the iris cannot pass through the pupil and pushes the iris forward, preventing aqueous drainage through the angle (pupillary block mechanism). Occurs in patients who have narrow anterior chamber angles.

   chronic angle closure: form of narrow angle glaucoma. Repeated attacks of angle obstruction over a long period (months to years) eventually block normal aqueous drainage channels permanently.

   chronic open angle: same as OPEN ANGLE (below).

   ciliary block: same as MALIGNANT (below).

   congenital: high intraocular pressures accompanied by hazy corneas and large eyes (buphthalmos) in newborn that result from developmental abnormalities in the anterior chamber angle obstructing the normal intraocular fluid drainage mechanism.

   hemorrhagic: same as NEOVASCULAR (below).

   hemolytic (hee-moh-LIT-ik): secondary glaucoma produced by bleeding into the eye.

infantile: same as CONGENITAL (above).

lens induced: same as PHACOLYTIC (below)

malignant: increase in intraocular pressure accompanied by a shallow anterior chamber and forward displacement of the iris and lens. Complication of surgery for acute angle closure glaucoma; may be caused by aqueous trapped behind vitreous. Also called ciliary block.

narrow angle: associated with anatomically narrow width of angle opening. Also called angle closure.

neovascular: caused by abnormal new blood vessel formation (neovascularization) in and on the iris that extends over the trabecular meshwork and closes angle drainage structures. Difficult to control; leads to a painful eye with high pressure, corneal swelling, and "cell and flare" in the anterior chamber. Associated with problems that cause blockage of the retinal blood vessels, e.g., diabetic retinopathy. Also called hemorrhagic.

open angle: most common type; gradual blocking of aqueous outflow from the eye despite an apparently open anterior chamber angle. If untreated, results in gradual, painless, irreversible loss of vision.

phacolytic: caused by mechanical blockage of the eye's drainage channels (trabecular meshwork) by cells carrying lens protein. Associated with advanced (hypermature) cataract or lens trauma.

pigmentary dispersion: type of open angle glaucoma caused by pigment granules gradually breaking free from the iris and ciliary epithelium and deposited on the back corneal surface, lens, zonules and pores of the trabecular meshwork.

primary open angle: same as OPEN ANGLE (above).

secondary: results from a known cause, such as inflammation, degeneration, trauma, or tumor growths within the eye.

glaucoma meds. *Drug.* Medications used for controlling intraocular pressure, to prevent visual loss. Types are:

adrenergic blocking agents (also known as beta blockers, sympatholytic drugs): block action of the sympathetic nerve fibers by blocking beta adrenergic receptor sites for nerve impulse transmission. Decrease aqueous fluid production and sometimes causes pupillary constriction.

adrenergic stimulating agents (also known as sympathomimetic drugs): mimic action of the sympathetic nervous system. Open the anterior chamber angle to increase aqueous outflow, decrease aqueous secretion, and help nerve transmission.

carbonic anhydrase inhibitors: systemically and topically administered drugs that decrease aqueous production and secretion.

miotics (also known as cholinergic stimulating agents, parasympathomimetic drugs): mimic actions of parasympathetic nerves by simulating acetylcholine chemically. Cause small pupils (miosis), increase aqueous outflow, and open trabecular meshwork.

osmotic agents: increase osmotic pressure in blood and tissues to draw fluid from the eye.

prostaglandin analogues: increase ease of aqueous outflow from the eye.

Glaucon (GLAW-kahn). *Drug.* Trade name of epinephrine; for treating glaucoma.

glaucoma suspect, ocular hypertensive. Patient whose intraocular pressure is elevated above 21 mm of mercury, with no obvious optic nerve damage or visual field defects. May or may not develop glaucoma with time.

glaucomatocylitic crisis (glah/ou-koh-muh-toh-si-KLIH-tik), **Posner-Schlossman syndrome**. *Pathologic condition.* Uveal inflammation, usually of one eye, resulting in an acute increase in intraocular pressure. Characterized by corneal swelling, decreased aqueous outflow, and an open anterior chamber angle. See also SECONDARY GLAUCOMA.

glaukomflecken (GLAH/OU-kohm-flekn). *Clinical sign.* Pale opacities on the front lens surface; may be a residual of acute angle closure glaucoma.

Glauctabs. *Drug.* Trade name of methazolamide pills, for treating glaucoma.

glia (GLEE-uh), **neuroglia.** *Anatomy.* Supporting cells of the central nervous system. Two types: astroglia, oligodendroglia.

glioma (glee-OH-muh). *Pathologic condition.* Tumor derived from neuroglial components.

> **optic nerve glioma**: slow-growing, non-malignant congenital tumor of the optic nerve or optic chiasm composed of glial supportive cells. Often presents with eye protrusion (proptosis), enlarged optic foramen and decreased vision. Often seen with neurofibromatosis. See also HAMARTOMA.

glipizide. *Drug.* For controlling blood sugar levels in diabetics. Trade name: Glucotrol. See also GLYBURIDE, TOLAZAMIDE, TOLBUTAMIDE.

globe, eyeball. *Anatomy.* Spherical sense organ that receives light imagery and transmits the visual information to the brain. Composed of three major structural layers (corneo-sclera, uvea and retina) and includes the lens, aqueous and vitreous.

Glucotrol. *Drug.* Trade name of glipizide; for controlling diabetes.

gluttata. Incorrect spelling of GUTTATA.

glyburide. *Drug.* For controlling blood sugar levels in diabetics. Trade names DiaBeta, Micronase. See also GLIPIZIDE, TOLAZAMIDE, TOLBUTAMIDE.

glycerin (GLIS-ur-un), **glycerol.** *Drug.* Sweet tasting agent used as an oral osmotic for lowering intraocular pressure in acute glaucoma. Trade names: Glyrol, Osmoglyn.

glycerol. See GLYCERIN.

Glyrol. *Drug.* Trade name of glycerine; for treating an acute glaucoma attack.

goblet cells. *Anatomy.* Large, superficial mucous glands in the conjunctiva that secrete mucin, which contributes to the pre-corneal tear film, moistening and protecting the conjunctiva and cornea. Absent or damaged in dry eye syndrome.

gold deposits, chrysiasis. *Pathologic condition.* Gold deposits in the eye, especially in the corneal and conjunctival epithelium. See also ARGYROSIS.

Goldenhar's syndrome, oculo-auriculo-vertebral dysplasia. *Congenital anomaly.* Characterized by ear and spine deformities, small jaw, and sometimes deafness. Associated eye findings include unilateral conjunctival and corneal dermoids, eyelid colobomas, and Duane's retraction syndrome.

Goldmann applanation tonometer (GOLD-mahn). *Instrument.* Measures intraocular pressure by flattening the cornea a small fixed amount. Usually attaches to a slit lamp.

Goldmann perimeter. *Instrument.* Bowl-like device for testing visual fields. Luminous kinetic targets of different sizes and intensities are projected onto standardized background illumination. Not computerized.

goniolens (GOH-nee-oh-lenz), **gonioscope.** *Optical device.* Specialized contact lens used for examining anterior chamber angle structures. See also KOEPPE LENS, THREE MIRROR LENS.

goniophotocoagulation (GOH-nee-oh-FOH-toh-koh-ag-yu-LAY-shun), **laser gonioplasty *(or)* trabeculoplasty.** *Surgical procedure.* Application of a laser beam to selectively burn trabecular meshwork area, to lower intraocular pressure. Used for treating open angle and neovascular glaucoma.

goniopuncture (GOH-nee-oh-punk-chur). *Surgical procedure.* Making a small opening in the trabecular meshwork for draining aqueous fluid into a subconjunctival filtration bleb. Used for treating congenital glaucoma.

gonioscope (GOH-nee-uh-skohp). See GONIOLENS.

gonioscopy (goh-nee-AHS-koh-pee). *Test.* Examination of the anterior chamber angle through a contact lens, using a slit lamp or modified hand-held microscope. See also GONIOLENS.

Goniosol (GOH-nee-oh-sol). *Drug.* Trade name of methylcellulose, used as a fluid bridge between the cornea and an examination contact lens, e.g., a goniolens.

goniosynechiae (GOH-nee-oh-sin-EE-kee-uh), **peripheral anterior synechia**. *Pathologic condition.* Abnormal adhesion binding the front surface of the peripheral iris to the back surface of the cornea, usually near the anterior chamber angle. Sign of previous iris inflammation. May cause glaucoma by blocking aqueous outflow through the anterior chamber angle. See also SYNECHIA.

goniotomy (goh-nee-AHT-uh-mee). *Surgical procedure.* Incision made in the trabecular meshwork. Used for treating congenital glaucoma.

    "blind": indicates there is no clear visualization of angle structures, e.g., when obscured by a cloudy cornea.

gonorrheal ophthalmia, ophthalmia neonatorum. *Pathologic condition.* Severe eye infection (gonococcal) of newborn infants acquired from the birth canal. Ophthalmia neonatorum is the preferred term. See also CREDE'S PROPHYAXIS.

Gradenigo's syndrome (grad-en-EE-gohz). *Pathologic condition.* Characterized by a 6th (abducens) cranial nerve palsy, which prevents the lateral rectus muscle from pulling the eye outward (away from nose), and unilateral headache. Occasionally involves the 7th (facial) cranial nerve. May follow middle ear infection.

graft. 1. *Surgical procedure.* Transfer of living tissue. 2. Donor eye tissue used for corneal transplants or for patching the sclera.

    autograft: transfer to a new site on the same individual.

    homograft: transfer from one individual to another.

gram-negative bacteria. *Microorganism.* Bacteria (e.g., *Pseudomonas*) that stain pink when Gram stain is applied.

gram-positive bacteria. *Microorganism.* Bacteria (e.g., *Streptococcus*) that stain dark blue when Gram stain is applied.

Gram stain. *Test.* Chemical solution applied to corneal and conjunctival tissue samples to detect and differentiate bacteria. Stains pink for negative (gram-negative), blue for positive (gram-positive). Used in all medical disciplines.

granular corneal dystrophy (DIS-truh-fee), **Groenouw type I dystrophy**. *Pathologic condition.* Corneal disorder with crumb-like, milky hyaline proteinaceous opacities in the corneal stroma. Does not usually affect vision; if it does, may require a corneal graft. Hereditary (dominant); begins in childhood.

granuloma (gran-yu-LOH-muh). *Pathologic condition.* Dense collection of cells (sometimes creating a nodule) consisting of various inflammatory types, including epithelioid, lymphoid and giant cells. May be associated with sarcoid, tuberculosis, syphilis, and some foreign bodies.

granulomatous uveitis (gran-yu-LOH-muh-tus yu-vee-I-tis). *Pathologic condition.* Non-purulent, chronic uveal inflammation characterized by cells and protein in the anterior chamber, fatty deposits on the back surface of the cornea, choroidal and retinal inflammation, dilated conjunctival vessels, ciliary flush, and small, irregular pupils; little pain or light sensitivity, no discharge. Causes include syphilis, tuberculosis, sarcoid, toxoplasmosis. See also BUSACCA NODULES, KOEPPE NODULES, "MUTTON FAT" KP'S.

graticule (GRAT-uh-kyul), **reticle, reticule**. *Measuring device.* Grid or scale in the eyepiece of some optical instruments (e.g., microscope, lensometer) as an aid to focusing, measuring or counting.

Graves' disease, Basedow's disease, endocrine *(or)* **Graves' exophthalmos** *(or)* **ophthalmopathy, thyroid eye disease, thyrotoxic** *(or)* **thyrotropic exophthalmos**. *Pathologic condition.* Eye signs that may occur with excessive thyroid-related hormone concentration. Includes eyelid retraction, eyelid lag on downward gaze, corneal drying, eye bulging (proptosis), fibrotic extraocular muscles, and optic nerve inflammation. See also DALRYMPLE'S SIGN, STELLWAG'S SIGN, VON GRAEFE SIGN.

Gray (Gy). *Measurement.* Unit of radiation, equal to 100 rads.

gray line, intra-marginal sulcus. *Anatomy.* Line that divides eyelid margins into outer and inner halves, separating eyelid skin from conjunctival mucous membrane. Eyelashes are positioned in front of the line, tarsal gland ducts behind.

Groenouw dystrophy (GRU-noh DIS-truh-fee); also spelled Grönouw. *Pathologic condition.* Rare corneal stromal disorder. Accumulation of opaque deposits in the cornea may produce a slowly progressive decrease in vision. Hereditary; begins in childhood. Rare.

>   **type I (granular corneal)**: characterized by crumb-like, milky hyaline proteinaceous opacities in the corneal stroma. Does not usually affect vision; if it does, may require a corneal graft.

>   **type II (macular corneal)**: characterized by a slowly progressive decrease in vision caused by an accumulation of opaque deposits (mucopolysaccharides) in the corneal cells.

Grönblad-Strandberg syndrome (GRIN-blat), **pseudo-xanthoma elasticum.** *Pathologic condition.* Elastic connective tissue disorder that gives skin a leathery quality and causes defects in major arteries. Eye findings include a network of pigmented lines (angioid streaks) under the retina due to damage in Bruch's membrane, and macular hemorrhages and scarring. Hereditary.

guanethidine (gwahn-ETH-ih-deen). *Drug.* Sympatholytic drug for treating hypertension. Also relieves eyelid retraction in thyroid eye disease and lowers intraocular pressure in glaucoma. Trade name: Ismelin.

Gullstrand's reduced eye (GOOL-strandz). *Optics.* Simplified geometrical drawing of the eye that serves as a model for teaching optical concepts. See also SCHEMATIC EYE.

Gunderson flap. *Surgical procedure.* Thin conjunctival overlay graft used for treating ulcerative corneal disease and corneal perforation.

Gunn pupil, Marcus-Gunn pupil, afferent *(or)* **relative afferent pupillary defect.** *Functional defect.* Diminished pupil reaction to light, usually secondary to optic nerve disease that causes slowed conduction in optic nerve fibers. In dim illumination, a sudden bright light stimulus to the normal eye will result in both pupils contracting briskly. When the light stimulus is shifted to the defective eye, the pupils contract less well, so they appear to enlarge. See also SWINGING FLASHLIGHT TEST.

Gunn's dots. *Clinical finding.* Tiny, bright metallic-looking dots, occasionally seen around the disc and macula during ophthalmoscopic examination. Represent light reflections from normally dimpled retinal surface.

Gunn syndrome, external pterygoid levator synkinesis, jaw winking *(or)* **Marcus-Gunn jaw winking syndrome.** *Congenital defect.* Droopy eyelid (ptosis) that opens wide when patient chews, sucks or moves mouth to the opposite side. Caused by abnormal innervation of the levator muscle by the 5th (trigeminal) cranial nerve.

guttata (gu-TAH-tuh). *Pathologic condition.* Small, whitish hyaline deposits on Descemet's membrane (on inner corneal surface). See also FUCHS' DYSTROPHY.

gyrate atrophy (JI-rayt). *Pathologic condition.* Rare disorder of amino acid metabolism that affects the choroid and retina in otherwise healthy adults. Degenerative patches begin near the equator and result in gradual loss of the visual field. Associated with night blindness, nearsightedness, and cataracts.

H

Haab's striae (hahbz STREE-uh). *Clinical sign.* Breaks or tears in Descemet's membrane (corneal layer). Associated with congenital glaucoma.

Haidinger brush (HI-din-jur). *Test.* Entopic phenomenon that is useful for examination and treatment of amblyopia and non-central (eccentric) fixation. Slowly rotating polarized filters create a propeller-like image that is visible to individuals with normal maculas.

Halberg clip. *Instrument.* Circular lens holder that clips onto a pair of eyeglasses. Used in refining a refraction.

Hallermann-Streiff syndrome, Francois syndrome, oculo-mandibulo-dyscephaly. *Congenital anomaly.* Bony deformity of the skull and face. Characterized by a bird-like face with small jaw and "parrot-beaked" nose, small eyes, dwarfism, congenital cataracts, and poor vision. Rare, hereditary. See also MANDIBULOFACIAL DYSOSTOSIS.

Haller's layer. *Anatomy.* Layer of large blood vessels in the outer choroid next to the sclera; forms part of the choroid.

halo. *Symptom.* Hazy ring around bright lights seen by some patients with a refractive error or optical defect (e.g., cataract, corneal swelling). See also ENTOPIC PHENOMENON.

hamartoma (ham-ahr-TOH-muh). *Congenital abnormality.* Non-cancerous tumor mass resulting from faulty embryonic development. Composed of cells normally found at that site. Example: cavernous hemangioma.

hand motion. See HAND MOVEMENT.

hand movement (HM). *Test.* Patient's ability to see movement of a waving hand at a specified distance, usually 1 ft. or less. Used when vision loss is too profound for counting fingers. See also LIGHT PERCEPTION.

Hand-Schuller-Christian disease. *Pathologic condition.* Characterized by overproduction of urine, forward displacement of eyes, and skull defects. Patient may exhibit optic nerve swelling and inability to move the eyes. Usually occurs by age 10.

haplopia. *Concept.* Perception of singleness generated when corresponding points in each retina are stimulated simultaneously.

haploscope (HAP-luh-skohp). *Instrument.* Presents separate visual targets to each eye simultaneously. Used in diagnosis and correction of binocular abnormalities. See also SYNOPTOPHORE, TROPOSCOPE.

haptic (HAP-tik). 1. Loop or foot of an intraocular lens implant that supports the lens against the iris. 2. Non-optical, supportive zone of a lenticular spectacle or contact lens.

Harada Ito (huh-RAH-duh EE-toh). *Surgical procedure.* Repositioning the anterior one-fourth of the superior oblique tendon, for reducing image tilt associated with 4th (trochlear) cranial nerve palsies.

Harada's syndrome, uveitis-vitiligo-alopecia-poliosis *(or)* **Vogt-Koyanagi-Harada syndrome.** *Pathologic condition.* Characterized by headache, hearing defect, hair loss, premature graying, patchy depigmentation of skin, lashes and retina, steamy corneas, vitreous opacities, and diffuse exudative choroiditis. Vision and hearing loss may occur, with incomplete recovery. Progressive; chronic. Rare; tends to affect young Italian or Japanese adults. See also POLIOSIS.

hard contact lens (HCL). *Optical device.* Rigid plastic lens that floats on the corneal tear film. Usually made of polymethyl methacrylate (PMMA). See also GAS PERMEABLE LENS, SOFT CONTACT LENS.

hard exudates (EKS-yu-daytz). *Pathologic condition.* Fat-like deposits in the retina caused by excessive vascular leakage and chronic, partial blockage of small retinal veins.

Hardy-Rand-Rittler plates (HRR). *Test charts.* Colored dots that appear as identifiable geometric figures (triangles, squares, circles); used for identifying color vision deficiencies. See also PSEUDO-ISOCHROMATIC CHART.

harmonious ARC (abnormal retinal correspondence). *Functional defect.* Binocular adaptation of the retinas to a long-standing eye deviation. The fovea of the straight (non-deviated) eye and a non-foveal point of the deviated eye (that corresponds to the deviation) work together, permitting single binocular vision of poor quality. See also NORMAL RETINAL CORRESPONDENCE, UNHARMONIOUS ARC.

Harrington-Flocks multiple pattern. *Test.* Screening device for the central visual field. Uses fluorescent dots of various sizes in different patterns on assorted plates. Obsolete.

Hashimoto's thyroiditis. *Pathologic condition.* Inflammitary thyroid disease that may have its basis in an autoimmune process. See also GRAVES DISEASE.

Hasner's valve, plica lacrimalis. *Anatomy.* Mucous membrane fold at the lower end of the nasolacrimal duct that prevents air from entering the lacrimal sac when the nose is blown.

Hassall-Henle bodies (HAS-ul-HEN-lee). *Degenerative change.* Small white hyaline outgrowths on Descemet's membrane, on the inside surface of the cornea at its periphery. Normal aging change. See also GUTTATA.

HATTS. *Lab test.* Blood test for syphilis.

HCTZ. *Drug.* Trade name of hydrochlorothiazide, a heart medication.

head tilt test, Bielschowsky head tilt test. For comparing eye deviations; the head is tilted to one shoulder, then the other, to distinguish between a truly weak vertical muscle in one eye and an apparently weak vertical muscle in the other eye. See also INHIBITIONAL PALSY OF THE CONTRALATERAL ANTAGONIST.

Healon (HEE-lon). *Drug.* Trade name for sodium hyaluronate, a thick, elastic gel. See also VISCOSURGERY.

heart attack, "coronary," myocardial infarction. *Pathologic condition.* Sudden blockage of a blood vessel that supplies nutrients to the heart. Results in death (infarction) of some of the heart muscle.

heat-treated lens. *Optical device.* Spectacle lens made safer by a hardening process. See also IMPACE RESISTANT LENS.

Heerfordt's disease (HEHR-fortz). *Pathologic condition.* Form of sarcoid disease characterized by iris, ciliary body and choroid inflammation (uveitis), fever, and parotid gland swelling.

Heimann-Bielschowsky phenomenon (HI-min-beel-SHA/O-skee). *Abnormal function.* Large, rhythmic up and down oscillations (nystagmus) that develop years after vision decreases in an eye. See also ANISOMETROPIC AMBLYOPIA, STRABISMIC AMBLYOPIA.

helicoid. *Description.* Spiral shaped; having a swirl-like pattern.

helicoid choroidopathy, serpiginous *(or)* geographic choroidopathy. *Pathologic condition.* Type of progressive, bilateral choroidal inflammation and degeneration that begins around the optic nerve head (peripapillary) and slowly, over months, extends in a creeping fashion.

HEMA (hydroxy-ethyl methacrylate). Plastic polymer used for making soft contact lenses. See also EDMA.

hemangioma (hee-man-jee-OH-muh). *Congenital abnormality.* Tumor comprised of blood vessels or vessel elements.

    capillary: composed of small dilated blood vessels. On the skin, it appears as small bright red spots.

    cavernous: deep purplish tumor composed of large vascular channels. Usually located in the eyelids or in the orbit above and behind the lids. Tends to regress somewhat with age.

hematocrit. *Lab test*. Measures quantity of blood cells as a percentage of total blood volume.

hematogenous (heem-uh-TAH-juh-nus). *Description*. Spread through the bloodstream.

heme (heem). *Anatomy*. Slang for blood.

hemeralopia (hem-ur-uh-LOH-pee-uh). *Symptom*. Vision that is normal in dim light which dramatically decreases in bright light.

hemi- Prefix: half.

hemianopia (hem-ee-uh-NOH-pee-uh). See HEMIANOPSIA.

hemianopsia (hem-ee-uh-NAHP-see-uh), **hemianopia**. *Functional defect*. Non-seeing area in the right or left half of the visual field.

hemifacial microsomia (hem-ee-FAY-shul mi-kroh-SOH-mee-uh). *Congenital abnormality*. Craniofacial asymmetry: half of the face is smaller than the other. Eye on affected side is smaller, deeper set in orbit and appears lower.

hemifacial spasm. *Pathologic condition*. Advanced form of essential blepharospasm, limited to one side of the face.

hemoglobin (HEE-moh-gloh-bin). *Anatomy*. Protein in red blood cells that carries oxygen from the lungs to the cells, and carries carbon dioxide from the cells to the lungs.

hemolytic glaucoma (hee-moh-LIT-ik glaw-KOH-muh). *Pathologic condition*. Secondary glaucoma that results from breakdown products of blood in the eye.

Hemophilus aegyptius (hee-MAH-fil-us ee-JIP-tee-us), **Koch-Weeks bacillus**. *Microorganism*. Gram-negative bacteria that causes an acute, pus-producing conjunctivitis.

hemoptysis (heem-AHP-tuh-sis). *Symptom*. Spitting or coughing up blood.

hemorrhage (HEM-rij). *Clinical sign*. Bleeding.

> **choroidal**: bleeding from ruptured choroidal blood vesssels after a sudden decrease in intraocular pressure; rare, serious complication of intraocular surgery that can result in the pushing out (extrusion) of intraocular contents through the surgical wound, with subsequent loss of vision. Also called expulsive.

hemorrhagic conjunctivitis (hem-ur-AJ-ik kun-junk-tih-VI-tus). *Pathologic condition*. Bright red patches of subconjunctival hemorrhages. Associated with some adenovirus infections.

hemorrhagic glaucoma (glaw-KOH-muh), **neovascular glaucoma**. *Pathologic condition*. Older term for severe, hard-to-control form of glaucoma that leads to a painful eye with high intraocular pressure, corneal swelling, and "cell and flare" in anterior chamber. Caused by abnormal new blood vessel formation (neovascularization) in and on the iris that extends over the trabecular meshwork and closes angle drainage structures. Associated with severe diabetic retinopathy and other problems that cause the blockage of retinal blood vessels, especially veins. See also RUBEOSIS IRIDES.

hemorrhagic retinopathy (ret-in-AHP-uh-thee), **"squashed tomato."** *Pathologic condition*. Massive intraretinal and nerve fiber layer hemorrhages with dilated and engorged veins (also swollen optic disc margins and retinal thickening). Caused by blockage of blood flow through the central retinal vein. Results in markedly decreased vision that rarely improves. May cause secondary glaucoma. Patients usually elderly. See also NEOVASCULAR GLAUCOMA, RUBEOSIS IRIDIS.

hemostasis (hee-moh-STAY-sis). Stoppage of bleeding.

Henle fiber layer (HEN-lee). *Anatomy*. Structure in the foveal area of retina where the axon fibers in the outer and inner plexiform layers run obliquely.

Henle's crypts. *Anatomy*. Microscopic pockets in the conjunctival fornices that, along with conjunctival goblet cells, secrete mucus into the tear film.

Henle's glands. *Anatomy*. Mucous membrane folds lined by epithelium. Part of the conjunctiva inside the eyelids.

hepato-lenticular degeneration (hep-AT-oh len-TIK-yu-lur), **Wilson's disease**. *Pathologic condition*. Characterized by abnormal copper accumulation. Causes brain cell and liver degeneration and copper deposits in the eye (Kayser-Fleisher ring in Descemet's membrane and sometimes a "sunflower" cataract). Rare; hereditary.

hepato-renal glycogenesis (REE-nul gli-koh-JEN-uh-sis), **Gierke's disease**. *Pathologic condition*. Characterized by the body's inability to store glycogen. Associated with cloudy corneal edges. Hereditary.

Herbert's pits. *Pathologic condition*. Small pit-like defects in the upper limbal edge of the cornea, caused by healed lymphoid follicles. Associated with trachoma.

hereditary. Genetic transmission of a quality or trait from parent to offspring.

heredopathia atactica polyneuritiformis (heh-reh-doh-PATH-ee-uh ay-TAK-tih-kuh pah-lee-nu-rih-tuh-FORM-is), **phylanic acid storage** *(or)* **Refsum's disease**. *Pathologic condition*. Enzymatic blockage of phytanic acid decomposition. Characterized by fatty acid accumulation, drop foot, increased cerebrospinal fluid, cerebral degeneration, inability to sleep, electrocardiogram changes, retinal pigment epithelium degeneration (causing defective dark adaptation and constricted visual fields), nystagmus, ptosis (droopy eyelids) and small pupils. Hereditary. See also RETINITIS PIGMENTOSA.

Hering's law. Innervation to one extraocular muscle to contract generates an equal innervation to contract its yoke muscle (muscle performing the same function in the other eye), e.g., right lateral rectus and left medial rectus. See also H_2S

herpes simplex virus (HSV). *Microorganism*. Virus that infects the nerves in the skin and mucous membranes. In the cornea it produces painful branch-like ulcers (dendritic keratitis). Frequently recurrent, causing corneal opacification. See also HERPETIC KERATITIS.

herpes zoster, shingles. *Pathologic condition*. Extremely painful, blisterlike skin lesions on the face, sometimes with inflammation of the cornea, sclera, ciliary body and optic nerve. Affects the 1st division (ophthalmic nerve) of the 5th (trigeminal) cranial nerve. Caused by the chickenpox virus.

herpetic keratitis (hur-PET-ik kehr-uh-TI-tis). *Pathologic condition*. Eye infection from herpes simplex virus. Results in recurrent corneal epithelial inflammations with branch-like lesions (dendritic keratitis), sometimes followed by formation of larger, irregularly shaped (geographic) ulcers. May progress to corneal stroma inflammation (disciform keratitis).

Herplex. *Drug*. Trade name of idoxuridine, anti-viral agent for treating herpetic corneal inflammations. See also HERPES SIMPLEX, HERPETIC KERATITIS.

Hess-Lees screen. *Instrument*. Test screen for recording relative positions of the eyes in the nine positions of gaze; used for diagnosing and documenting weak extraocular muscles. See also LANCASTER RED-GREEN.

heterochromia of iris (HET-ur-uh-KROH-mee-uh). *Anatomic defect*. Having a different color iris in each eye.

heterochromic uveitis (het-ur-uh-KROH-mik yu-vee-I-tis), **Fuchs' heterochromic cyclitis**. *Pathologic condition*. Unilateral, low grade inflammation of the ciliary body and iris; the iris appears lighter in color than in the other eye. Secondary cataract or glaucoma may develop.

heteronymous (het-ur-AHN-uh-mus). *Description*. Located on the opposite side. See also HOMONYMOUS.

heteronymous diplopia, crossed diplopia. *Symptom.* Double vision in which the image seen by the right eye appears to be to the left of the image seen by the left eye. Associated with outward eye deviation (exotropia). See also UNCROSSED DIPLOPIA.

heterophoria (het-ur-uh-FOR-ee-uh), **phoria.** *Functional defect.* Latent tendency of the eyes to deviate that is prevented by fusion. Thus, a deviation occurs only when a cover is placed over an eye; when uncovered, the eye straightens.

heterophoric position (het-ur-uh-FOR-ik), **dissociated** *(or)* **fusion-free position, physiologic position of rest.** *Function.* Position assumed by the eyes, relative to each other, when one eye is covered or its vision obstructed. See also PHORIA.

heterotopia, ectopia. *Pathologic condition.* Misplacement of parts. Commonly refers to dragged macula in ROP or other conditions that create retinal scars.

heterotropia (het-ur-uh-TROH-pee-uh), **deviation, squint, strabismus, tropia.** *Functional defect.* Eye misalignment caused by extraocular muscle imbalance: one fovea is not directed at the same object as the other. Present when both eyes are uncovered. See also PHORIA.

hippus (HIP-us). *Function.* Spasmodic, rhythmic dilating and contracting pupillary movements, particularly noticeable when pupil function is tested with a light. Usually normal.

Hirschberg test. Determines relative position of corneal light reflexes on both eyes, to allow estimation of a misaligned eye's deviation.

histiocytic lymphoma. *Pathologic condition.* Form of non-Hodgkins lymphoma. Malignant tumor of the immune system that affects the eye and central nervous system. Most commonly affects the posterior segment, producing bilateral chronic uveitis, vitritis, retinal bleeding, and cotton wool spots. Difficult to diagnose and often fatal. Seen in middle to old age. Previously called reticulum cell sarcoma.

histocompatibility. *Function.* State of mutual tolerance between tissues that allows them to be grafted effectively.

histoplasmosis (hiss-toh-plaz-MOH-sus). *Pathologic condition.* Fungus infection caused by inhalation of *Histoplasma capsulatum.* Effects begin in the lungs and spread to other organs. Eye findings occur years later and are characterized by small scattered choroidal and pigment epithelial scars ("punched out" lesions), irregular pigment changes around the optic disc, and a central lesion at or near the macula (initially a gray-green spot; eventually results in retinal swelling and hemorrhage with visual distortion and loss). See also HISTO SPOTS, PRESUMED OCULAR HISTOPLASMOSIS SYNDROME.

histo spots (HISS-toh). *Clinical sign.* Small "punched out" lesions, usually without a pigmented border, representing pigment epithelial and chorioretinal scars. Sign of ocular histoplasmosis.

HLA (human leukocyte antigens). *Anatomy.* Series of genetically determined antigens (carried on surfaces of white blood cells) that are related to tissue compatibility and help account for acceptance or rejection of transplanted tissue. Some are associated with uveitis.

HLA typing. *Test.* Classification of histocompatibility of the antigens found on nucleated cells. Differences among types influence graft rejections.

Hobb's striae. Incorrect spelling of HAAB'S STRIAE.

Hollenhorst plaque. *Clinical sign.* Orange-yellow cholesterol clump, usually found at branching sites of retinal arterioles. Rare cause of blood vessel blockage. Associated with severe atherosclerosis of the carotid arteries, from which they usually arise.

Holmgren's test. Color vision test for industrial use; requires patient to match strands of colored yarn.

homatropine (hoh-MAT-roh-peen). *Drug.* Cycloplegic eyedrop that blocks parasympathetic nerves, producing pupillary enlargement and paralysis of focusing ability (accommodation). Similar to atropine, but less active. Effect lasts 2–4 days.

homeostasis (hoh-mee-oh-STAY-sis). *Function.* Various processes that work to maintain a stable environment within the body, such as for keeping temperature and chemical composition within a narrow range for optimal biological functioning.

Homer-Wright rosettes. *Pathologic change.* Microscopic rosette (histopathologic arrangement of cells) in retinoblastoma, with less differentiation than the Flexner-Wintersteiner rosette; the form is indistinguishable from the rosettes in neuroblastoma and medulloblastoma.

homocystinuria (hoh-moh-sis-ten-YU-ree-uh). *Congenital defect.* Metabolic disorder of excessive homocystine secretion into the urine (due to liver deficiency of the enzyme cystathionine synthetase). Characterized by mental retardation, seizures, blood clotting difficulties, lens dislocation, secondary glaucoma, cataracts, and peripheral retinal degeneration. Hereditary.

homograft. *Surgical procedure.* Transfer of living tissue from one individual to another. See also AUTOGRAFT.

homologous. *Description.* Corresponding in structure or position.

homonymous (hoh-MAHN-ih-mus). *Description.* Located on the same side.

homonymous diplopia (dih-PLOH-pee-uh), **uncrossed diplopia.** *Symptom.* Double vision in which the image from the right eye appears to be to the right of the left eye's image. Typically associated with an inturning eye (esotropia).

homonymous hemianopia (hem-ee-uh-NOH-pee-uh), **homonymous hemianopsia**. *Functional defect.* Visual field defect caused by a visual pathway abnormality behind the chiasm. Affects the same half of each eye's field.

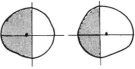

LEFT HOMONYMOUS HEMIANOPSIA

Honan balloon, Honan cuff. *Instrument.* Balloon-like device with a pressure gauge; may be used before surgery to press on the eye, to reduce intraocular pressure in a controlled way.

hook. *Surgical instrument.* Curved tool used for holding, lifting or pulling on tissue.

hordeolum (hor-DEE-oh-lum). *Pathologic condition.*

    external (stye): pustular infection of the oil glands of Zeis, located in the eyelash follicles at the eyelid margins.

    internal: infection or inflammation in a meibomian gland (of the eyelid). If chronic, it is called a chalazion.

horizontal cells. *Anatomy.* Retinal neurons in the inner nuclear layer that connect bipolar cells and cone cells and spread neural information within in the retina.

horizontal gaze center, pontine gaze center, paramedian pontine reticular formation. *Anatomy.* Region near the center of the brainstem (in the pons) at the level of the 6th (abducens) cranial nerve nucleus; believed to organize and integrate saccades (fast, horizontal parallel eye movements).

horizontal meridian. *Optics.* Position of the plane that divides the eyeball into upper and lower halves. Referred to as the 0° or 180° meridian.

horizontal nystagmus (ni-STAG-mus). *Abnormal function.* Involuntary, simultaneous, rhythmic side-to-side movements of both eyes.

horizontal raphe (ruh-FAY). *Anatomy.* Dividing line on the temporal retina between the upper and lower nerve fiber layer patterns. Corresponds to a horizontal line on the nasal side of the visual field.

horizontal strabismus. *Functional defect.* Inward or outward eye misalignment. See also ESOTROPIA, EXOTROPIA.

horizontal tightening procedure. *Surgical procedure*. For horizontally shortening a lower eyelid that does not rest against the eyeball (ectropion). Examples: Bick procedure, pentagonal excision, "lazy T" procedure.

Horner's syndrome. *Pathologic condition*. Constricted pupil (miosis), droopy eyelid (ptosis) and reduced facial sweating (anhydrosis), usually on one side of the face. Caused by damage to sympathetic nerves to the head. See also CESTAN'S SYNDROME, RAEDER'S SYNDROME.

horopter (hor-AHP-tur). Imaginary figure in space that contains all object points whose images fall on corresponding retinal points when a central object point is imaged on both foveae.

horror fusionis. *Clinical sign*. The avoidance of bifoveal fixation.

horseshoe tear. *Pathologic condition*. Crescent-shaped retinal tear. Most common type associated with retinal detachment.

HOTV. *Test chart*. Uses these four letters for assessing vision in pre-school children. Responses consist of matching an identified letter with the same letter on a card.

Howard-Dolman apparatus. *Instrument*. Long box containing two vertical rods. Patient tries to place one rod at same distance from the eyes as the other rod. Used for evaluating binocular depth perception.

Hruby lens (RU-bee). *Instrument*. Lens of −55 diopters that neutralizes the optical power of the cornea, to enable the examiner to view the vitreous and retina with illumination and magnification. Attaches to slit lamp.

H₂S. Mnemonic: Hering's law applies to innervation of extraocular muscles in 2 eyes while Sherrington's law refers to innervation of extraocular muscles in 1 eye.

Hudson-Stahli line. *Pathologic condition*. Linear, brown sub-epithelial iron pigment deposit in the cornea.

hue. *Optics*. Aspect of color that gives it its name. For spectral colors, correlates with the wavelength of the visual stimulus.

Hughes procedure. *Surgical procedure*. Two-step technique for reconstructing the inner or central section of the lower eyelid. Section of tarsus and conjunctiva from the upper lid is dissected on three sides and pulled down to fill the defect. Tissue is shared for a few months, then surgically separated. See also CUTLER-BEARD PROCEDURE.

human leukocyte antigens. See HLA.

Hummelsheim procedure (HUM-ul-shime). *Surgical procedure*. For helping correct a lateral rectus palsy; the inferior and superior rectus muscles are split, with half of each muscle reattached beside the lateral rectus insertion. See also JENSEN PROCEDURE.

Humorsol. *Drug*. Trade name of demecarium bromide, anticholinesterase eyedrops. Used rarely for treating glaucoma.

Humphrey Analyzer. *Instrument*. Trade name of a bowl-shaped automated perimeter; works with a computerized program to map field of vision.

Hunter syndrome. *Pathologic condition*. Metabolic dysfunction characterized by skeletal abnormalities, mental retardation and cloudy corneas, all appearing after age 30. Mucopolysaccharidosis (Type II) from deficiency in enzyme iduronidate sulfate sulfatase. Hereditary.

Hurler's syndrome, gargoylism. *Pathologic condition*. Characterized by severe skeletal abnormalities, dwarfism, short spinal column, short fingers, depressed bridge of nose, joint stiffness, heart problems, severe mental retardation, retinal degeneration and corneal clouding. Form of mucopolysaccharidosis caused by enzyme alpha-L-iduronidase deficiency. Hereditary.

Hutchinson's pupil. *Functional defect*. Fixed dilated pupil that occurs with 3rd (oculomotor) cranial nerve compression, usually from increasing intracranial pressure.

Hutchinson's sign. *Sign.* Small lesions on side of nose seen in herpes zoster ophthalmicus. Characteristic of involvement of the nasociliary branch of the ophthalmic division of the 5th (trigeminal) cranial nerve.

Hutchinson's triad. *Pathologic condition.* Three signs of congenital syphilis: ghost vessels in inner corneal layers, notched permanent teeth and incisors with narrow edges lacking an enamel coating, and nerve deafness.

hyaline masses (HI-uh-lin), **disc drusen**. *Pathologic condition.* Glistening nodules within the optic nervehead. May blur disc margins. Sometimes mistaken for chronic papilledema.

hyalitis (hi-uh-LI-tus), **vitritis**. *Clinical sign.* Inflammatory intraocular reaction (with clouding and cells) in the vitreous. Often accompanies inflammation of the ciliary body, iris, choroid or retina.

hyalocytes. *Anatomy.* Structural cells of the vitreous.

hyaloid artery (HI-uh-loyd). *Embryology.* Branch of the dorsal ophthalmic artery that nourishes the lens during embryologic development. Disintegrates before birth.

hyaloid canal, Cloquet's canal. *Anatomy.* Pathway within the vitreous that extends from the optic disc to the lens. In the fetus, contains the hyaloid artery, which disappears before birth, though canal remains. See also PHPV.

hyaloideo-capsular ligament, Egger's line, Weiger's ligament. *Anatomy.* A weak line of adherence between the anterior vitreous and the posterior surface of the lens, in the form of a ring 8–9 mm in diameter.

hyaloid membrane. *Anatomy.* Membranous sheets of condensation within the vitreous.

> **anterior**: front surface layer; extends from the ora serrata to a ringlike insertion on the back of the lens. Separates vitreous from aqueous in the posterior chamber.

> **posterior (PHM)**: back surface layer that is firmly attached to the internal surface of the retina (limiting membrane).

hyaluronidase (hi-el-yu-RON-ih-dace). *Chemical.* Enzyme that is added to anesthetic agents to hasten and spread their effect. See also WYDASE.

hyaluronate (sodium). *Drug.* Thick elastic gel used during eye surgery to help stabilize structures in their normal positions and protectively coat them. Trade names: Amvisc, Healon. See also VISCOELASTIC AGENT.

Hydeltrasol (hi-DEL-truh-sol). *Drug.* Trade name of prednisolone, an anti-inflammatory steroid.

hydraulic retinal reattachment. *Surgical procedure.* The use of air fluid gas exchange in repair of a retinal detachment, to push the retina back into place (by exerting pressure from inside the eye).

hydrochlorothiazide. *Drug.* Heart medication that increases urination so that excess body fluid is removed. May cause retinal hemorrhages. Trade name: HCTZ. See also CHLOROTHIAZIDE, FUROSEMIDE.

hydrocortisone, cortisone. Drug. Steroid medication used for treating inflammatory and allergic diseases.

hydrogel. Rigid plastic used in the manufacture of contact lenses and intraocular lenses.

hydrogel lens (HI-droh-jel). See HYDROPHILIC LENS.

hydrogen peroxide sterilization. Method of sterilizing soft contact lenses.

Hydronol. *Drug.* Trade name of isosorbide; for lowering intraocular pressure.

hydrophilic (hi-droh-FIL-ik). *Characteristic.* Combines with, or attracts, water. See also HYDROPHOBIC.

hydrophilic lens, hydrogel lens. *Optical device.* Soft contact lens that absorbs and binds with water. Made from various plastic polymers.

hydrophobic (hi-droh-FOH-bik). *Characteristic.* Repels water; will not mix with water. See also HYDROPHILIC.

hydrophthalmos, buphthalmos. *Pathologic condition.* Abnormally large eyeball ("ox-eye") caused by glaucoma in a young, stretchable eye. See also CONGENITAL GLAUCOMA, MACROPHTHALMOS, MEGOPHTHALMOS.

hydrops (HI-drahps), **corneal hydrops**. *Pathologic condition.* Sudden, abnormal fluid accumulation within corneal tissue, resulting in clouded vision. Seen in keratoconus.

hydropic degeneration. *Pathologic condition.* Glycogen accumulation in pigmented iris epithelium. Associated with diabetes.

hydroxyamphetamine (hi-DRAHKS-ee-am-FET-uh-meen). *Drug.* Eyedrop that stimulates sympathetic nerves, causing mild pupillary dilation. Used as aid in diagnosis of Horner's syndrome. Trade name: Paredrine.

hydroxyapatite. Porous material modified from coral reefs. Sometimes used as an orbital implant to replace an enucleated eyeball.

hydroxychloroquine (hi-DRAHKS-ee-KLOR-uh-kwin). *Drug.* Used in treating malaria, lupus erythematosus and rheumatoid arthritis. May cause pigment clumping in macular area and result in visual loss. Trade name: Plaquenil.

hydroxy-ethyl methacrylate (hi-DRAHK-see, meth-AK-ril-ayt). See HEMA.

hydroxypropylmethylcellulose (hi-DRAHK-see-PROH-pil-METH-ul-SEL-yu-lohs). *Drug.* Form of methylcellulose viscoelastic. Trade name: Occucoat.

hyper- Prefix: above, higher, or excessive.

hyperemia (hi-pur-EE-mee-uh). *Clinical sign.* Increased blood flow. Usually refers to eye redness caused by congestion of conjunctival blood vessels. See also INJECTION.

hyperfluorescence. *Clinical sign.* In a fluorescein angiogram, increased fluorescence. Can result from abnormal blood vessels, leaking vessels, or increased fluorescein transmission.

hyperlipoproteinemia (HI-pur-LI-poh-proh-tih-NEE-mee-uh). *Pathologic condition.* Abnormality of fat (lipid) metabolism. Associated with milky colored retinal vessel blood (lipemia retinalis), pinkish choroid, yellowish lipid deposits along the corneal edge (limbus) and in the skin near the nose, and systemic artery abnormalities.

hypermature cataract, Morgagnian cataract. *Pathologic change.* Totally opaque lens that has begun to shrink and liquify, so that the remaining hard nucleus floats about within the lens capsule. Degraded lens protein molecules may leak into the aqueous through the lens capsule. See also PHACOLYTIC GLAUCOMA.

hypermetropia (hi-pur-muh-TROH-pee-uh). See HYPEROPIA.

hyperopia (hi-pur-OH-pee-uh), **farsightedness, hypermetropia.** *Refractive error.* Focusing defect in which an eye is underpowered. Thus light rays coming from a distant object strike the retina before coming to sharp focus; true focus is said to be "behind the retina." Corrected with additional optical power, which may be supplied by a plus lens (spectacle or contact) or by excessive use of the eye's own focusing ability (accommodation).

    absolute: cannot be neutralized completely by accommodation.

    axial: caused by abnormal shortness of the eye's anteroposterior diameter.

    facultative: same as MANIFEST (below).

    high: measures 6 diopters or more.

    index (subgroup of refractive hyperopia): caused by decrease in the index of refraction of the eye's lens. Usually associated with diabetes or aging.

    latent: portion of total hyperopia that cannot be relaxed with plus lenses. The difference between manifest and total hyperopia, not apparent to the individual. Identified by cycloplegia.

    manifest: amount indicated by the strongest convex spectacle or contact lens a patient will accept while retaining his best visual acuity.

    refractive: caused by relatively low optical power of the eye.

    total: entire amount of hyperopia (latent and manifest).

hyperopic (hi-pur-AHP-ik). *Description.* Farsighted.

hyperopic astigmatism. *Refractive error.* Optical defect in which light rays entering the eye are bent unequally in different meridians, preventing a sharp focus on the retina. The rays form two focal lines perpendicular to each other. Corrected by a cylindrical (toric) eyeglass or contact lens.

    simple: one focal line forms on the retina and the other forms behind the retina.

    compound: both focal lines form behind the retina.

hyperphoria (H) (hi-pur-FOR-ee-uh). *Function.* Tendency toward upward deviation that occurs only when the eye is covered; when uncovered, the eye straightens. See also HYPERTROPIA.

hyperplasia (hi-pur-PLAY-zhuh). *Anatomic defect.* Increased number of one type of cell. Associated with increased frequency of cell division.

hypertelorism (hi-pur-TEE-lur-izm). *Congenital anomaly.* Abnormally wide distance between the bony orbits, resulting in the eyes being widely separated. Often associated with mental deficiency and an outward eye deviation (exotropia). See also TELECANTHUS.

hypertensive retinopathy. *Pathologic condition.* Retinal changes that accompany high blood pressure. May include narrow arterioles, dull light reflections from blood vessel surfaces ("copper wiring"), vein irregularities, nicking where arteries cross veins, flame-shaped retinal hemorrhages, cotton-wool spots, and optic disc swelling when the process is advanced.

hyperthyroidism (hi-pur-THI-royd-izm). *Pathologic condition.* Neuromuscular changes and increased tissue metabolism caused by excessive thyroid hormone concentration. Common signs include fatigue, weight loss (in spite of increased appetite), fine tremors, excessive sweating, and a rise in blood pressure. If eye signs occur (lid lag, lid retraction, strabismus), the disorder is called Basedow's disease, Graves' disease, endocrine exophthalmos, endocrine ophthalmopathy, thyrotoxic exophthalmos or thyrotropic exophthalmos.

hypertonic. *Characteristic.* Refers to a solution that contains salts more concentrated than normally found in the body.

hypertonic saline, hypertonic sodium chloride. *Drug.* Salt water of higher concentration (usually about 5%) than "normal" saline (0.9%). Used in ointment for dehydrating a cornea that is swollen with water in diseases that damage the endothelial water pump system, e.g., Fuchs' dystrophy. Trade name: Absorbonac.

hypertrophy (hi-PUR-truh-fee). *Anatomic defect.* Increased size of one type of cell leading to enlargement of a cell, tissue, or organ.

hypertropia (HT) (hi-pur-TROH-pee-uh). *Abnormal function.* Upward deviation of one eye while the other remains straight and fixates normally. See also HYPERPHORIA.

RIGHT HYPERTROPIA

hyperviscosity syndrome (hi-pur-vis-KAHS-ih-tee). *Pathologic condition.* Group of systemic problems associated with abnormally viscid (thick) blood, which slows blood flow. Causes retinopathy in both eyes, with dilated veins, retinal hemorrhages, and ischemia.

hypervitaminosis A. *Pathologic condition.* Caused by excessive vitamin A. May result in thickened dry skin over the body. May be associated with orbital swelling (pseudo-tumor) and a swollen optic nerve.

hypervitaminosis D. *Pathologic condition.* Caused by excessive vitamin D. Abnormal calcium deposits may occur in many body organs and tissues, including the conjunctiva and cornea.

hypesthesia (hi-piz-THEE-zhuh). *Symptom.* Impaired or decreased sensitivity to touch, as caused by damage to the nerve supplying that region.

hyphema (hi-FEE-muh). *Clinical sign.* Blood in the anterior chamber, such as following blunt trauma to the eyeball.

hypo- Prefix: below, lower, deficient.

hypofluorescence. *Clinical sign.* In a fluorescein angiogram, decreased fluorescence. Can result from blocked blood vessels, decreased blood flow, or fewer vessels for the fluorescein to flow through.

hypophysectomy. *Surgical procedure.* Removal of the pituitary gland.

hypophysis (hi-PAH-fih-sis), **pituitary body.** *Anatomy.* Master gland of the body that makes several hormones and controls activity of other glands. Hangs sac-like from the base of the brain, between and behind the orbits and below the optic chiasm. See also SELLA TURCICA.

hypoplasia (hi-poh-PLAY-zhuh). *Congenital anomaly.* Incomplete development of a tissue or organ.

hypoplastic disc (hi-poh-PLAS-tik). *Congenital defect.* Small optic disc. May or may not cause poor vision or be associated with other eye or brain malformations.

hypopyon (hi-POH-pee-un). *Pathologic condition.* Accumulation of pus in the anterior chamber.

HypoTears. *Drug.* Trade name of polyvinyl alcohol eyedrops or ointment; for relieving dry eye symptoms.

hypotony (hi-PAH-tuh-nee). *Functional defect.* Low intraocular pressure often related to chronic intraocular inflammation (uveitis), wound leaks after eye surgery, or a retinal detachment. Prolonged low pressure can lead to irregular choroidal and retinal pigment epithelium folding, engorged retinal vessels, and swollen optic discs.

hypotropia (hi-poh-TROH-pee-uh). *Functional defect.* Downward deviation of one eye while the other remains straight and fixates normally.

LEFT HYPOTROPIA

hypoxia (hi-PAHK-see-uh). *Pathologic condition.* Oxygen deficiency in any body tissue. See also ANOXIA.

hysterical amblyopia (am-blee-OH-pee-uh). *Psychological disorder.* Apparent vision loss in eye(s) that have normal visual potential; patient believes he cannot see. See also MALINGERER.

hysterical field. *Functional defect, psychological disorder.* Visual field abnormalities, usually in both eyes, that have a psychological or emotional cause. The result is a tunnel field (normal central vision, constricted periphery); may constrict during the test, producing a spiral field.

I

iatrogenic (ee-at-roh-JEN-ik). *Description.* Refers to an adverse condition inadvertently caused by a physician as a result of a treatment or diagnostic procedure.

ICE (irido corneal endothelial) syndrome. *Pathologic condition.* Anterior chamber disorder resulting in adhesions (from abnormal proliferation of corneal and iris endothelium) that bind the iris to the cornea, clogging drainage from the anterior chamber and producing a rise in intraocular pressure. See also CHANDLER'S SYNDROME, COGAN'S SYNDROME, ESSENTIAL IRIS ATROPHY.

icthyosis (ik-thee-OH-sis). *Pathologic condition.* Skin disorder; abnormal production of keratin (fingernail-like tissue) causes skin to be dry, scaly, and rough. May be accompanied by conjunctivitis, corneal opacities or cataracts.

idiopathic (id-ee-oh-PATH-ik). *Description.* Having an unknown cause; not derived from a recognized disease or treatment.

idiopathic arteritis of Takayasu (ar-tur-I-tis, tak-uh-YASH-oo), **pulseless *(or)* Takayasu's disease.** *Pathologic condition.* Inflammatory disorder of the large arteries, caused by obstruction. Characterized by insufficient blood flow reaching the brain, upper extremities and eyes. Most frequently affects children and young people.

idoxuridine (I-dahks-YUR-ih-deen). See IDU.

IDU (idoxuridine). *Drug.* Anti-viral eyedrops or ointment used for treating herpetic corneal infections. Trade names: Herplex, Stoxil. See also HERPES SIMPLEX, HERPETIC KERATITIS.

IgA. Immunoglobulin having antibody activity. Found in mucous tissues such as tears, saliva and nasal fluids.

Ig D. Immunoglobulin having antibody activity.

Ig E. Immunoglobulin having antibody activity; associated with allergic and hypersensitivity reactions.

IgG. Major immunoglobulin having antibody activity; associated with bacterial and viral infections.

IgM. Immunoglobulin having antibody activity; associated with bacterial and viral infections. Found largely in the bloodstream.

illiterate E, tumbling E. *Test.* The letter E presented in different sizes and rotated to different directions; used for testing visual acuity in illiterates and children who do not know the alphabet.

illuminance. *Optics.* Luminous flux (light) falling on a unit area of a surface.

Ilotysin (i-loh-TI-sin). *Drug.* Trade name of erythromycin ointment, an antibiotic.

image. Visual impression of an object formed by a lens or mirror.

　　false: in diplopia, the image arising in the deviating eye.

　　Purkinje: four sets of reflected images, from front and rear surfaces of the cornea and front and rear surfaces of the lens.

　　real: in optics, the image formed by converging light rays, which can be focused onto a screen.

　　true: in diplopia, the image received by the non-deviating eye.

　　virtual: in optics, an image created by light rays diverging from an optical system. These rays do not pass through image points, hence they cannot be focused directly onto a screen.

image displacement. *Optics.* Apparent displacement of an object from its true position when viewed through the peripheral portion of a spectacle lens, especially a high-powered lens.

image jump. *Optics*. Sudden movement of an image that occurs when prism power is abruptly introduced into an optical system, e.g., at the top edge of some bifocals. Occurs when gaze is shifted between the upper (distance) portion of a bifocal lens and the lower (reading) segment.

image point, focus. *Optics*. Point where light rays are brought to a sharp image point by a lens.

immature cataract. *Pathologic condition*. Cloudy lens that has some clear zones remaining. Vision loss depends on extent and density of clouding. See also CATARACT.

immune response. *Function*. The body's cellular and chemical response to protect itself from foreign proteins, microorganisms, parasites and toxins.

immune system. *Microanatomy*. Body's elaborate defense system against injury from foreign proteins, microorganisms, parasites, and toxins.

immunocompromised, immunosuppressed. *Description*. Refers to an immune system that has been weakened or impaired, as by illness (e.g., HIV) or drugs (unintentionally or intentionally) so as to help prevent organ transplant rejection or to treat cancer. This state markedly reduces the body's resistance to infection. Some immunosuppressants are azathioprine, cyclosporine, cyclophosphamide, dexamethasone, methotrexate, prednisone, tamoxifen.

immunoglobulin (Ig). *Anatomy*. One of five classes of protein (IgA, IgD, IgE, IgG, IgM) having specific antibody activities. Found in body fluids.

immunosuppressed. See IMMUNOCOMPROMISED.

impact-resistant lens. *Optical device*. Spectacle lens treated with a hot potassium salt solution to harden it and meet safety standards for impact resistance. See also HEAT-TREATED LENS.

implant.

    intraocular. *Optical device*. Plastic lens that is surgically implanted to replace the eye's natural lens. Also called intraocular lens (IOL) or pseudophakos.

    intrascleral. *Surgical device*. Foreign material (usually solid silicone or silicone sponges) sutured under a flap of sclera to indent the globe, to help seal a retinal break or tear. See also SCLERAL BUCKLE.

    orbital. Plastic or glass sphere placed in the eye socket after surgical removal of an eyeball. Buried under Tenon's capsule and conjunctiva. See also ENUCLEATION, PROSTHESIS.

Imuran. *Drug*. Trade name of azathioprine; for treating cancer.

incident ray. *Optics*. Any ray of light that strikes a substance.

incipient cataract. *Pathologic condition*. Cataract in its early stages, or one that has sectors of opacity with clear spaces intervening. Has little impact on visual acuity.

incise (in-SIZE). *Surgical technique*. To cut into, without removal. See also EXCISE.

incision (in-SIH-zhun). *Surgical procedure*. Cut into. See also EXCISION.

inclusion bodies. *Pathology*. Structures within certain body cells that indicate viral or chlamydial infection. Can be found in samples of conjunctival or corneal epithelial tissue.

incomitant strabismus (struh-BIZ-mus), **noncomitant strabismus**. *Functional defect*. Eye deviation whose amount varies in different positions of gaze.

incongrous (in-KAHN-gru-us). *Description*. Refers to dissimilarity (extent and intensity) of visual field loss in each eye.

incongruous field defects. *Functional defect*. Dissimilar visual field loss in the two eyes.

incontinentia pigmenti (in-kahn-tin-EN-shuh pig-MEN-ti). *Pathologic condition*. Skin pigmentation disorder associated with skeletal, dental, central nervous system and eye abnormalities. Eye signs include cataracts, optic atrophy, retrolental mass, and patchy, mottled, diffuse depigmented retin-opathy. Rare; hereditary.

incycloduction (in-si-kloh-DUK-shun), **intorsion**. *Function*. Rotation of an eye's 12 o'clock meridian toward the nose.

incyclovergence. *Function*. Rotation of the 12 o'clock meridians of both eyes toward the nose while maintaining single binocular vision.

indentation tonometer (tuh-NAHM-ih-tur). *Instrument*. Determines intraocular pressure from amount the cornea is indented by a fixed weight. Somewhat less accurate than an applanation tonometer. Trade name: Schiotz.

indentation tonometry (tuh-NAHM-ih-tree). *Test*. Determination of intraocular pressure by indenting the cornea with a known weight. See also SCLERAL RIGIDITY, TONOMETRY.

Inderal. *Drug*. Trade name of propanolol, heart medication.

index hyperopia (hi-pur-OH-pee-uh). *Refractive error*. Underpowered optical system of an eye caused by a decrease in index of refraction of its lens. Usually associated with diabetes or aging. Corrected with plus lenses.

index myopia (mi-OH-pee-uh). *Refractive error*. Overpowered optical system of an eye caused by an increase in index of refraction of its lens. Usually associated with diabetes or early cataract. Corrected with minus lenses.

index of refraction, refractive index. *Measurement*. Ratio of speed of light in a vacuum to the speed of light traveling through a particular substance. The greater the index, the more optical effect a material produces.

indirect ophthalmoscope (ahf-THAL-muh-skohp). *Instrument*. For visualizing the interior of the eye (fundus). Creates an inverted image of the fundus projected in front of the eye, with a wide field of view. Consists of a bright light source and a hand-held high-plus lens. Binocular model allows stereo-scopic depth perception of the retina. See also DIRECT OPHTHALMOSCOPE.

indocyanine green angiography (ICG). *Test*. Used for evaluating retinal, choroidal and iris blood vessels, as well as any eye problems affecting them. Indocyanine green dye is injected into an arm vein, then rapid, sequential photographs are taken of the eye as the dye circulates. Differs from fluorescein angiography in that ICG allows visualization of leaks under a layer of blood, which is opaque to fluorescein.

induced tropia test (ITT). For detection of fixation preference in non-mis-aligned eyes; a prism is used (10^Δ vertically or 25^Δ horizontally) to induce a misalignment in corneal reflex position.

infantile esotropia (ee-soh-TROH-pee-uh), **congenital esotropia**. *Functional defect*. Inward (toward nose) eye deviation seen at birth or within first 6 months. Usually a large misalignment that requires surgery to straighten the eyes; unaffected by eyeglasses. See also CROSS-FIXATION.

infantile glaucoma (glaw-KOH-muh), **congenital glaucoma**. *Congenital defect*. High intraocular pressure accompanied by hazy corneas and large eyes (buphthalmos) in the newborn, resulting from developmental abnor-malities in the anterior chamber angle that obstruct the intraocular fluid drainage mechanism. Characteristic symptoms are tearing, light sensitivi-ty (photophobia) and uncontrolled blinking (blepharospasm). Requires early surgical correction. See also CYCLO-CRYO, GONIOTOMY, TRABECULECTOMY AB EXTERNO.

infarct. *Pathologic condition*. Death of tissue from insufficient blood supply.

infection. *Pathologic condition*. Invasion of disease-producing microorgan-isms, resulting in localized cell injury, toxin secretion, or antigen-antibody reaction.

inferior. *Location*. On or near the lower part of an organ or of the body. See also SUPERIOR.

inferior arcade. *Anatomy.* Arch of the inferior temporal retinal arterioles and venules, leading from the optic disc and extending to the retinal periphery. See also SUPERIOR ARCADE.

inferior canaliculus (kan-uh-LIK-yu-lus). *Anatomy.* Part of the tear drainage system; thin duct in the lower eyelid near the nose, connecting the inferior punctum to the common canaliculus. Plural: canaliculi.

inferior colliculi. *Anatomy.* Pair of mounds on the roof of the midbrain. Contain centers for responses to sound. See also SUPERIOR COLLICULI.

inferior longitudinal fasiculus (fuh-SIK-yu-lus). *Anatomy.* Nerve fiber tract in the brain through which visual fibers from the association areas in the occipital cortex pass to the temporal lobe.

inferior nasal artery. *Anatomy.* One of the four main branches of the central retinal artery; nourishes the lower inner retinal quadrant from the optic disc to the ora serrata.

inferior nasal vein. *Anatomy.* One of four main tributaries of the central retinal vein; drains the lower inner retinal quadrant from the ora serrata to the optic disc.

inferior oblique (IO) (oh-BLEEK or oh-BLIKE). *Anatomy.* Extraocular muscle attached to the lower, outer side of the eyeball behind the equator. Three functions: extorsion (rotating top of eye away from nose, especially on outward movement), elevation (especially on inward movement); and abduction (outward eye movement). Innervated by the 3rd (oculomotor) cranial nerve.

inferior ophthaimic vein (off-THAL-mik). *Anatomy.* Blood vessel that drains the floor of the orbit back toward the cranial cavity. Receives tributaries from veins in the inferior and lateral extraocular muscles, conjunctiva and lacrimal sac, and two inferior vortex veins from the eye. Extends backward with the inferior rectus, joining the superior ophthalmic vein usually before exiting the orbit through the superior orbital fissure to the cavernous sinus.

inferior orbital fissure. *Anatomy.* Canal in the bony orbital floor behind the eye (at junction of the greater wing of the spheroid bone and the maxillary bone), through which pass the infraorbital nerve, zygomatic nerve and infraorbital artery.

inferior punctum, lower punctum. *Anatomy.* Tiny opening in the papilla (elevation on lower eyelid margin near nose). Marks the lower entrance site of tear drainage (lacrimal) system into the nose. See also SUPERIOR PUNCTUM.

inferior rectus (IR). *Anatomy.* Extraocular muscle attached to underside of the eyeball (globe). Three functions: depression (moves eye downward, especially when it is turned ou); extorsion (rotates eye outward, especially on inward gaze), and adduction (inward eye movement). Innervated by the 3rd (oculomotor) cranial nerve.

inferior temporal artery. *Anatomy.* One of four main branches of the central retinal artery. Nourishes the lower, outer retinal quadrant from the optic disc to the ora serrata.

inferior temporal vein. *Anatomy.* One of four main branches of the central retinal vein. Drains the lower outer retinal quadrant from the ora serrata to the optic disc.

inferonasal. *Location.* Situated below a reference position (e.g., the eyeball or optic disc) and toward the nose. See also SUPERONASAL.

inferotemporal. *Location.* Situated below a reference position (e.g., the eyeball or optic disc) and toward the ear. See also SUPEROTEMPORAL.

infiltrate (IN-fil-trayt). *Sign.* Abnormal accumulation of cells and fluid in tissue where they are not normally found (such as by tumor cells or inflammatory cells). See also EXUDATE.

infinity. *Optics.* Distance from which light rays arrive or leave in parallel bundles. For clinical purposes, this distance is 20 ft. (6 m) or greater.

Inflamase (IN-fluh-mayz). *Drug.* Trade name of prednisolone, an anti-inflammatory steroid.

inflammation, inflammatory response. *Pathologic condition.* Body's localized protective response to injury, infection or irritation by enclosing the involved area. Characterized by pain, heat, redness and swelling.

infraduction (IN-fruh-DUK-shun). *Function.* Movement of an eye downward from the straight-ahead position. See also DEORSUMVERSION, DEPRESSION.

infranuclear pathway (in-fruh-NU-klee-ur). *Anatomy.* Nerve fiber bundles that lead from a cranial nerve's nucleus in the brainstem to the eye and/or body. See also SUPRANUCLEAR PATHWAYS.

infraorbital artery (in-fruh-OR-bih-tul). *Anatomy.* Branch of the internal maxillary artery (which branches from the external carotid artery) that supplies blood to the inferior eyelid area. Enters the orbit through the inferior orbital fissure and exits through the infraorbital foramen.

infraorbital nerve. *Anatomy.* Branch of the maxillary nerve (2nd division of the 5th [trigeminal] cranial nerve) that enters the orbit through the inferior orbital fissure and exits through the infraorbital foramen. Some of its branches supply the skin and conjunctiva of the lower eyelid.

infrared radiation. *Optics.* Infrared portion of the electromagnetic spectrum that has a wavelength between about 750 -1,000 nm.

infusion-aspiration (I/A). See IRRIGATION-ASPIRATION.

inhibitional palsy of the contralateral antagonist. *Functional defect.* Confusing condition associated with long-standing extraocular muscle palsies. Weakness of the affected muscle allows its stronger, direct antagonist to overact when innervated normally, causing its yoke muscle (contralateral antagonist in the fellow eye) to appear weak (e.g., right superior oblique weakness mistaken for left superior rectus weakness).

injection. *Clinical sign.* Tissue redness and swelling from dilated blood vessels. Caused by infection or inflammation. See also HYPEREMIA.

inner canthus (KAN-thus), **medial canthus**. *Anatomy.* Angle formed by the inner (near nose) junction of upper and lower eyelids.

inner nuclear layer. *Anatomy.* Retinal region composed of bipolar, Mueller, horizontal, and amacrine cell bodies. See also OUTER NUCLEAR LAYER.

inner plexiform layer. *Anatomy.* Retinal region containing neural connections (synapses) between bipolar and amacrine cell axons and ganglion cell dendrites.

inner retina (RET-in-uh). *Anatomy.* Retinal layers that lie nearest the vitreous.

inner segment (of rods and cones). *Anatomy.* Section of a retinal photoreceptor cell (rod or cone) that contains an ellipsoid portion with mitochondria, and a myoid portion with a Golgi complex and ribosomes. Its function is not understood.

input nerve, afferent *(or)* sensory nerve. *Anatomy.* Nerve that carries impulses toward the brain or spinal cord, e.g., the 2nd (optic) cranial nerve. See also OUTPUT NERVE.

insertion. *Anatomy.* Site of attachment of a muscle to the tissue it moves.

insert (ophthalmic). *Drug.* Slowly dissolving membrane containing medication; placed in the lower conjunctival sac (fornix) to provide continuous release of medication over several hours. Trade name: Ocusert.

in situ (in-SI-tu). *Description.* In place (Latin). Used for describing surface cancers that are still within their site or layer of origin (e.g., skin) and have not invaded any surounding tissue.

inspissated (IN-spih-say-tud). *Description.* Refers to a secretion or exudate that has become dried or hardened.

intercanthal distance (ICD). *Anatomy.* Distance across the bridge of the nose, between the inner canthi of right and left eyelids.

interference. *Optics*. Consequence of phase interaction of light waves creating alternating bands or rings of increased and decreased light intensities.

intermediate curve. *Optics*. On the back surface of a tricurve hard contact lens, the curve between the central base curve and the peripheral curve.

intermittent esotropia [E(T)] (ee-suh-TROH-pee-uh). *Functional defect*. Eye deviation in which the eyes sometimes look straight ahead and work together, and other times one eye deviates inward (toward nose) while the other fixates normally.

intermittent exotropia [X(T)] (ek-suh-TROH-pee-uh). *Functional defect*. Eye deviation in which the eyes sometimes look straight ahead and work together, and other times one eye deviates outward (away from nose) while the other fixates normally.

intermittent strabismus (struh-BIZ-mis). *Functional defect*. Any eye deviation in which eyes are sometimes straight, and other times one eye is straight and the other deviates.

intermuscular membrane. *Anatomy*. Thin fibrous membrane connecting the sheaths that envelop the extraocular muscles. Prevents the muscles from slipping sideways.

internal carotid artery (kuh-RAH-tid). *Anatomy*. Major blood vessel to the head, whose 1st branch supplies blood to the front portion of the brain, including the eyes.

internal hordeolum (hor-DEE-oh-lum). *Pathologic condition*. Pustular infection in a meibomian gland (of the eyelid). If chronic, it is called a chalazion. See also EXTERNAL HORDEOLUM.

internal levator resection (posterior approach) (luh-VAY-tur). *Surgical procedure*. For repair of a moderately drooping eyelid. A conjunctival incision (on underside of lid) is made through the tarsus, muscle is removed, and the eyelid is repositioned to the desired height. See also EXTERNAL LEVATOR RESECTION.

internal limiting membrane. *Anatomy*. Innermost layer of sensory retina, incorporating the outer (cortical) fibers of the vitreous and the internal footplates of retinal Mueller cells.

internal ophthalmoplegia (ahf-thal-moh-PLEE-juh). *Functional defect*. Loss of function of certain muscles inside the eye, with loss of accommodation and pupillary constriction. Caused by paralysis of parasympathetic nerve fibers affecting the iris sphincter and ciliary muscle.

internal strabismus (struh-BIZ-mus), **convergent deviation, cross-eyes, esotropia**. *Functional defect*. Eye misalignment in which one eye deviates inward (toward nose) while other fixates normally. Deviation is present even when both eyes are uncovered. See also ESOPHORIA.

internal tarsal-orbicularis resection, tarsoconjunctival resection. *Surgical procedure*. For repair of an inward turning eyelid due to aging. Part of the tarsus and the underlying orbicularis muscle are removed. See also SENILE ENTROPION.

internal tarsoconjunctival Müllerectomy, Fasenella-Servat procedure. *Surgical procedure*. Repair of a mildly drooping upper eyelid (ptosis) by removal of a section of conjunctiva, Müller's muscle, and tarsus from the underside of the lid.

internuclear. *Location*. Between nerve cell groups. For eye function, refers to nerve tissue interconnecting the nuclei of the cranial nerves within the brainstem. See also MEDIAL LONGITUDINAL FASCICULUS.

internuclear ophthalmoplegia (INO) (ahf-thal-muh-PLEE-juh), **Bielschowsky-Lutz-Cogan syndrome**. *Pathologic condition*. Eye movement abnormalities attributed to a brainstem lesion. Eye on same side of body as the lesion has limited inward movement (adduction); other eye has jerky movements on outward gaze (abduction); convergence ability is normal. Frequently accompanied by vertical oscillations (nystagmus), especially on up-gaze, and skew deviations. Associated with multiple sclerosis.

interocular. *Location.* Between the eyes.

interpupillary distance (IPD), pupillary distance. *Measurement.* Distance from the center of one pupil to the center of the other pupil. Used for proper positioning of eyeglass lenses.

interrupted sutures. *Surgical technique.* Type of suturing in which each stitch is tied separately. See also CONTINUOUS SUTURES.

interstitial keratitis (IK) (in-tur-STISH-ul ker-uh-TI-tis). *Pathologic condition.* Inflammatory disease of the cornea that results in abnormal growth of blood vessels (neovascularization) in the middle corneal layers. Often associated with congenital syphilis. See also COGAN'S SYNDROME.

interval of Sturm. *Optics.* Space lying between the two focal line images formed by a cylindrical (astigmatic) lens.

"in-the-bag." *Description.* Slang for placement of an intraocular lens in the capsular bag after an extracapsular cataract extraction.

"in-the-sulcus" (SUL-kus). *Description.* Slang for placement of an intraocular lens in the posterior chamber with its haptics wedged in the ciliary sulcus.

intorsion, incycloduction. *Function.* Rotation of the eye's 12 o'clock meridian toward the nose.

intracameral. *Location.* Situated or occurring within (or administered into) an organ or chamber, e.g., the eye. Usually pertains to site of an injection.

intracapsular cataract extraction (ICCE). *Surgical procedure.* Removal of a cloudy lens (cataract) with its surrounding capsule. Formerly a standard procedure; now rare. See also EXTRACAPSULAR CATARACT EXTRACTION.

intraepithelial epithelioma (IN-truh-eh-pih-THEE-lee-ul ep-ih-thee-lee-OH-muh), **Bowen's disease, corneoconjunctival intrepithelial neoplasia.** *Pathologic condition.* Slow-growing malignant tumor, commonly arising at multiple sites near the corneo-scleral junction (limbus) but limited to the epithelial layer. Precursor to squamous cell carcinoma. May be caused by chronic sun exposure.

intra-marginal sulcus (SUL-kus), **gray line.** *Anatomy.* Line that divides the eyelid margins into outer and inner halves, separating eyelid skin from conjunctival mucus membrane. Eyelashes grow in front, tarsal gland ducts open behind the line.

intramuscular (IM). *Location.* Within (or administered into) a muscle.

intraocular (in-truh-AHK-yu-lur). *Location.* Inside the eye.

intraocular lens: see IOL.

intraocular muscles, intrinsic ocular muscles. *Anatomy.* Muscles inside the eye: the ciliary muscle and the iris sphincter and dilator.

intraocular pressure (IOP). 1. *Function.* Fluid pressure inside the eye. 2. *Measurement.* Assessment of pressure inside the eye with a tonometer. Also called tension. See also GLAUCOMA, TONOMETRY.

intraretinal microvascular abnormalities (IRMA) (in-truh-RET-ih-nul mi-kroh-VAS-kyu-lur). *Pathologic condition.* Development of abnormal blood vessels with tiny aneurysms along with connections (shunts) from arterioles to venules. Occurs in hypertensive and diabetic retinopathy, when blood is unable to flow through the normal capillaries, resulting in retinal anoxia and possible retinal swelling (edema).

intrascleral implant. *Surgical device.* Foreign material (usually solid silicone or silicone sponges) sutured under a flap of sclera to indent the globe, to help seal a retinal break or tear. See also SCLERAL BUCKLE.

intrascleral nerve loops, loops of Axenfeld. *Anatomy.* Loops of a long ciliary nerve into the anterior sclera; appear as a tiny dark spot of uveal tissue on the sclera near the limbus.

intrasheath tenotomy (ten-AH-tuh-mee). *Surgical procedure.* Weakening a superior oblique muscle by dissecting and then severing its tendon from the sheath. See also FREE TENOTOMY.

Intrastromal Corneal Ring (ICR). *Surgical device.* Trade name for material placed within the corneal stroma to create a reversible, adjustable method for changing the shape and optical power of the cornea. For correcting refractive errors.

intravenous (IV) (in-truh-VEEN-us). *Location.* Within (or administered into) a vein.

intravenous fluorescein angiography (IVFA) (FLOR-uh-seen an-jee-AHG-ruh-fee). *Test.* For evaluating retinal, choroidal and iris blood vessels, as well as eye problems affecting them. Fluorescein dye is injected into an arm vein, then rapid sequential photographs are taken of the eye as the dye circulates. See also ARTERIAL PHASE, CHOROIDAL FLUSH, INDOCYANINE GREEN ANGIOGRAPHY.

intravitreal. *Location.* Within the vitreous cavity, such as for an injection (of drugs, gas or air).

intrinsic ocular muscles. See INTRAOCULAR MUSCLES.

intumescent cataract (in-tu-MES-ent). *Pathologic condition.* Lens that has swollen and enlarged in the process of becoming cloudy. May lead to secondary acute angle closure glaucoma.

invisible-segment progressive power lens, progressive addition lens. *Optical device.* Type of near-vision eyeglass lens designed so that power for near increases gradually from zero (in the center) to maximum add (in the lower portion); there is no telltale bifocal demarcation line.

involutional ectropion, senile ectropion. *Functional defect.* Eyelid that sags away from normal contact with the eyeball because of stretched, weakened portions. Usually in the elderly.

involutional entropion, senile entropion. *Functional defect.* Eyelid that turns inward against the eyeball because of anatomic changes associated with aging.

iodopsin (i-oh-DAHP-sin). *Chemical.* Photosensitive visual pigment found in the cones of chickens. Necessary for conversion of light to neuro-electrical impulses.

IOL (intraocular lens), implant, pseudophakos. *Optical device.* Plastic lens that may be surgically implanted to replace the eye's natural lens.
> **anterior chamber**: implanted into anterior chamber (in front of the iris).
> **iris fixation**: implanted in the plane of the pupil and held in place by lens feet (haptics) clipped to the iris.
> **posterior chamber**: implanted into posterior chamber (behind the iris).

Iopidine (i-AW-pih-deen). *Drug.* Trade name of apraclonidine; for treating glaucoma.

ipsilateral. *Description.* Refers to the same eye or same side of body. See also CONTRALATERAL.

ipsilateral antagonist, direct antagonist. *Anatomy.* Extraocular muscle whose action opposes that of another muscle in the same eye, (e.g., right medial rectus and right lateral rectus).

iridectomy (ir-ih-DEK-tuh-mee). *Surgical procedure.* Cutting out (removing) a portion of iris tissue. See also IRIDOTOMY.
> **basal**: removal at the far periphery (near the iris root).
> **peripheral**: removal at the periphery.
> **sector**: removal of a wedge-shaped section that extends from the pupil margin to the iris root, leaving a keyhole-shaped pupil.

iridencleisis (ir-ih-den-KLI-sis), **iridocorneosclerectomy**. *Surgical proce-dure*. Creation of a permanent drainage route from the anterior chamber by wedging iris tissue into the wound to act as a wick. Obsolete treatment for glaucoma.

iridocapsulotomy (ir-id-oh-kap-suh-LAH-tuh-mee). *Surgical procedure*. Creation of a new pupillary opening after an extracapsular cataract extraction by incising the residual membrane.

irido corneal endothelial syndrome. See ICE SYNDROME.

iridocorneosclerectomy (IR-id-oh-KOR-nee-oh-skler-EK-toh-mee). See IRIDENCLEISIS.

iridocyclectomy (ir-id-oh-si-KLEK-tuh-mee). *Surgical procedure*. Removal of a segment of ciliary body and contiguous peripheral iris, e.g., for excising a localized tumor.

iridocyclitis (ir-id-oh-si-KLI-tis), **anterior uveitis**. *Pathologic condition*. In-flammation the of iris, anterior chamber or ciliary body. Causes pain, tear-ing, blurred vision, constricted pupil, and a red (congested) eye. See also CILIARY INJECTION, POSTERIOR UVEITIS.

iridodialysis (ir-id-oh-di-AL-ih-sis). 1. *Pathologic condition*. Circular tear of the base of the iris that pulls it from the ciliary body, usually from blunt trauma to the eye. 2. *Surgical procedure*. Tear in the iris made with surgical instru-ments; may be intentional or unintentional.

iridodonesis (IR-ih-doh-duh-NEE-sis). *Functional defect*. Iris that flops loose-ly due to lack of normal support from the lens. Follows lens dislocation or removal.

iridoplegia (ir-id-oh-PLEE-juh). *Functional defect*. Iris sphincter paralysis; pre-vents the pupil from moving in response to light or near stimulation.

iridoschisis (ir-ih-doh-SKEE-sis). *Pathologic condition*. Splitting of the iris structure (stroma) into layers, with the anterior fibers containing the blood vessels. Often leads to angle closure glaucoma. See also ICE SYNDROME.

iridotomy (ir-ih-DAHT-uh-mee). *Surgical procedure*. Puncture-like opening made through the iris without removal of any iris tissue. Allows aqueous to drain freely from the posterior chamber to the anterior chamber.

    laser i: application of a laser light beam to burn a hole through the iris near its base.

iris. *Anatomy*. Pigmented tissue lying behind the cornea that gives color to the eye (e.g., blue eyes) and controls amount of light entering the eye by varying the size of the pupillary opening. Most forward extension of the middle (uveal) layer of the eye; separates the anterior chamber from the posterior chamber. Plural: irides.

iris bombe (bahm-BAY). *Pathologic condition*. Iris that balloons forward, block-ing aqueous outflow channels through the angle. Usually caused by adhe-sions of the iris-pupillary border to the lens, which creates fluid pooling behind the iris and a sudden rise in intraocular pressure. See also ACUTE ANGLE CLOSURE GLAUCOMA .

iris coloboma (kah-luh-BOH-muh). *Anatomic defect*. Defect of the iris that leaves a gap in iris tissue. May be a congenital abnormality or result from iridectomy.

iris crypts, crypts of Fuchs. *Anatomy*. Pit-like depressions in the front surface of the iris.

iris dilator, dilator muscle *(or)* **pupillae, pupil dilator** (DI-lay-tur). *Anatomy*. Smooth iris muscle that contracts to enlarge the pupillary opening. Ex-tends like wheel spokes from the pupillary margin to the iris periphery. Innervated by sympathetic nerve fibers.

iris fixation lens. *Optical device*. Type of intraocular lens implanted in the plane of the pupil and held in place by lens feet (haptics) clipped to the iris.

iris prolapse. *Anatomic defect*. Protrusion of iris tissue into a corneal wound.

iris root. *Anatomy*. Junction of iris and ciliary body; located just under the limbus.

iris sphincter (SFINK-tur), **sphincter pupillae**. *Anatomy*. Circle of iris muscle that surrounds the pupillary margin. Receives innervation from parasympathetic nerves to contract pupil size (miosis) in response to bright light.

iris stroma (STROH-muh). *Anatomy*. Bulk of the iris structure. Consists of a loose collagenous supporting network that contains the iris sphincter and dilator muscles, pigment, blood vessels and nerves.

iris tuck. *Surgical procedure*. During cataract extraction, the iris is tucked behind the nucleus before the lens nucleus is removed.

iritis (i-RI-tis). *Pathologic condition*. Inflammation of the iris. Can cause pain, tearing, blurred vision, small pupil (miosis) and a red congested eye. See also CILIARY INJECTION, UVEITIS.

irradiance. *Measurement*. Density of radiant flux incident on a surface.

irregular astigmatism (uh-STIG-muh-tizm). *Refractive error*. Distorted imagery caused by warped optical surfaces. Warping is usually corneal and the result of scarring from trauma, inflammation or developmental anomalies. May be corrected by contact lenses but not by standard eyeglasses.

irreversible amblyopia (am-blee-OH-pee-uh), **organic amblyopia**. *Functional defect*. Poor vision in one or both eyes caused by nonapparent damage to the visual system. No effective therapy. See also AMBLYOPIA, NEUTRAL DENSITY FILTER.

irrigation-aspiration (I/A), infusion-aspiration. *Surgical instrument/technique*. Simultaneously cutting and removing tissue by suction (aspiration) while fluid is injected (infusion) to maintain ocular volume, using an instrument with two ports. Used in phacoemulsification and in vitreous surgery.

Irvine-Gass syndrome. *Pathologic condition*. Consists of cysts that form in the macula after cataract surgery, impairing vision; sometimes temporary. May be associated with vitreous adhesion to the corneal wound. See also CYSTOID MACULAR EDEMA.

ischemia (ih-SKEE-mee-uh). *Pathologic condition*. Inadequate blood supply to a body part caused by partial blockage of a blood vessel. If not reversed, surrounding tissue dies from lack of nutrients. See also INFARCT.

ischemia (retinal) (is-KEE-mee-uh). *Pathologic condition*. Abnormal reduction of retinal blood supply from varying degrees of blood vessel blockage. May result in retinal edema, cotton-wool spots, microaneurisms, venous engorgement, and neovascularization.

ischemic (is-KEE-mik). *Description*. Tissue that has been deprived of blood supply.

ischemic optic neuropathy (ION) (nur-AHP-uh-thee). *Pathologic condition*. Loss of structure and function of a portion of optic nerve, caused by blood flow obstruction (atherosclerotic or inflammatory). Produces sudden, painless loss of vision in the elderly.

iseikonic lens (i-suh-KAHN-ik). *Optical device*. Eyeglass lens that magnifies or minifies image size. Used for correcting image size difference between the two eyes. See also ANEISEKONIA.

Ishihara test plates (ish-ee-HAH-ruh). *Test chart*. Colored dots that appear as identifiable numbers or patterns to individuals who have various types of color vision defects. Used for color vision evaluation. See also PSEUDO-ISO-CHROMATIC CHARTS.

Ismotic. *Drug*. Trade name of isosorbide; for treating glaucoma.

isobutyl 2-cyanacrylate. *Surgical material*. Plastic glue-like substance that can attach tissues to each other. Used in the cornea to fill a superficial defect or in the punctum to occlude it.

isometropia (I-soh-meh-TROH-pee-uh). *Refractive error*. Equal refractive errors in both eyes; differences less than one-half diopter are insignificant and are considered equal.

isopia (i-SOH-pee-uh). *Function.* Equal vision in both eyes.

isoproterenol (i-soh-proh-TEHR-ih-nol). *Drug.* Stimulates sympathetic nerve fibers, causing decrease in aqueous secretion. Used rarely for treating glaucoma. Trade name: Isuprel.

isopter (i-SAHP-tur). *Measurement.* In a visual field test, the line connecting points denoting areas of equal sensitivity to light. Analogous to contour lines denoting equal elevations on a map.

Isopto-Atropine (i-SAHP-toh-AT-roh-peen). *Drug.* Trade name of atropine eyedrops; for treating iritis.

Isopto-Carbachol (KAHR-buh-kol). *Drug.* Trade name of carbachol.; for treating glaucoma.

Isopto-Carpine (KAHR-peen). *Drug.* Trade name of pilocarpine eyedrops; for treating glaucoma.

IsoptoFrin. *Drug.* Trade name of weak solution of phenylephrine; eyedrops that constrict blood vessels to "whiten" the eye.

Isopto-Homatropine (hohm-AT-roh-peen). *Drug.* Trade name of homatropine eyedrops; used as a cycloplegic.

Isopto-Hyoscine (HI-oh-seen). *Drug.* Trade name of scopolamine eyedrops; for treating anterior uveitis.

Isopto-Tears. *Drug.* Trade name of methylcellulose eyedrops; for treating dry eyes.

isosorbide (i-soh-SOR-bide). *Drug.* Oral osmotic agent that lowers intraocular pressure by pulling fluid out of the eye. Short term use. Trade names: Hydronol, Ismotic. See also OSMOTIC AGENT.

Isuprel (I-suh-pril). *Drug.* Trade name of isoproterenol; for treating glaucoma.

J

jack-in-the-box phenomenon. *Optical illusion*. Objects located in the periphery of the visual field appear to jump suddenly into view as the eye or head is moved. Occurs while wearing eyeglasses for high hyperopia, including cataract glasses.

Jackson cross cylinder. *Optical device*. Single lens composed of a plus cylinder and a minus cylinder of equal optical strength, placed perpendicular to one another. Used in a refraction to determine the axis and power of an astigmatic correction.

Jaeger test (YAY-gur or JAY-gur). Assessment of near visual acuity using numbers and symbols in a graded series of type sizes.

Jakob-Creutzfeldt disease (YAH-kohb KROYTS-feld). *Pathologic condition*. Rare, infectious, progressive neurological disease caused by a slow-acting virus. Can be transmitted by donor tissue, e.g., corneal transplant. Fatal.

Jansen's syndrome. *Pathologic condition*. Vitreoretinal degeneration, with lattice and retinoschisis in the peripheral retina. May lead to retinal detachment. Prognosis for vision is poor. Hereditary. Variant of Wagner's disease.

Jansky-Bielschowsky syndrome (beel-SHAH/OH-skee). *Congenital defect*. Childhood form of amaurotic familial idiocy. Characterized by nervous system and retinal disease affecting central vision.

jaw winking syndrome, external pterygoid-levator synkinesis, Marcus Gunn jaw winking syndrome. *Congenital defect*. Droopy eyelid (ptosis) that opens wide upon chewing, sucking, or moving the mouth to the opposite side. Caused by abnormal innervation of the levator muscle by the 5th (trigeminal) cranial nerve.

Jensen procedure. *Surgical procedure*. Tying the lateral loops of halved inferior and superior rectus muscles to the upper and lower loops of a halved lateral rectus muscle, to correct lateral rectus palsy. See also HUMMEL-SHEIM PROCEDURE.

Jensen's choroiditis juxtapapillaris (kor-oyd-l-tis juks-tuh-pap-ih-LEHR-is). *Pathologic condition*. Severe inflammation of choroid and retina adjacent to the optic disc. May result in optic nerve damage.

jerk nystagmus (ni-STAG-mus). *Functional defect*. Involuntary, rhythmic side-to-side or up-and-down eye movements that are faster in one direction than the other. Types are listed under nystagmus.

jerrum. *Incorrect spelling of BJERRUM*.

Johnson syndrome, adherence syndrome. *Congenital anomaly*. Limitation of outward eye movement (abduction) caused by adhesions between the lateral rectus and inferior oblique muscle sheaths, or limitation of upward eye movement caused by adhesions between the superior rectus and superior oblique muscle sheaths.

Jones test. For evaluating tear drainage system function; measures the time for fluorescein dye to appear inside the nose after being dropped onto the cornea. See also FLUORESCEIN DYE DISAPPEARANCE TEST.

　　Jones I: for detecting an obstruction in the tear drainage system or poor pumping of tears. Test is positive when fluorescein instilled in lower conjunctiva does not drain through to the nose.

　　Jones primary dye test: same as JONES I (above).

Jones secondary dye test: same as JONES II (below).

Jones II: for distinguishing partial from complete obstruction, localizing site of blockage, and determining appropriate surgical repair; involves injection of fluid into the tear drainage system. Performed after an abnormal Jones I.

Jones tube. *Surgical device*. Glass tube that is inserted into the conjunctiva, through the orbital bone and into the nose to permit tear drainage. Used when there is a severe obstruction of the natural drainage channels.

Joubert's syndrome. *Pathologic condition*. Characterized by central nervous system defects, retinal dystrophy, severe psychomotor retardation, and breathing problems. Ocular findings are similar to Leber's amaurosis (abnormal saccades and pursuit), but visual evoked responses are normal. Hereditary.

joule (J). *Measurement*. Unit of energy; used in comparing lasers or laser beams.

jump (image). *Optics*. Sudden movement of an image that occurs when prism power is abruptly introduced into an optical system, e.g., at the top edge of some bifocals. Occurs when gaze is shifted between the upper (distance) portion of a bifocal lens and the lower (reading) segment.

junction scotoma (skuh-TOH-muh). *Functional defect*. Visual field defect characterized by a central scotoma (area of vision loss) in one eye and temporal hemianopia (vision loss in outer half of field) in the other eye. Caused by a chiasmal lesion that interrupts the lower nasal fibers from one eye and the macular fibers of the other eye, just after crossing the chiasm. See also VON WILLEBRANDT'S KNEE.

Just Tears. *Drug*. Trade name of polyvinyl alcohol eyedrops; for treating dry eyes.

juvenile corneal epithelial dystrophy, Meesmann's dystrophy. *Pathologic condition*. Non-progressive early childhood disorder characterized by fine, dot-like, glycogen-containing opacities in the corneal epithelium. Treatment usually unnecessary. Hereditary.

juvenile Gm$_1$ gangliosidosis (gang-lee-oh-si-DOH-sis). *Pathologic condition*. Metabolic disorder (of enzyme beta-galactosidase) characterized by weakness, incoordination, seizures, and an inward eye deviation (esotropia). Appears about age 1, with death at about 3–8 years. Hereditary. See also GANGLIOSIDOSIS, SPHINGOLIPIDOSES.

juvenile Gm$_2$ gangliosidosis. *Pathologic condition*. Metabolic disorder (of the enzyme hexosaminidase A) characterized by nervous system abnormalities and cherry red spots in the macula. Results in blindness. Appears from ages 2–6, with death at about 5–15 years. Hereditary. See also GANGLIOSIDOSIS, SPHINGOLIPIDOSES.

juvenile retinoschisis (ret-in-oh-SKEE-sis), **congenital retinoschisis**. *Congenital anomaly*. Splitting of the retina into inner and outer layers, usually involving the macular area. Hereditary, X-linked. See also RETINOSCHISIS.

juvenile rheumatoid arthritis, Still's disease. *Pathologic condition*. Uncommon childhood connective tissue disease. Often associated with inflammation of the iris and ciliary body (uveitis) and a band-shaped calcium deposit on the cornea (band keratopathy).

juvenile xanthogranuloma (JXG) (ZAN-thoh-gran-yu-LOH-muh). *Pathologic condition*. Consists of small yellowish lesions in the skin and in the eyes (iris and ciliary body) that may produce intraocular hemorrhages and cause glaucoma. Affects infants and children.

juxtapapillary. *Location*. Next to the optic nerve head.

K

K. Abbreviation for curvature; in clinical usage, the flattest corneal curvature. The corneal meridian having the least amount of optical power, measured with a keratometer. Important in contact lens fitting. See also FLATTEST MERIDIAN, K-READINGS, STEEPEST MERIDIAN.

Kandori's syndrome. *Pathologic condition*. Characterized by night blindness and multiple, irregular, large yellowish flecks in the equatorial retina. Nonprogressive. Hereditary.

kappa (angle). *Optics*. Angle formed at the nodal point of an eye between the visual axis and the mid-pupillary line.

Kaufman vitrector (vit-REK-tur). *Surgical instrument*. For anterior vitreous removal; has suction and cutting components. Disposable.

Kayser-Fleischer ring (KI-zur-FLI-shur). *Clinical sign*. Brownish-yellow ring visible around the corneo-scleral junction (limbus). Consists of copper deposits in Descemet's membrane, extending into the trabecular meshwork. Sign of Wilson's disease.

Kearns-Sayre syndrome (kurnz-sehr). *Pathologic condition*. Characterized by a gradual inability to move the eyes (progressive external ophthalmoplegia), retinal pigmentary degeneration, heart block (delays of electrical conductivity), increased protein in the cerebrospinal fluid, and minute spaces within the brain and brainstem. Childhood onset.

Keflex. *Drug*. Trade name of cephalexin, an antibiotic.

Keflin. *Drug*. Trade name of cephalothin, an antibiotic used for treating some infections inside the eye (endophthalmitis).

Kefzol. *Drug*. Trade name of cephazolin, an antibiotic used for treating some infections inside the eye (endophthalmitis).

kelazion. Incorrect spelling of CHALAZION.

Kellner's law. Incorrect spelling of KOLLNER'S LAW.

Kennedy syndrome, Foster Kennedy syndrome. *Pathologic condition*. Characterized by optic nerve degeneration (atrophy) on the same side as a frontal lobe brain tumor, and optic nerve swelling on the opposite side, due to increased pressure in the brain.

Keppy nodules. Incorrect spelling of KOEPPE NODULES.

keratabrasion (kehr-uh-tuh-BRAY-zhun). *Surgical procedure*. Smoothing the corneal surface (epithelium) with a diamond dental burr. Used for treating a pterygium or removing a corneal elevation.

keratectasia (kehr-uh-tek-TAY-zhuh), **corneal ectasia**. *Pathologic condition*. Abnormal bulging forward of thinned cornea, as with keratoconus.

keratectomy (kehr-uh-TEK-tuh-mee). *Surgical procedure*. Removal of a piece or segment of the cornea.

    photorefractive (PRK): use of high intensity laser light (e.g., with an excimer laser) to reshape the corneal curvature for correcting refractive errors. Includes laser sculpting, LASIK. Also called laser keratorefractive surgery, photorefractive surgery.

    phototherapeutic: use of an excimer laser on the cornea to remove scars and smooth an irregular surface.

keratic precipitates (kehr-AT-ik). See KP'S.

keratitis (KEHR-uh-TI-tis). *Pathologic condition*. Corneal inflammation, characterized by loss of luster and transparency, and cellular infiltration.

    dendritic k: superficial corneal infection characterized by branch-shaped corneal ulcers. Characteristic of herpes simplex virus infection.

disciform k: corneal stromal inflammation, probably related to an immune response. Appears as a disc-shaped, gray lesion; usually related to herpes simplex virus infection.

exposure k: corneal drying or inflammation, from incomplete closure of the eyelid.

filamentary k: strands of coiled, superficial corneal cells (epithelium) loosely attached to the cornea that when broken free, leave small painful ulcers. Associated with keratoconjunctivitis sicca and trachoma.

herpetic k: eye infection from herpes simplex virus. Results in recurrent corneal epithelial inflammations with branch-like lesions (dendritic keratitis), sometimes followed by the formation of larger, irregularly shaped (geographic) ulcers. May progress to corneal stroma inflammation (disciform keratitis).

neurotrophic k (nu-roh-TROH-fik): results from trauma or corneal exposure following damage to corneal nerves; accompanied by loss of corneal sensitivity (corneal anesthesia).

punctate k: characterized by small superficial corneal lesions. Symptoms include foreign body sensation and sensitivity to bright light. Sometimes recurs after spontaneous remissions. Cause unknown.

superficial punctate (SPK): same as PUNCTATE (above).

k. sicca (SIK-uh): corneal and conjunctival dryness due to deficient tear production, mostly in menopausal and post-menopausal women. Causes foreign body sensation, burning eyes, filamentary keratitis, and erosion of the conjunctival and corneal epithelium. Also called dry eye syndrome and keratoconjunctivitis sicca. See also SJÖGREN'S SYNDROME.

kerato- (KEHR-uh-toh). Prefix: pertaining to the cornea.

keratoacanthoma (KEHR-uh-toh-ay-kan-THOH-muh), **molluscum sebaceum**. *Pathologic condition.* Benign, rapid-growing, cup-shaped skin lesion with a central crater; tends to form on lids and face. Often regresses spontaneously.

keratocele (KEHR-uh-toh-seel), **descemetocele**. *Pathologic condition.* Protrusion of Descemet's membrane into the cornea to "plug" a defect after an ulcer has eroded away the overlying stroma. Protects the eye from "blowing out."

keratocentesis (KEHR-uh-to-sen-TEE-sis), **anterior chamber tap, paracentesis**. *Surgical procedure.* Corneal puncture with removal of some aqueous fluid for laboratory analysis or to lower eye pressure temporarily.

keratoconjunctivitis (KEHR-uh-toh-kun junk-tih-VI-tis). *Pathologic condition.* Inflammation involving both the cornea and conjunctiva.

keratoconjunctivitis sicca (KCS). See KERATITIS SICCA.

keratoconus (kehr-uh-toh-KOH-nus). *Pathologic condition.* Degenerative corneal disease affecting vision. Characterized by generalized thinning and cone-shaped protrusion of the central cornea, usually in both eyes. Becomes apparent during 2nd decade of life. Hereditary.

keratoglobus (kehr-uh-toh-GLOH-bus). *Congenital anomaly.* Enlarged, protruding, spherical cornea accompanied by thinning of the middle corneal layer (stroma) near the corneo-scleral junction (limbus).

keratolysis (kehr-uh-toh-LI-sis), **corneal melt**. *Pathologic condition.* Superficial corneal layers that "melt" away. May be associated with severe inflammatory disease of the sclera or peripheral cornea, dry eyes (keratitis sicca), and rheumatoid arthritis. See also FURROWS.

keratomalacia (kehr-uh-toh-muh-LAY-shuh). *Degenerative change.* Corneal softening and opacification, associated with vitamin A deficiency.

keratome (KEHR-uh-tohm). *Instrument.* Knife designed for making a corneal incision; usually has a triangular blade.

keratometer (kehr-uh-TAH-mih-tur). *Instrument.* Used for measuring corneal curvature (K-readings) and for detecting and measuring astigmatism. See also MIRES.

keratometry (kehr-uh-TAH-mih-tree). *Technique.* Obtaining corneal curvature measurements with a keratometer. Unequal meridional powers indicate astigmatism. See also FLATTEST MERIDIAN, STEEPEST MERIDIAN.

keratomileusis (kehr-uh-toh-mih-LU-sis). *Surgical procedure.* Method of reshaping the cornea to change its optical power. A disc of cornea is shaved off, quickly frozen, lathe-ground to flatten its front surface, then returned to its original position. Used for correcting very high refractive errors, especially myopia. See also LASIK.

keratomycosis (kehr-uh-toh-mi-KOH-sis), **fungal keratitis**. *Pathologic condition.* Gray pus-producing corneal ulcer with irregular borders. Develops after eye injury from vegetable matter (e.g., tree branch, fingernail). See also CANDIDA ALBICANS, FUSARIUM.

keratopathy (kehr-uh-TAH-puh-thee). *Pathologic condition.* Any abnormality of the cornea.

keratophakia (kehr-uh-toh-FAY-kee-uh). *Surgical procedure.* Insertion of a preserved lathe-cut donor corneal disc into the cornea. Used for correcting severe degrees of farsightedness (hyperopia).

keratoplasty (KEHR-uh-toh-plas-tee). *Surgical procedure.* Surgery on the cornea. Usually refers to replacement of scarred or diseased cornea with clear corneal tissue from a donor (corneal graft or transplant).

    autokeratoplasty: a discrete opacity is excised, rotated and resutured to shift its position; type of penetrating keratoplasty.

    automated lamellar (ALK): excision of the lamellae with a computer-controlled keratome, usually as part of a refractive keratoplasty procedure.

    lamellar: involves outer corneal layers (lamellae). Also called lamellar graft, partial-thickness graft.

    penetrating: the full thickness of the cornea is replaced.

    refractive: surgery on the cornea to change the optical power of the eye, e.g., epikeratophakia, keratomileusis, LASIK.

keratoprosthesis (kehr-uh-toh-prahs-THEE-sis). *Optical device.* Plastic optical implant surgically placed in the cornea and through the closed eyelid to restore vision in patients with severe anterior segment opacification, when a corneal graft alone is insufficient. Rarely successful.

keratorefractive surgery. See REFRACTIVE SURGERY.

keratoscope (KEHR-uh-tuh-skohp). *Instrument.* Used for evaluating smoothness, regularity and power across the corneal surface. See also PLACIDO DISK, PHOTOKERATOSCOPE.

keratoscopy (kehr-uh-TAHS-kuh-pee). Use of a keratoscope to observe surface reflections (created by focusing guides called mires) from the anterior corneal surface. See also CORNEAL TOPOGRAPHY, PHOTOKERATOSCOPY.

keratotomy (kehr-uh-TAH-tuh-mee). *Surgical procedure.* 1. Any incision into the cornea. 2. Obsolete procedure for limiting the spread of an ulcer. Plural: keratotomies.

    arcuate: method of flattening the steeper corneal meridian with a curved corneal incision, for reducing astigmatism after corneal surgery.

    radial (RK): series of spoke-like (radial) cuts (usually 4 to 8) made in the corneal periphery to allow the central cornea to flatten, reducing its optical power and thereby correcting nearsightedness.

    transverse: incision into the cornea parallel to the limbus, usually to reduce astigmatism after corneal surgery.

keratouveitis (KEHR-uh-toh-yu-vee-I-tis). *Pathologic condition.* Inflammation of the cornea and uveal tract (iris, ciliary body and choroid).

Kestenbaum procedure. *Surgical procedure*. Method of strengthening or weakening both medial rectus and lateral rectus muscles, so an individual with nystagmus (side-to-side eye movements) will not need to hold head in an abnormal position to see well. The position with least eye movement (null point) is repositioned straight ahead.

Kestenbaum rule. *Formula*. Approximates the power needed for a low vision aid (magnifying lens) based on distance acuity (1/visual acuity = dioptric power needed).

ketoconazole. *Drug*. Oral mediation used for treating fungal eye infections. Trade name: Nizoral. See also: AMPHOTERICIN B, CLOTRIMAZOLE, FLUCYTOSINE, MICONAZOLE, NATAMYCIN.

ketorolac tromethamine. *Drug*. Eyedrops used for treating allergic conjunctivitis. Trade name: Acular. See also CROMOLYN, LODOXAMIDE.

keyhole pupil. *Anatomic defect*. Pupil shape following a sector iridectomy in which an iris section extending from the pupillary margin to the iris periphery is excised.

Keystone cards. *Test object*. Set of picture cards used for testing vision and depth perception.

kiazum. *Incorrect spelling of* CHIASM.

kinetic perimetry (kin-ET-ik puh-RIM-ih-tree). *Test*. Type of visual field test in which stimuli are moved from a non-seeing area until they are first perceived. See also GOLDMANN PERIMETER, STATIC PERIMETRY.

kinetics. *Science*. Study of movement.

kiroscope. *Incorrect spelling of* CHEIROSCOPE.

"kissing choroidals" (kor-OY-dulz). *Pathologic condition*. Choroidal detachment that is so large that both convex surfaces touch in the vitreous cavity. Usually occurs as a post-operative complication.

Klebsiella pneumoniae (kleb-see-EL-uh nu-MOH-nee-ee). *Microorganism*. Gram-negative rod-shaped bacteria. May cause corneal ulcers.

Klippel-Fiel syndrome (FI-ul). *Pathologic condition*. Characterized by deafness, mental deficiency, and upper spine and neck problems. Sometimes associated with Duane's syndrome or choroidal and retinal degeneration. Hereditary.

Klumpke's paralysis. *Pathologic condition*. Brachial plexus damage from injury to the armpit, usually from birth trauma. Any damage to sympathetic nerves may result in Horner's syndrome on that side.

Knapp procedure. *Surgical procedure*. Transposition of lateral and medial rectus muscles to either side of the superior rectus to correct a downward eye deviation (hypotropia).

Knapp's rule. *Optics*. When a refractive error is caused by excessively long or short eyeball length (axial ametropia), corrective eyeglasses positioned 15 mm in front of the eyes will create retinal images of the same size, no matter what the degree of error. See also ANTERIOR FOCAL LENGTH, AXIAL LENGTH.

Koch-Weeks bacillus (kok-weekz buh-SIL-us), *Hemophilus aegyptius*. *Microorganism*. Gram-negative bacteria that causes acute, pus-producing conjunctivitis.

Koellner's Law. See KÖLLNER'S LAW.

Koeppe lens (KEH-pee). *Instrument*. Specially designed high-plus contact lens that is placed on an anesthetized cornea for a direct view of anterior chamber angle structures, to help in evaluation of glaucoma. Used with a hand-held illuminating source and microscope. See also GONIOSCOPY.

Koeppe nodules. *Clinical sign*. Accumulation of inflammatory cells at the pupillary margin of the iris. Seen with uveitis. See also BUSACCA NODULES.

Köllner's law (KEL-nurz), **Koellner's law.** Retinal diseases cause blue and yellow color vision defects primarily, whereas optic nerve diseases affect red and green. Controversial.

Koplik's spots. *Clinical sign.* Measles spots; pale white, small rounded lesions appearing on the mucus membranes of the buccal cheek, conjunctiva and caruncle.

koroid. Incorrect spelling of CHOROID.

KPs (keratic precipitates). *Clinical sign.* Inflammatory cells and white blood cells from the iris and ciliary body that enter the aqueous and adhere to the innermost corneal surface (endothelium). Called "mutton fat" if KPs are large clusters (granulomatous) or "punctate" if smaller (nongranulomatous). Typical finding in various types of uveitis.

Krabbe's disease (KRAB-eez), **galactosyl ceramide lipidosis**. *Pathologic condition.* Hereditary defect in fat (lipid) metabolism caused by enzyme beta-galactosidase deficiency. Characterized by irritability, progressive motor and mental deterioration, optic nerve degeneration, deafness, and death. Onset during first 6 months of life. See also SPHINGOLIPIDOSES.

Krause glands. *Anatomy.* Accessory tear glands located under the lids at the upper and lower conjunctival cul-de-sacs.

K-readings. *Measurement.* Corneal curvature measurements obtained with a keratometer. Unequal measurements indicate astigmatism. See also FLATTEST MERIDIAN, STEEPEST MERIDIAN.

Krimsky method. *Test.* Assessment of eye deviation by using prisms to equalize the position of the corneal light reflex within each pupil.

Kroenlein procedure. See KRÖNLEIN PROCEDURE.

Krönlein procedure (KROHN-line), **lateral orbital decompression**; also spelled Kroenlein. *Surgical procedure.* Partial removal of the bony orbital wall (zygoma) and/or floor (maxillary sinus roof) to relieve forward pressure on the eye when the orbital contents have increased in size (e.g., in Graves' disease). See also THYROID EYE DISEASE.

Krukenberg's spindle (KRU-ken-burgz). *Clinical sign.* Vertical pigment deposit in the center of the innermost corneal surface (endothelium). Found with pigment dispersion glaucoma and following uveitis.

Krupin tube (KRU-pin). *Surgical device.* Valve implanted under the sclera for draining aqueous from the anterior chamber into the subconjunctival space. For controlling intraocular pressure in glaucoma.

Krupin valve. *Instrument.* Unidirectional, pressure-sensitive filtering valve implanted through the cornea into the anterior chamber (with a scleral flap closure over it) to allow fluid to drain from the eye and control intraocular pressure. Especially useful in neovascular glaucoma.

Kufs' disease (koofs). *Pathologic condition.* Adult form of amaurotic familial idiocy, characterized by behavioral disturbance and unsteady gait. Vision usually unaffected.

Kuhnt-Junius disease (koont-JYU-nee-us), **disciform degeneration of the macula**. *Pathologic condition.* Retinal degeneration leading to permanent loss of central vision; peripheral vision stays intact. Begins with a fluid leak under the retinal pigment epithelium in the macular area, usually followed by hemorrhage and scarring. Most common cause of blindness over age 50. See also MACULAR DEGENERATION.

Kuhnt-Szymanowski procedure (zi-man-AH/OU-skee). *Surgical procedure.* Outdated method of repairing a lower eyelid that does not rest against the eyeball (ectropion). See also SENILE ECTROPION.

    Smith modification: horizontal eyelid shortening technique for repair of an ectropion.

L

labile (LAY-bile). *Description.* Easily or frequently changing; characterized by wide fluctuations.

Labrador keratopathy, climatic droplet keratopathy, spheroid degeneration. *Pathologic condition.* Corneal disorder caused by chronic inflammation and by exposure to ultraviolet light. Characterized by amber fatty-like protein droplets from collagen degeneration in the cornea. Seen in older patients who have led an outdoor life.

labyrinthine nystagmus (lab-ih-RIN-theen ni-STAG-mus), **caloric *(or)* vestibular nystagmus.** *Function.* Involuntary, jerky eye movements in any direction caused by a disturbance in normal innervation from the labyrinths in the ears. Unrelated to visual stimuli. See also COWS.

lacquer cracks. *Clinical sign.* Linear breaks in Bruch's membrane (in macular area of the retina) that occur when an eyeball is stretched. Associated with progressive myopic degeneration.

Lacril (LAK-rul). *Drug.* Trade name of methylcellulose eyedrops; for treating dry eyes.

Lacrilube (LAK-rih-loob). *Drug.* Trade name of polyvinyl alcohol ointment; for treating dry eyes.

lacrimal apparatus (LAK-rih-mul), **tear drainage system.** *Anatomy.* Orbital structures for tear production and drainage. Tears (produced in lacrimal gland above eyeball) flow across the corneal surface, drain into the upper and lower puncta (openings at inner eyelid margins), through the upper and lower canaliculi to the common canaliculus, into the tear sac, then through the nasolacrimal duct into the nose.

lacrimal artery. *Anatomy.* Branch of the ophthalmic artery that supplies blood to the lacrimal gland.

lacrimal bone. *Anatomy.* Small bone forming the front part of the medial orbital wall. One of seven bones forming the orbit (eye socket).

lacrimal canaliculus (kan-uh-LIK-yu-lus). *Anatomy.* Tiny channel in each eyelid; part of the tear drainage system. Begins at the lacrimal punctum in both upper and lower lids, joining to form the common canaliculus, which leads to the tear (lacrimal) sac and then through the nasolacrimal duct into the nose. Plural: canaliculi. See also PUNCTUM.

lacrimal duct, nasolacrimal *(or)* tear duct. *Anatomy.* Tear drainage channel that extends from the lacrimal sac to an opening in the mucous membrane of the nose.

lacrimal gland. *Anatomy.* Almond-shaped structure that produces tears. Located at the upper outer region of the orbit, above the eyeball.

lacrimal lake. *Anatomy.* Pool of tears in the lower conjunctival cul-de-sac that drains into the openings (puncta) of the tear drainage system.

lacrimal nerve. *Anatomy.* Smallest branch of the ophthalmic division of the 5th (trigeminal) cranial nerve. Supplies sensation to the conjunctiva and skin of the outer half of the upper eyelid and innervates the lacrimal gland.

lacrimal papilla (puh-PIL-uh). *Anatomy.* Small conical elevations on the upper and lower eyelids at the inner canthus (near nose), pierced by an opening (punctum) to the tear drainage system. Particularly evident in the elderly.

lacrimal probe. *Instrument.* Thin rod used for clearing obstructions in the tear drainage system.

lacrimal sac, tear sac. *Anatomy.* Tear collecting structure under the skin near the bridge of the nose. Tears enter from the common canaliculus and leave through the lacrimal duct into the nose.

lacrimation (lak-rih-MAY-shun). *Function.* Tear production; crying.

lacunae (luh-KOON-ee). *Anatomic defect.* Microscopic puddles (e.g., in retinal edema or glaucomatous optic nerve).

lagophthalmos (lag-ahf-THAL-mus). *Functional defect.* Difficult or impossible complete eyelid closure. Can be caused by 7th (facial) cranial nerve palsy, an abnormally enlarged or protruding eye, or eyelid retraction from thyroid eye disease. See also EXPOSURE KERATITIS.

lambda (angle). *Optics.* Angle formed at the center of a pupil between the visual axis and the optic axis.

lambert. *Measurement.* Unit of luminance.

lamella. *Anatomy.* A layer of tissue, usually one of multiple similar layers, as in the corneal stroma. Plural: lamellae.

lamellar (luh-MEL-ur). *Description.* In layers.

lamellar cataract, zonular cataract. *Pathologic condition.* Form of cataract in which concentric thin layers (lamellae) of opacities are surrounded by zones of clear lens. Usually in both eyes. Vision may remain good.

lamellar graft. See LAMELLAR KERATOPLASTY.

lamellar keratoplasty (LKP) (KEHR-uh-toh-plas-tee), **lamellar *(or)* partial-thickness graft.** *Surgical procedure.* Removal of the outer corneal layers (lamellae) and replacement with normal corneal tissue from a donor. See also CORNEAL TRANSPLANT, PENETRATING KERATOPLASTY.

lamina cribrosa (LAM-in-uh krih-BROH-suh), **cribiform plate.** *Anatomy.* Thin, sieve-like portion of sclera at the base of the optic disc through which retinal nerve fibers leave the eye to form the optic nerve. See also LAMINA DOTS.

lamina dots. *Anatomy.* Holes in the lamina cribrosa that are visible in the optic disc portion of the fundus; particularly noticeable when there is optic nerve degeneration. May also be found in normal eyes.

lamina fusca sclerae (FOOS-kuh SKLEH-ree). See LAMINA SUPRACHOROIDEA.

lamina papyracea (pah-pih-RAY-shee-uh). *Anatomy.* Refers to the extremely thin medial orbital wall (ethmoid bone).

laminar flow (LAM-in-ur). *Function.* Phenomenon of blood moving along the wall of a blood vessel and tending not to mix with the blood in the center. Visible in the arterio-venous phase of fluorescein angiography.

lamina suprachoroidea (su-pruh-kor-OYD-ee-uh), **suprachoroid, lamina fusca sclerae.** *Anatomy.* Thin, brown outermost layer of choroid lying against the sclera.

lamina vitrea (VIT-ree-uh), **basal lamina, Bruch's membrane.** *Anatomy.* Membrane underlying the retinal pigment epithelium. Innermost layer of choroid.

Lancaster red-green. *Test.* For identifying eye deviations that vary in the nine positions of gaze. Wearing 1 red and 1 green lens, patient attempts to superimpose a green streak of light onto a red streak projected on a grid. See also HESS-LEES SCREEN.

Lancaster-Regan dial #1, clock *(or)* "sunburst" dial. *Test chart.* Radial arrangement of black lines used for subjectively refining the axis of an astigmatic refractive error. See also ASTIGMATIC CLOCK, FAN DIAL, LANCASTER-REGAN DIAL #2.

Lancaster-Regan dial #2. *Test chart.* Two perpendicular lines on a movable disc, used for subjectively refining the amount of astigmatic refractive error. See also ASTIGMATIC CLOCK, CLOCK DIAL

Landolt "broken ring" chart, Landolt "C" *(or)* Landolt ring chart. *Test chart.* Visual acuity chart with C-like symbols in graded Snellen sizes, rotated so that the break appears up, down, right, or left.

Langhans giant cell. *Pathologic change*. Large macrophage cell seen in some granulomatous processes. Has abundant cytoplasm and a row of multi-nuclei arranged along the cell periphery.

Lanthony's desaturated 15 hue test. Sensitive color vision test for detecting congenital or acquired color deficiencies. See also MUNSELL SCALE.

laser. *Instrument*. Acronym: Light Amplification by Stimulated Emission of Radiation. High energy light source that uses light emitted by the natural vibrations of atoms (of a gas or solid material) to cut, burn or dissolve tissues for various clinical purposes: in the retina, to treat diabetic retinopathy and macular degeneration, to destroy leaking and new blood vessels (neo-vascularization); on the iris or trabecular meshwork, to decrease pressure in glaucoma; after extracapsular cataract extraction, to open the posterior lens capsule.

> **argon**: filled with argon gas; for placing minute burns to selectively destroy bits of iris, retina, abnormal blood vessels (neovascularization), tumors, etc.

> **carbon dioxide**: filled with carbon dioxide gas; for photocoagulation using an infrared emission for cutting tissue through heat absorption.

> **excimer**: emits an ultraviolet light beam that cuts by rupturing molecules and ejecting molecular fragments, rather than by heat. In refractive corneal surgery, controlled by computer to make precise pre-programmed shavings of eye tissue to produce a given optical correction.

> **krypton**: filled with krypton gas; uses similar to ARGON (above).

> **Nd:YAG** (acronym: yttrium-aluminum-garnet): produces short pulsed, high energy light beam to cut, perforate or fragment tissue.

laser assisted intrastomal keratoplasty. See LASIK.

laser gonioplasty, goniophotocoagulation. See LASER TRABECULOPLASTY.

laser interferometer (in-tur-fur-AHM-uh-tur). *Instrument*. Diagnostic laser used for predicting visual acuity potential when an opacity (e.g., cataract) is present. See also POTENTIAL ACUITY METER.

laser iridectomy. Incorrect term for LASER IRIDOTOMY.

laser iridotomy (ir-ih-DAHT-uh-mee). *Surgical procedure*. Application of a laser light beam to burn a hole through the iris near its base. Used for controlling eye pressure in angle-closure glaucoma.

laser keratorefractive surgery, laser refractive corneal surgery, photorefractive keratectomy (PRK). *Surgical procedure*. Use of high intensity laser light (e.g., an excimer laser) to reshape the corneal curvature; for correcting refractive errors. Includes laser sculpting, LASIK.

laser pupillomydriasis (pyu-pil-oh-mih-DRI-uh-sis). *Surgical procedure*. Application of a laser light beam to the edge of the pupil to enlarge pupil size. See also COREOPLASTY.

laser refractive corneal surgery. See laser KERATOREFRACTIVE SURGERY.

laser sculpting, laser sculpturing. *Surgical procedure*. Use of a computer-controlled excimer laser to remove a thin layer from the cornea, changing its shape and optical power. See also EXCIMER LASER, KERATOREFRACTIVE SURGERY.

laser trabeculoplasty (LTP) (truh-BEK-yu-loh-plas-tee), **laser gonioplasty, goniophotocoagulation**. *Surgical procedure*. Application of a laser beam to selectively burn the trabecular meshwork area, to lower intraocular pressure. Used for treating open angle and neovascular glaucoma.

Lasex. *Drug*. Trade name of furosemide, which increases urination; heart medication.

LASIK (LAY-sik). *Surgical procedure*. Acronym: LAser in SItu Keratomileusis, also Laser ASsisted Intrastromal Keratoplasty. Type of lamellar refractive surgery in which the cornea is reshaped to change its optical power. A disc of cornea ("button") is raised as a flap, then an excimer laser is used to reshape the intrastromal bed, producing surgical flattening of the cornea. Used for correcting very high refractive errors, especially myopia. (Differs from keratomileusis, in which reshaping is done by lathe-cutting the corneal button.) See also LASER SCULPTING.

latanoprost . *Drug.* Class of drugs that increases ease of aqueous drainage to lower pressure inside the eye. Used for treating glaucoma. Has side effect of changing eye color. Trade name: Xalatan.

latent. *Description.* Masked or hidden. See also MANIFEST.

latent hyperopia (hi-pur-OH-pee-uh). *Refractive error.* Portion of total hyperopia (underpowered eye) that cannot be relaxed with plus lenses; the difference between manifest and total hyperopia. Not apparent to the individual; identified by cycloplegia.

latent nystagmus (ni-STAG-mus). *Functional defect.* Jerky, rhythmic oscillations in one eye that occur when the other eye is covered. May be more marked in one eye than in the other. See also NYSTAGMUS.

lateral. *Location.* Toward the side of the body, away from the midline. See also MEDIAL.

lateral canthotomy (kan-THAH-tuh-mee). *Surgical procedure.* Horizontal incision at the outer (lateral) junction of the upper and lower eyelids (canthi) to temporarily enlarge lid separation, or as part of reconstructive lid plastic surgery.

lateral canthus (KAN-thus), **outer canthus.** *Anatomy.* Angle formed by the outer (away from nose) junction of the upper and lower eyelids.

lateral geniculate body (LGB) (jen-IK-yu-lit), **external geniculate body, lateral geniculate nucleus.** *Anatomy.* Paired prominences at the sides of the midbrain (upper end of brainstem); neural way-station where optic tract fibers connect (synapse) to optic radiations and transmit visual information.

lateral geniculate nucleus (LGN). See LATERAL GENICULATE BODY.

lateral horn. *Anatomy.* 1. End of the levator muscle in the upper eyelid that attaches to the lateral palpebral ligament near the outer canthus. Partially supports the lacrimal gland against the orbital roof. See also APONEUROSIS OF THE EYELID. 2. Part of internal fluid system of the brain (ventricles), located within the temporal lobe.

lateral medullary syndrome (MED-yu-lehr-ee), **Wallenberg syndrome.** *Pathologic condition.* Most common brainstem stroke. Characterized by eye overshoot (dysmetria), Horner's syndrome, rotary nystagmus, skew deviations on the same side of the body, and facial and body weakness on the opposite side of the body.

lateral orbital decompression, Krönlein procedure. *Surgical procedure.* Partial removal of the bony orbital wall (zygoma) and/or floor (maxillary sinus roof) to relieve forward pressure on the eye when the orbital contents have increased in size, as in Graves' disease. See also THYROID EYE DISEASE.

lateral palpebral ligament (pal-PEE-brul). *Anatomy.* Strong fibrous band of tissue that anchors the upper and lower eyelid tarsi to the orbital tubercle on the zygomatic bone. Much weaker than the medial palpebral ligament.

lateral rectus (LR). *Anatomy.* Extraocular muscle that moves the eye outward (abduction) from the straight-ahead position. Attached to outer side of eyeball; innervated by the 6th cranial (abducens) nerve.

lateral rectus palsy, abducens *(or)* 6th nerve palsy. *Pathologic condition.* Partial or total loss of function of the 6th (abducens) cranial nerve. The affected eye deviates inward (esotropia) and has defective ability to turn out beyond the midline (abduct) since it no longer receives adequate innervation; thus the deviation becomes more apparent when both eyes rotate toward the affected side.

lathe-cut lens. *Optical device.* Contact lens produced by the lathe method of cutting and grinding.

lattice dystrophy. *Pathologic condition.* Corneal stroma disease due to amyloid deposition in the stroma. Characterized by fine, branching central corneal opacities that spread peripherally, giving cornea the appearance of ground glass. Appears in childhood, with marked visual impairment by middle age. Treatment is by corneal transplant. Hereditary (dominant).

lattice retinal degeneration, equatorial degeneration. *Degenerative change.* Retinal thinning with dense vitreous traction in a degenerative zone near the retinal equator. May lead to retinal tears and detachment. Common.

Laurence-Moon-Biedl syndrome (bee-DEL). *Pathologic condition.* Characterized by obesity, mental deficiency, extra fingers and toes, underdeveloped sex organs, and retinitis pigmentosa. Rare, hereditary.

"lazy eye," amblyopia. *Functional defect.* Decreased vision in one or both eyes without detectable anatomic damage in the eye or visual pathways. Uncorrectable by optical means (e.g., glasses). Types listed under AMBLYOPIA.

"lazy T" procedure, medial ectropion operation. *Surgical procedure.* For repair of a lower eyelid and punctum that do not rest against the eyeball. Wound resembles a letter T on its side. See also PUNCTAL ECTROPION, MEDIAL ECTROPION.

leash. *Functional defect.* Tethering effect of an extraocular muscle that restricts eyeball movement in a particular direction. The muscle is on the side of the eyeball opposite the restriction.

Lebensohn chart (LAY-ben-sun). *Test chart.* Size-graded letters and numbers used for testing near visual acuity.

Leber's cells (LAY-burz). *Pathologic change.* Large macrophage cells with debris found in the conjunctiva. Common in trachoma.

Leber's congenital amaurosis (am-uh-ROH-sis). *Congenital defect.* Blindness or near-blindness in both eyes. May be accompanied by nystagmus, sensitivity to light and sunken eyes. Marked reduction in retinal function seen on an electroretinogram.

Leber's disease, Leber's optic atrophy. *Pathologic condition.* Characterized by rapidly progressive optic nerve degeneration affecting both eyes. No known treatment; vision stabilizes and is not totally lost. Occurs in young men ages 20–30. Rare; hereditary.

Leber's idiopathic neuroretinitis. *Pathologic condition.* Acute swelling of the optic disc; may occur after a viral infection. Can lead to retinal edema with development of a macular star and hard exudates in and around the macula. Causes vision loss, with a central or centrocecal scotoma that improves over time. Affects children and young adults. See also OPTIC NEURITIS, PAPILLITIS.

Leber's miliary aneurisms, retinal telangectasia. *Pathologic condition.* Malformed, irregularly dilated retinal blood vessels in one eye that leak proteineaceous fatty exudates into and under the retina. Congenital; early stage of Coats' disease. Affects mostly males, with leakage occurring in late youth. Preferred term is retinal telangectasia.

left-beating nystagmus (ni-STAG-mus). *Functional defect.* Rhythmic, side-to-side eye oscillations with the fast phase toward left gaze.

left deorsumvergence, positive vertical vergence *(or)* **divergence, right sursumvergence.** *Function.* Upward movement of the right eye relative to the left, usually to maintain single binocular vision, e.g., when increasing amounts of base-up prism are placed over the right eye. See also SURSUMVERGENCE.

left gaze. Eye position to the left of straight-ahead, as the head remains stationary. The eyes are moved by contraction of the right medial rectus and left lateral rectus.

left-gaze verticals. *Anatomy.* Extraocular muscles (left inferior rectus, left superior rectus, right inferior oblique, right superior oblique) that move an eye up or down when in left gaze.

left sursumvergence, negative vertical vergence *(or)* **divergence, right deorsumvergence.** *Function.* Upward movement of the left eye relative to the right, usually to maintain single binocular vision, e.g., when increasing amounts of base-down prism are placed over the left eye.

legal blindness. Best-corrected visual acuity of 20/200 or less, or reduction in visual field to 20° or less, in the better seeing eye.

lens. *Anatomy.* Natural crystalline lens of the eye. Transparent, biconvex intraocular tissue that helps bring rays of light to focus on the retina. Suspended by fine ligaments (zonules) attached between ciliary processes.

> **capsule**: elastic bag enveloping the lens; helps control shape of lens for accommodation.

> **cortex**: jelly-like main part of the lens, composed of millions of thin lens fibers. Located between the denser inner nucleus and elastic outer capsule.

> **nucleus**: optically defined zone in the center. Becomes denser with age, eventually hardening and filling the entire lens.

lens. *Optics.* Any piece of glass or other transparent material that can bend light rays predictably. See also REFRACTION.

> **biconcave**: thinner in the center and thicker at the edges, with inward curvature of both surfaces. Minus powered.

> **biconvex**: thicker in the center and thinner at the edges, with outward curvature of both surfaces. Plus powered.

> **concave**: thicker at the edges than in the center, increasing divergence of incoming light rays; corrects nearsightedness. Same as minus lens.

> **concavo-convex (meniscus)**: has an outward-curving (convex) front surface and an inward-curving (concave) back surface.

> **convex**: thicker in the center than at the edges, adding optical power to incoming light rays. Corrects farsightedness (hyperopia).

lens axis: imaginary line passing through the optical centers of both surfaces of a lens. Also called optical axis, principal axis.

lensectomy. *Surgical procedure.* Removal of a lens. See also CATARACT EXTRACTION.

lens-induced glaucoma (glaw-KOH-muh), **phacolytic glaucoma**. *Pathologic condition.* Increased intraocular pressure caused by mechanical blockage of the eye's drainage channels (trabecular meshwork) by cells carrying lens protein. Associated with advanced (hypermature) cataracts or lens trauma.

lens-induced uveitis (yu-vee-I-tis). *Pathologic condition.* Inflammation of the iris, ciliary body and choroid caused by an immune reaction to lens protein. Occurs after lens capsule is torn from trauma or after cataract extraction.

lensometer (lenz-AH-mih-tur). *Instrument.* Used for determining the refractive power of an eyeglass or contact lens.

lens power (formula). *Optics.* Dioptric power of a lens is equal to 1 divided by its focal length in meters ($P = I/f$). For example, if the focal length is 1/2 meter, the power is 2 D.

lenticonus (len-tih-KOH-nus). *Congenital defect.* Characterized by an abnormal cone-shaped protrusion of the lens, usually on the front surface. Rare.

lenticular astigmatism (len-TIK-yu-lur uh-STIG-muh-tiz-um). *Refractive error.* Optical defect caused by different curvatures of one or both surfaces of the eye's lens.

lenticular. *Description.* Pertaining to or shaped like a lens.

lenticular lens. *Optical device.* Eyeglass or contact lens constructed of a carrier flange of no power or low power in the periphery and a central bowl with power. Bowl may be a high-plus lens (cataract glasses) or a high-minus lens (e.g., Myodisc), allowing reduced edge thickness. See also ASPHERIC LENTICULAR SPECTACLES.

lenticule. *Optical device*. Lens-shaped material, often corneal donor tissue, used in some types of refractive surgery. See also EPIKERATOPHAKIA, KERATOMILEUSIS.

lentiglobus (len-tih-GLOH-bus). *Congenital defect*. Characterized by an abnormal spherical protrusion of the lens, usually on the back surface. Rare.

lentigo (LEN-tih-goh). 1. Small pigmented spot in the skin that is unrelated to sun exposure; potentially malignant. 2. A freckle. Plural: lentigines.

lesion. *Pathologic condition*. Localized, abnormal change in tissue formation due to injury or disease.

> **benign**: does not threaten health or life. Non-cancerous.

> **malignant**: having uncontrolled growth; may produce death or deterioration. Cancerous.

leukocoria (lu-koh-KOR-ee-uh). *Clinical sign*. Any eye condition that whitens the pupil. See also CATARACT, CAT'S EYE REFLEX, PHPV, RETINOBLASTOMA.

leukocyte. *Anatomy*. White blood cell; part of the body's immune system. Five types: basophil, eosinophil, lymphocyte, monocyte and neutrophil.

leukocytosis (lu-koh-si-TOH-sus). *Pathologic condition*. Having an increased number (above normal levels) of white blood cells in the circulating bloodstream.

leukoma (lu-KOH-muh). *Anatomic defect*. Dense corneal opacity (a less dense opacity is called a macula; the least dense is a nebula).

> **adherent l**: corneal opacity to which the iris is attached.

leukopenia (lu-koh-PEEN-ee-uh). *Clinical sign*. Abnormally low number of white blood cells in the blood.

levator aponeurosis (luh-VAY-tur uh-pahn-yur-OH-sis), **aponeurosis of the eyelid**. *Anatomy*. Fan-shaped membranous expansion of the end of the levator muscle. Spans the entire width of the upper orbit and attaches to the skin of the upper eyelid and to the tarsal plate. Its two extremities are called horns. See also LATERAL HORN, MEDIAL HORN.

levator muscle. See LEVATOR PALPEBRAE SUPERIORIS.

levator palpebrae superioris (pal-PEE-bree su-pih-ree-OR-is), **levator muscle**. *Anatomy*. Muscle that raises the upper eyelid. Innervated by the upper division of the 3rd (oculomotor) cranial nerve. Originates at the rear of the orbit in the annulus of Zinn, comes forward above the superior rectus to insert into the upper eyelid.

levator resection (luh-VAY-tur). *Surgical procedure*. Repair of a drooping eyelid (ptosis) by shortening the levator muscle in the upper lid.

> **internal (posterior approach)**: for a moderately ptosis, a conjunctival incision (on underside of lid) is made through the tarsus, muscle is removed, and the lid is repositioned to the desired height.

> **external (anterior approach)**: for a moderate-to-severe ptosis, a skin incision is made in the lid in the desired position for removing excess muscle and reconstructing the fold in the lid.

levobunolol (LEE-voh-BYU-nuh-lawl). *Drug*. Beta-one and beta-two blocking agent that reduces aqueous secretion. Eyedrops for treating glaucoma. Trade name: Betagan. See also BETAXOLOL, CARTEOLOL, METIPRANOLOL, TIMOLOL.

levoversion (LEE-voh-vur-zhun). *Function*. Parallel movement of both eyes to the left.

Lhermitte's sign. *Clinical sign*. Electric-like shocks in the limbs and trunk when the neck is flexed forcibly forward. Suggests multiple sclerosis.

lid-bracing sutures, Quickert 3-suture operation. *Surgical procedure*. For repair of an inturned lower eyelid (entropion). Three horizontal stitches are placed just below the tarsal edge of the lower eyelid at its inner, central and outer portions. See also SENILE ENTROPION.

lid cellulitis, pre-septal cellulitis. *Pathologic condition*. Swelling or infection of eyelid tissue in front of the orbital septum. Does not affect the eyeball. See also ORBITAL CELLULITIS.

lid fold, superior palpebral furrow. *Anatomy*. Fold seen in the upper eyelid when the eye is open.

lid lag, von Graefe sign. *Clinical sign*. Delay (lag) in downward movement of the upper eyelid as it follows the eye into down-gaze. Common sign of thyroid eye disease.

lid retraction. *Clinical sign*. A "pulled up" upper eyelid that exposes more white of the eye (sclera) than normal, resulting in a "stare" appearance. Common sign of thyroid eye disease. See also COLLIER'S SIGN.

lid speculum (SPEK-yu-lum). *Instrument*. Used for holding the eyelids open and apart for examination or surgery.

lidocaine (LI-doh-kayn). *Drug*. Anesthetic agent given by injection for eye surgery. Trade name: Xylocaine.

lids, eyelids. *Anatomy*. Structures covering the front of the eye. Their function is to protect the eye, limit amount of light entering the pupil, and distribute tear film over the exposed corneal surface.

ligament of Lockwood. See LOCKWOOD'S LIGAMENT.

ligamentum pectinatum iridis (lig-uh-MEN-tum pek-tih-NAH-tum IR-ih-dis), **cribiform ligament, scleral trabeculae, trabecular meshwork**. *Anatomy*. Mesh-like structure inside the eye at the iris-scleral junction of the anterior chamber angle. Filters aqueous fluid and controls its flow into the canal of Schlemm, prior to its leaving the anterior chamber.

light. Portion of the electromagnetic spectrum that gives rise to a sensation of brightness through stimulation of the retina.

light adaptation. *Function*. Physiologic process (mainly retinal and photochemical) that adjusts eye to bright light levels. See also DARK ADAPTATION, PHOTOPIC VISION.

light-near dissociation. *Clinical sign*. Absence of pupillary constriction to a direct light stimulus in combination with normal constriction to a near target (about 14 in.). See also ARGYLL-ROBERTSON PUPILS.

light perception (LP). *Test measurement*. Lowest level of acuity based on the patient's ability to distinguish light from dark. Used when vision loss is profound. See also COUNTS FINGERS, HAND MOVEMENTS.

light perception and projection (LP + P). *Test measurement*. Low level of visual acuity denoting the ability to distinguish light from darkness and to determine the direction of a light source.

light pipe (fiberoptic), endoilluminator. *Instrument*. Light source used for illuminating the inside of the eye during surgical procedures. Comprised of a flexible bundle of closely packed transparent fibers that conduct light.

light projection. *Test measurement*. Low level of acuity (slightly better than light perception) based on the patient's ability to determine the direction of a light source. Used when vision loss is profound.

Lignac-Fanconi's syndrome (LEEN-yak fan-KOH-nees), **nephropathic cystine storage disease**. *Pathologic condition*. Characterized by rickets, cystine crystal accumulation in the kidneys, liver, spleen, bone marrow, lymph nodes, conjunctiva, cornea and choroid, and sensitivity to light (photophobia). Rare; hereditary.

limbal approach. *Surgical procedure*. Method of gaining access to the eyeball by cutting through conjunctiva at corneo-scleral junction (limbus).

limbal-based flap. *Surgical procedure*. Type of conjunctival flap. Cutting the conjunctiva several millimeters behind the limbus (corneo-scleral junction) to cover a limbal incision site into eye, e.g., during a cataract extraction. See also FORNIX-BASED FLAP.

limbus, corneo-scleral junction. *Anatomy*. Transitional zone about 1–2 mm wide, where the cornea joins the sclera and the bulbar conjunctiva attaches to the eyeball.

limulus lysate test (LIM-yu-lus LI-sayt). Sensitive indicator of gram-negative endotoxins. For determining if a gram-negative organism is involved in an eye infection when previous medication has interfered with usual culture media.

Lindau's disease. See LINDAU-VON HIPPEL DISEASE.

Lindau-von Hippel disease, angiomatosis retinae, Lindau's disease. *Pathologic condition.* One of several hereditary disorders called phakomatoses. Characterized by tumors of the retina, central nervous system and visceral organs. Primary eye findings are blood-filled retinal tumors (hemangiomas) fed by large, tortuous blood vessels; may also be associated with exudate leakage into the retina and retinal detachment.

linear perspective, geometric perspective. As parallel lines and planes recede into the distance, they appear to approach each other at the horizon. One of several monocular cues to depth perception. See also MONOCULAR DEPTH PERCEPTION.

line of direction. Imaginary line connecting an object in space with the retinal point where it is imaged. See also LINE OF FIXATION.

line of fixation, primary line of sight, principal line of direction, visual axis *(or)* **line**. Imaginary line connecting a viewed object and the fovea. See also FIXATION.

lipemia retinalis (li-PEE-mee-uh ret-ih-NAL-is). *Clinical sign.* Creamy coloring of retinal blood vessels due to high retinal blood fat (lipid) level. Associated with hyperlipidemia, pancreatitis, and diabetes mellitus.

lipid. Fat and fat-like substances.

lipofuscin (li-poh-FYU-sin). *Anatomy.* Fatty substance found in the retinal pigment epithelium. Excessive amounts are abnormal.

Liquifilm forte (LIK-wuh-film FOR-tay). *Chemical.* Trade name of polyvinyl alcohol eyedrops; for treating dry eyes.

Liquifilm tears. *Chemical.* Trade name of polyvinyl alcohol eyedrops; for treating dry eyes.

Lisch nodules. *Pathologic condition.* Multiple lightly pigmented elevations that occur on the iris of patients who have neurofibromatosis.

Listing's law. *Function.* As an eye moves to any oblique position from a primary position, the amount of torsion present is independent of how the eye traveled to get there.

Listing's plane. Imaginary plane passing through the equator and the center of rotation of an eye when the eye is in the primary position.

lithiasis (lith-I-uh-sis). *Degenerative change.* Calcified spots on the conjunctiva covering the inner surfaces of the eyelids. Usually asymptomatic, but may act as a foreign body, scratching the eyeball.

Livostin. *Drug.* Trade name of levocabastine, an antihistamine. For treating allergic conjunctivitis.

localization, spatial localization. *Function.* Perception of an object's position in space. Determined by which retinal elements are stimulated: nasal elements localize in temporal space, temporal elements in nasal space, and the fovea straight ahead. See also VISUAL DIRECTION.

Lockwood's ligament. *Anatomy.* Lower, thickened portion of Tenon's capsule; fascial band under the eye formed by the blending of the sheaths of the inferior oblique and inferior rectus muscles. Has extensions to the orbital walls, orbital septum and lower tarsus. Forms a hammock-like support beneath the eyeball.

lodoxamide. *Drug.* Eyedrops used for treating allergic conjunctivitis. Trade name: Alomide. See also CROMOLYN, KETOROLAC TROMETHAMINE.

long ciliary nerves (SIL-ee-eh-ree). *Anatomy.* Two branches of the nasociliary nerve that enter the sclera and pass between it and the choroid to supply sensory fibers to the iris, cornea and ciliary muscle; also send some sympathetic nerve fibers to the pupil dilator muscle. See also CILIARY NERVES.

longitudinal axis of Fick, anteroposterior *(or)* **sagittal** *(or)* **y axis of Fick.** Imaginary line running through the center of rotation of the eye, connecting the geometric center of the cornea (anterior pole) with the geometric center of the back of eye (posterior pole). Tilting (torsional) eye rotations occur around this axis.

long posterior ciliary arteries (SIL-ee-eh-ree). *Anatomy.* Two blood vessels that branch from the ophthalmic artery in the orbit and enter the eye near the optic nerve, running forward between the sclera and choroid to the ciliary muscle, where they join the anterior ciliary arteries and form the major arterial circle of iris. See also CILIARY ARTERIES.

loops of Axenfeld, intrascleral nerve loops. *Anatomy.* Loops of a long ciliary nerve into the anterior sclera; appear as a tiny dark spot of uveal tissue on the sclera, near the limbus.

Lopressor. *Drug.* Trade name of metaprolol; for controlling high blood pressure (hypertension).

Louis-Bar syndrome (LU-ee), **ataxia telangiectasia.** *Pathologic condition.* Characterized by small, spidery blood vessels (telangiectasia) on the skin, conjunctiva, optic nerve and brain. Associated with immunoglobulin and lymphoproliferative abnormalities. Hereditary. See also PHAKOMATOSIS.

loupes (loopz). *Instrument.* Magnifying lenses mounted over eyeglasses. Often worn by doctors while performing eye surgery.

lovastatin. *Drug.* Heart medication, for decreasing cholesterol levels. Trade name: Mevacor. See also CHOLYSTYRAMINE, CLOFIBRATE.

lower punctum, inferior punctum. *Anatomy.* Tiny opening in the papilla (slight elevation on lower eyelid margin near nose) that marks the entrance site of the tear drainage (lacrimal) system into the nose.

Lowe's syndrome, oculo-cerebro-renal syndrome. *Pathologic condition.* Characterized by mental retardation, renal problems, cataracts, and congenital glaucoma. Rare. Hereditary, X-linked (affects males; female carriers have only cataracts).

low-vision aids (LVA). *Optical device.* High-powered plus lenses and telescopes with high magnification, to help patients who have poor vision.

LR$_6$ (SO$_4$)^3. Mnemonic: the Lateral Rectus is innervated by the 6th (abducens) cranial nerve, the Superior Oblique by the 4th (trochlear) cranial nerve, and the rest of the extraocular muscles by the 3rd (oculomotor) cranial nerve.

lues (LU-eez). *Pathologic condition.* Slang for syphilis.

lumbar puncture. *Diagnostic test, procedure.* Removal of cerebrospinal fluid or injection of anesthetic drugs through a needle inserted into the lumbar portion of the spinal canal. See also SPINAL TAP.

lumen (LU-muhn). 1. *Anatomy.* Cavity of a hollow organ or blood vessel. 2. *Optics.* Unit of measure of luminous flux. See also APOSTILB.

luminance. *Optics.* Amount of light emanating from an object and producing a sensation of brightness.

luminous flux. *Optics.* Total quantity of light flowing in all directions from a light source.

luminous intensity. *Optics.* Amount of light emitted from a light source in a given direction. Measured in candelas.

lupus erythematosus (LU-pus er-ih-thee-muh-TOH-sis), **systemic lupus erythematosus.** *Pathologic condtion.* Autoimmune collagen disease characterized by fever, facial rash in a "butterfly" pattern, and heart and kidney problems. May be associated with double vision, decreased vision, nystagmus, swollen and puffy eyelids, dry eyes, cotton-wool retinal deposits and, rarely, optic nerve degeneration, retinal hemorrhages and retinal blood vessel blockages.

lux. *Optics.* Amount of light falling on a surface. Older term for lumens per square meter.

luxation. *Pathologic condition.* Displacement of tissue from its normal position. 1. Usually refers to the eye's crystalline lens; caused by broken or absent zonules that normally provide support. 2. "Popped out" appearance of the eyeball as caused by an abnormally shallow orbit. See also SUBLUXATION.

lymphadenopathy (lim-fad-en-AHP-uh-thee). *Clinical sign.* Abnormal enlargement of lymph nodes.

lymphangioma (lim-fan-jee-OH-muh). *Pathologic condition.* Tumor formed from dilated (enlarged) lymphatic vessels.

lymph node (limff). *Anatomy.* Mass of lymphocytes that filter tissue fluids; found along lymph vessels in many locations in the body. Part of body's immune system. Swelling and tenderness may indicate infection in that region.

lymphocyte (LIM-foh-site). *Anatomy.* Type of white blood cell. May be large or small, B-cell or T-cell. Important in immune system and inflammatory system responses.

lymphoma (lim-FOH-muh). *Pathologic condition.* Tumor of lymphoid tissue; often malignant.

Lyon's hypothesis. *Theory.* Explains the variable partial expression of an X-linked recessive disease in the female carrier.

lyophilize (li-AHPH-uh-lise). *Lab technique.* Freeze-dry method of removing water (dehydration) from tissue or chemical products.

lyse (lice). Rupturing of a cell wall, with release of intracellular contents.

lysozyme (LI-soh-zime). *Chemical.* Anti-bacterial enzyme found in normal tears. Dissolves outer coating of some bacteria.

M

MacKay-Marg tonometer (toh-NAHM-ih-tur). *Instrument.* Applanation tonometer that electronically measures and records intraocular pressure from the force required to flatten 2.5 mm of cornea. See also TONOMETRY.

macroglobulinemia (Waldenstrom's). *Pathologic condition.* Very large protein globulin molecules in the blood. May cause blockage of blood vessels because of increased viscosity of the blood. Cause unknown.

macrophage (MAK-roh-fayj). *Anatomy.* Type of white blood cell. Scavenger cell that removes microorganisms, debris, dead tissue and foreign proteins from the tissues. Part of the body's immune system.

macrophthalmos (mak-ruf-THAL-mus), **megophthalmos**. *Anatomic defect.* Abnormally large eyeball. See also BUPHTHALMOS, MEGALOCORNEA.

macropsia (mak-RAHP-see-uh). *Functional defect.* Distorted vision in which objects appear larger than normal. See also METAMORPHOPSIA, MICROPSIA.

macula (MAK-yu-luh). 1. *Anatomy.* See MACULA LUTEA. 2. *Pathologic condition.* Moderately dense corneal opacity. See also LEUCOMA, NEBULA.

macula lutea (LU-tee-uh), **macula**. *Anatomy.* Literally, "yellow spot." Small (3°) central area of the retina surrounding the fovea; area of acute central vision.

macular corneal dystrophy (MAK-yu-lur KOR-nee-ul DIS-truh-fee), **Groenouw type II dystrophy**. *Pathologic condition.* Rare disorder of the corneal stroma characterized by a slowly progressive decrease in vision caused by an accumulation of opaque deposits (mucopolysaccharides) in the corneal cells. Hereditary (recessive); begins in childhood.

macular degeneration (ARMD, AMD), age-related *(or)* **senile macular degeneration**. *Pathologic condition.* Group of conditions that include deterioration of the macula, resulting in a loss of sharp central vision. Two general types: "dry," which is usually evident as a disturbance of macular pigmentation and deposits of yellowish material under the pigment epithelial layer in the central retinal zone; and "wet" (sometimes called Kuhnt-Junius disease), in which abnormal new blood vessels grow under the retina and leak fluid and blood, further disturbing macular function. Most common cause of decreased vision after age 60.

macular pucker, cellophane maculopathy, epimacular proliferation, epiretinal membrane. *Pathologic condition.* Retinal wrinkling in the macular area caused by contraction of the transparent membrane lying on the retinal surface. Distorts vision.

macular sparing. *Functional defect.* Refers to the unaffected central 10° zone of vision within a blind area of the visual field.

macular splitting. *Functional defect.* Loss of the right or left half of each eye's visual field (homonymous hemianopsia), including loss of half of the central part. Occurs when central visual fibers have been severely damaged behind the chiasm.

macular star. *Pathologic condition.* Residual inflammatory deposits in the area of central vision (macula) that appear to radiate outward in a star-like pattern. Occurs in any retinal condition associated with a fluid logged macula, such as severe hypertensive retinopathy or papillitis.

maculopathy (mak-yu-LAH-puh-thee). *Pathologic condition.* Nonspecific abnormality of the macula.

Maddox rod. *Test instrument.* Series of small high-powered cylinders set into a disk that converts a spot of light into an apparent streak of light. See also MADDOX ROD TEST.

Maddox rod test. For quantifying misalignment in phoric or tropic eyes. As the patient views a fixation light with both eyes, a Maddox rod is held before one eye. Two images (an apparent line and a spot of light) are created. Prism power is added until the two images are superimposed; the amount indicates the degree of misalignment.

Maddox wing. *Test instrument.* Measures vertical, horizontal or cyclophorias at near. Requires patient to align arrows along scales that represent the amount of the deviation.

madarosis (mad-uh-ROH-sus). *Abnormal condition.* Loss of eyelashes or eyebrows.

magnetic resonance imaging (MRI). *Test.* Type of imaging technique using high intensity magnets and computers. Permits examination of soft tissues inside the body that cannot be seen with x-rays. Newer term for NMR (nuclear magnetic resonance). See also CT SCAN.

magnification. *Optics.* 1. Increased image size obtained by using optical devices. 2. Change in image size created by a given lens system as compared to the size of an object located 25 cm away as seen without a lens.

major amblyoscope (AM-blee-uh-skohp). *Instrument.* Binocular viewing system that permits simultaneous presentation of separate fixation targets (usually on slides) for each eye. Used in evaluation and treatment of strabismus and other binocularity problems. See also SYNOPTOPHORE, TROPOSCOPE.

major arterial circle of the iris. *Anatomy.* Primary blood distribution system to the front half of the eye. Seven anterior ciliary arteries and two long posterior ciliary arteries form a circular configuration at the junction of the iris and ciliary body.

major meridians. *Optics.* Refers to the meridians of highest and lowest optical power in an optical system that is astigmatic. Meridians are situated perpendicular to each other.

malformation. *Congenital anomaly.* Defect of part or all of an organ or area as a result of abnormal development.

malignant glaucoma (glaw-KOH-muh), **aqueous mis-direction syndrome, ciliary block glaucoma**. *Pathologic condition.* Increase in intraocular pressure accompanied by a shallow anterior chamber and forward displacement of the iris and lens. Complication following surgery for acute angle closure glaucoma; may be caused by aqueous trapped behind the vitreous.

malignant lesion, cancer. *Pathologic condition.* Tissue of potentially unlimited growth that expands locally by invasion and throughout the body by metastasis. See also CARCINOMA, SARCOMA.

malignant myopia (mi-OH-pee-uh), **degenerative myopia**. *Pathologic condition.* Uncommon form of nearsightedness (myopia) accompanied by progressive stretching changes and gradual damage to the retina, choroid, vitreous, sclera and optic nerve. See also FUCHS' SPOT, LACQUER CRACKS.

malingerer (muh-LING-ur-ur). Patient who feigns illness; tries to "fail" the eye examination by giving incorrect answers, not answering, or claiming to see less than he does. See also HYSTERICAL AMBLYOPIA.

malprojection. *Functional defect.* Faulty perception of an object's location resulting from extraocular muscle weakness of recent onset. Object viewed by the involved eye in the affected muscle's field of action appears to be farther from the midline than it actually is. Temporary.

mandibulofacial dysostosis (man-dih-byu-loh-FAY-shul dis-ahs-TOH-sis), **Franceschetti *(or)* Treacher-Collins syndrome**. *Congenital anomaly.* Skull and face deformity characterized by birdlike appearance, with small jaw and "parrot-beak" nose, indistinct orbital margins, notching of lower lids (coloboma), and antimongoloid slant of eyelids. Rare, hereditary. See also HALLERMANN-STREIFF SYNDROME.

manifest. *Description*. Obvious or apparent. See also LATENT.

manifest hyperopia (hi-pur-OH-pee-uh), **facultative hyperopia**. *Refractive error*. Farsighted defect in the eye's optical system. Corrected by a plus lens (spectacle or contact) or by the eye's own focusing ability (accommodation).

manifest latent nystagmus (ni-STAG-mus). *Functional defect*. Involuntary eye movements (nystagmus) in which the fast phase of the movement is toward the fixing eye. Occurs in early onset eso and exo deviations. When one eye has poor vision, e.g., with amblyopia, that eye acts as an occluder, resulting in a latent nystagmus in the normal seeing eye becoming apparent (manifest). Congenital.

manifest refraction (M), refined refraction. 1. *Test*. Presentation of a series of test lenses in graded powers to determine without using eyedrops (cycloplegics) which corrective lenses provide the sharpest, clearest vision. 2. Prescription for eyeglasses or contact lenses resulting from this test.

mannitol. *Medication*. Sugar solution. Given intravenously (IV) to temporarily increase osmotic pressure of the blood. For breaking an acute glaucoma attack. Trade name: Osmitrol. See also ANGLE CLOSURE GLAUCOMA, OSMOTIC AGENT.

Manz (glands of). *Anatomy*. Microscopic bulbar conjunctival mucin-secreting glands; arranged in a ring around the cornea, near the limbus.

map-dot-fingerprint dystrophy, corneal epithelial basement membrane disease, Cogan's microcystic dystrophy. *Pathologic condition*. Common corneal epithelial basement membrane disease characterized by cysts, dots or lines that may change in pattern and distribution over time and resemble a map. Bilateral; may be asymptomatic or may lead to recurrent corneal erosions. Degenerative; hereditary.

map dystrophy. Term sometimes used for MAP-DOT-FINGERPRINT DYSTROPHY.

Marcaine. *Drug*. Trade name of bupivacaine, an anesthetic agent used in eye surgery.

Marchesani's syndrome (mahr-chez-AN-eez). *Pathologic condition*. Characterized by rare skeletal and ocular abnormalities, including a short, stocky body, spade-shaped hands and feet, round dislocated lenses, nearsightedness (myopia), wobbling irides (iridodonesis), and glaucoma. Hereditary.

Marcus-Gunn jaw winking syndrome, external pterygoid-levator synkinesis, Gunn *(or)* jaw winking syndrome. *Congenital defect*. Droopy eyelid (ptosis) that opens widely when chewing, sucking or moving the mouth to the opposite side of the body. Caused by abnormal innervation of the levator muscle by the 5th (trigeminal) cranial nerve.

Marcus-Gunn pupil (MG), Gunn pupil, afferent *(or)* relative afferent pupillary defect. *Functional defect*. Diminished pupil reaction to light, usually secondary to optic nerve disease that causes slowed conduction in optic nerve fibers. In dim illumination, a sudden bright light stimulus to the normal eye will result in both pupils contracting briskly. When the light stimulus is shifted to the defective eye, the pupils contract less well, so they appear to enlarge. See also SWINGING FLASHLIGHT TEST.

Marfan's syndrome, arachnodactyly. *Pathologic condition*. Connective tissue disease characterized by "spidery" fingers and toes (due to extra-long, slender bones), relaxed ligaments, spine and joint deformities, congenital heart disease, and dislocated lenses. Patient may be very nearsighted (myopic) and have large corneas, cataracts, droopy eyelids (ptosis), eye deviations (strabismus), or incomplete choroidal formation. Rare; hereditary.

marginal blepharitis (blef-uh-RI-tis). *Pathologic condition*. Inflammation of the eyelid margin, with redness, swelling, itching and scaly skin.

marginal catarrhal ulcer (kuh-TAHR-ul). *Pathologic condition.* Small, super-ficial ulcer (loss of corneal epithelium) near the limbus (corneo-scleral junction), usually associated with blepharitis or conjunctivitis. Attributed to hypersensitivity to *staphylococcus aureus* bacteria toxins.

marginal myotomy (mi-AH-tuh-mee). *Surgical procedure.* Weakening an extraocular muscle with two staggered incisions from opposite edges; for correcting an eye deviation.

margin reflex distance (MRD). *Measurement.* Distance from the upper eye-lid margin to the position of the corneal reflex.

Marinesco-Sjogren syndrome (mahr-in-ES-koh SHOH-grin). *Pathologic con-dition.* Characterized by mental retardation, slow growth, unsteady gait, congenital cataracts, inability to chew, thin and brittle fingernails, and sparse, incompletely keratinized hair. Hereditary.

Maroteaux-Lamy syndrome (MAHR-uh-toh LAH-mee). *Pathologic condition.* Hereditary form of mucopolysaccharoidosis (type VI). Characterized by skeletal abnormalities and corneal clouding, with no degeneration of the retinal pigment epithelium.

Martegiani's area (mahr-tuh-GHAHN-eez). *Anatomy.* Area over the surface of the optic nerve head where there is an absense of vitreous adherence. This area is surrounded by a ring of firm vitreous adherence to the rim of the optic nerve head.

masquerade syndrome. *Pathologic condition.* Refers to certain tumors that are a diagnostic dilemma. A malignant eye tumor may simulate conjunc-tivitis, uveitis or vitritis. Sebaceous cancer of the eyelid may first appear as a blepharoconjunctivitis. Retinoblastoma, malignant melanoma or reticular cell sarcoma may initially appear as inflammation.

massive periretinal proliferation (MPP), massive preretinal retraction (MPR), massive vitreous retraction (MVR). Obsolete terms; replaced by PROLIFERATIVE VITREORETINOPATHY.

mature cataract. *Pathologic condition.* Opaque lens with no clear zones re-maining but not yet shrunken. Causes marked decrease of vision. Used to be called "ripe."

Maxidex (MAK-see-deks). *Drug.* Trade name of dexamethasone, an anti-in-flammatory steroid suspension.

maxilla, maxillary bone (mak-SIL-uh). *Anatomy.* One of the seven bones forming the orbit (eye socket). Located on nasal side of orbital floor.

maxillary nerve (MAK-sil-eh-ree). *Anatomy.* Second branch of the 5th (tri-geminal) cranial nerve; provides sensation to the skin on the upper and lower eyelids, cheek muscles, and mucous membranes of cheeks, gums, sinuses and lower part of nose. Branches into the infraorbital and zygomatic nerves before exiting the orbit through the inferior orbital fissure.

maxillary sinus. *Anatomy.* Mucus-lined air cavity within the maxillary bones; one of the nasal sinuses that drains into the nose. Others are ethmoid, frontal and sphenoid.

maxima. 1. Plural of maximum. 2. In geometric optics, the peak of a wave-length of light.

Maxitrol (MAKS-ih-trol). *Drug.* Trade name of medication combining neomy-cin and polymixyn (antibiotics), and dexamethasone (steroid); for treating non-viral eye infections.

Maxwell's spot. *Test.* Perception of a bluish spot surrounded by a halo, seen when a blue filter is placed before the eye. Sometimes used as a test for macular function. See also ENTOPTIC PHENOMENON.

McCannel suturing. *Surgical technique.* Method of tying an intraocular lens haptic (loop) to the iris without opening the eye; the suture is passed through the cornea.

measles, rubeola. *Pathologic condition*. Common, systemic viral disease that may be accompanied by acute conjunctivitis or superficial corneal inflammation. See also KOPLIK'S SPOTS.

Mecholyl (MEK-oh-lihl). *Drug*. Trade name of methacholine eyedrops, used in the diagnosis of Adie's pupil. See also MECHOLYL TEST.

Mecholyl test. Instillation of Mecholyl 2.5% eyedrops to diagnose an Adie's pupil; it will constrict; normal pupil will not be affected. See also DENER-VATION SUPERSENSITIVITY.

medial. *Location*. Toward the midline of the body. See also LATERAL.

medial canthus (MEE-dee-ul KAN-thus), **inner canthus**. *Anatomy*. Angle formed by the junction of the upper and lower eyelids, near the nose.

medial horn. *Anatomy*. The end of the levator muscle closest to the nose. Attaches to the medial palpebral ligament. See also APONEUROSIS OF THE EYELID.

medial longitudinal fasciculus (MLF) (fuh-SIK-yu-lis). *Anatomy*. Nerve fiber tract extending from the upper midbrain to the cervical region of the spine, interconnecting ocular motor and vestibular nerve nuclei and cortical centers.

medial palpebral ligament (pal-PEE-brul). *Anatomy*. Strong fibrous band that anchors the medial end (near nose) of the upper and lower tarsi (eyelid structures) to the lacrimal bone.

medial rectus (MR). *Anatomy*. Extraocular muscle that moves the eye inward from the straight-ahead position (adduction). Attached to the outside of the eyeball on the nasal side. Innervated by the 3rd (oculomotor) cranial nerve.

mediate. Aid in the occurrence of, or foster the development of.

medium. *Optics*. Substance through which light travels. Plural: media. See also REFRACTIVE MEDIA.

medulla (muh-DUH-luh), **medulla oblongata**. *Anatomy*. Lowest part of the brainstem, connecting the pons with the spinal cord. Responsible for many involuntary activities, e.g., breathing, heartbeat.

medulated nerve fibers, myelinated nerve fibers. *Congenital anomaly*. Nerve fibers in the retina that are covered with patches of myelin. Non-progressive, asymptomatic. Requires no treatment.

medulloblastoma (MED-yu-loh-blas-TOH-muh). *Pathologic condition*. Highly malignant cerebellar tumor, usually found in children.

medulloepithelioma (MED-yu-loh-ep-ih-thee-lee-OH-muh). *Pathologic condition*. Invasive unilateral tumor arising from nonpigmented ciliary epithelium. Occurs in childhood; not hereditary. See also PHPV, RETINOBLASTOMA.

Meesmann's dystrophy, juvenile corneal epithelial dystrophy. *Pathologic condition*. Non-progressive early childhood disorder, characterized by fine, dot-like, glycogen-containing opacities in the corneal epithelium. Treatment usually unnecessary. Hereditary.

megalocornea (MEG-uh-loh-KOR-nee-uh). *Congenital anomaly*. Non-progressive, developmental abnormality: front third of the eye is larger than normal. See also BUPHTHALMOS.

megophthalmos (meg-ahf-THAL-mus), **macrophthalmos**. *Anatomic defect*. Abnormally large eyeball. See also BUPHTHALMOS, MEGALOCORNEA.

meibomian gland (mi-BOH-mee-un), **tarsal gland**. *Anatomy*. Oil gland (one of a series) within eyelid tissue (tarsus) whose duct opens onto the eyelid margin just behind the gray line. Secretions supply the outer portion of tear film, preventing rapid tear evaporation and tear overflow and providing tight eyelid closure.

meibomian gland dysfunction (MGD) (*Pathologic condition*). Abnormality in the composition of the secretion from the meibomian glands in the tarsus of the eyelids. One cause of blepharitis (eyelid inflammation).

meibomianitis. *Pathologic condition*. Inflammation of the meibomian glands in the eyelids.

Meige syndrome (mehj). *Pathologic condition.* Blepharospasm accompanied by lower facial twitches and contortions.

melanin (MEH-luh-nin). *Cellular component.* Primary pigment in body; responsible for normal and abnormal color variations in skin and iris.

melanocytes (meh-LAN-oh-sites). *Anatomy.* Mature pigment-forming cells found in the surface epithelium, uvea and pigment epithelium of the retina, ciliary body and iris.

melanocytoma (MEH-luh-noh-si-TOH-muh). *Congenital abnormality.* Pigmented (black) non-malignant tumor, usually found on the surface of the optic disc. Extremely slow-growing; usually asymptomatic.

melanoma (meh-luh-NOH-muh). *Pathologic condition.* Malignant tumor derived from pigment cells. In the eye, can initiate in the choroid, ciliary body or iris, though any eye tissue can be affected by metastases or invasive growth from a melanoma elsewhere in the body.

membrane peeling. *Surgical procedure.* Separation of an abnormal epiretinal membrane from the retinal surface.

meninges. *Anatomy.* Three layers of tissue that cover and protect the brain.

meningioma (men-in-jee-OH-muh). *Pathologic condition.* Slow-growing tumor arising from the meninges (tissue covering brain). May exert pressure on the brain, optic nerve or chiasm, or extend into the orbit.

meningomyelocoele (men-in-goh-MI-uh-loh-seel). *Congenital abnormality.* Protrusion of the spinal cord and membrane covering it through a bony defect in the spinal column.

meniscus (men-IS-kus). 1. *Description.* Crescent or crescent-shaped body, e.g., the tear-filled space between a contact lens and the surface of the cornea. 2. Concavo-convex lens shape. 3. *Anatomy.* The cartilage present in some joints, e.g., the knee. Plural: menisci, meniscuses.

meniscus lens, concavo-convex lens. *Optical device.* Lens that has an outward-curving (convex) front surface and an inward-curving (concave) back surface.

mepivacaine. *Drug.* Injectable anesthetic agent used for eye surgery. Trade name: Carbocaine. See also BUPIVACAINE, LIDOCAINE, PROPARACAINE, XYLOCAINE.

meridian. *Optics.* Signifies a specific direction in an optical system. See also ASTIGMATISM, CYLINDER.

meridians (major). *Optics.* Refers to the meridians of highest and lowest optical powers in an optical system that is astigmatic. Situated perpendicular to each other.

meridional amblyopia. *Functional defect.* Reduced vision in one or both eyes, in children who have at least 1 diopter of uncorrected astigmatism. Vision often improves after eyeglasses are worn for several months.

mesodermal dysgenesis of cornea (mez-oh-DUR-mul, dis-JEN-uh-sis). See PETER'S ANOMALY.

mesodermal dysgenesis of iris. See RIEGER'S ANOMALY.

mesopic vision (meh-ZAH-pik). *Function.* Refers to vision at dim light levels, between daylight and night vision; e.g., at full moonlight. See also PHOTOPIC VISION, SCOTOPIC VISION.

Mestinon. *Drug.* Trade name of pyridostigmine bromide; long-lasting anticholinesterase agent used in the treatment of myasthenia gravis.

metachromatic leukodystrophy (met-uh-kroh-MAT-ik lu-koh-DIS-truh-fee), **sulfatide lipidosis.** *Pathologic condition.* Group of genetic defects in fat (lipid) metabolism producing disruption in nerve tissue. Characterized by weakness, mental retardation, eye muscle palsies, optic nerve degeneration, and blindness. Affects young children; death occurs within a few years. See also SPHINGOLIPIDOSES.

metaherpetic lesion (met-uh-her-PEH-tik). *Pathologic condition.* Epithelial corneal ulcer that persists or recurs after a herpes virus infection.

metamorphopsia (met-uh-mor-FAHP-see-uh). *Symptom.* Shape of objects appears distorted. Usually caused by macular disturbances that disrupt normal retinal position or thickness.

metaplasia (met-uh-PLAY-zhuh). *Pathologic condition.* Non-malignant transformation of one type of cell or tissue into another.

metastasis (muh-TAS-tuh-sus). *Pathologic condition.* Transfer of disease-producing cells or microorganisms from disease site to another part of the body, producing similar disease in the new location. Often refers to cancer cells.

metastatic retinitis (reh-tih-NI-tis), **septic retinitis**. *Pathologic condition.* Infection of the retina caused by microorganisms that reach it through the bloodstream.

meter angle. *Measurement.* Angular unit of convergence. One meter angle is the amount of convergence required to binocularly fixate an object 1 m away; equal to the reciprocal of the distance (in meters) between the object and the bridge of the nose. Obsolete. See also PRISM DIOPTER.

methacholine (meth-uh-KOH-leen). *Drug.* Eyedrop that stimulates parasympathetic nerve fibers, producing small pupils (miosis) and increasing aqueous outflow. Used in diagnosis of Adie's pupil. See also MECHOLYL.

methazolamide (meth-uh-ZOH-luh-mide). *Drug.* Oral medication that lowers intraocular pressure by decreasing aqueous secretion. For treating glaucoma. Trade names: Glauctabs, Neptazane, MZM. See also CARBONIC ANHYDRASE INHIBITOR.

methicillin. *Drug.* Antibiotic used for treating ocular infections.

methotrexate. *Drug.* Anti-cancer drug, also used for uveitis or cyclitis that does not respond to steroids. Trade names: Folex, Mexate.

Methulose (METH-uh-lohs). *Drug.* Trade name of methylcellulose eyedrops; for relieving dry eyes.

methylcellulose (meth-ul-SEL-yu-lohs). *Drug.* Artificial tears solution used for relief of dry eye symptoms (itching, burning, foreign body sensation), thickening tears, reducing corneal drying, and in drug solutions to prolong their contact with the cornea; some products used for treating recurrent corneal erosion. Trade names: Bion Tears, Methulose, Murocel, Refresh Plus, Ultra Tears. See also POLYVINYL ALCOHOL, TEAR FILM BREAKUP TIME.

methylprednisolone (METH-ul-pred-NIH-seh-lohn). *Drug.* Anti-inflammatory steroid. Trade names: Depo Medrol, Solumedrol.

Metimyd (MET-ih-mid). *Drug.* Trade name of eyedrop containing sodium sulfacetamine and prednisolone; for treating inflammations and allergies.

metipranolol. *Drug.* Beta-one and beta-two blocking agent that reduces aqueous secretion. Used as eyedrops for treating glaucoma. Trade name: Optipranolol. See also BETAXOLOL, CARTEOLOL, LEVOBUNOLOL, TIMOLOL.

"mets." *Pathologic condition.* Slang for metastatic cancerous lesions.

Mevacor. *Drug.* Trade name of lovastatin; for lowering cholesterol levels.

Mexate. *Drug.* Trade name of methotrexate; for treating cancer.

Meyer's loop, temporal loop. *Anatomy.* Portion of optic radiations in the temporal lobe of the brain that circles the lateral ventricles before continuing to the occipital lobe. See also "PIE IN THE SKY" DEFECT.

miconazole (mi-KAHN-uh-zol). *Drug.* Topical agent used for treating ocular *Acanthomoeba* infections. Also injected intravenously to treat fungal eye endophthalmitis. Trade name: Monistat. See also AMPHOTERICIN B, CLOTRIMAZOLE, FLUCYTOSINE, KETOCONAZOLE, NATAMYCIN.

microaneurysm (mi-kroh-AN-yur-izm). *Pathologic condition.* Minute bubble in the wall of a small blood vessel. Appears in the retinal vessels as a small round red spot resembling a deep hemorrhage. Typical finding in long-standing diabetes mellitus.

microcornea (mi-kroh-KOR-nee-uh). *Congenital anomaly.* Abnormally small cornea (less than 10 mm diameter). May be accompanied by farsightedness, nystagmus and, in adulthood, glaucoma. See also MEGALOCORNEA.

microcystic edema (MCE) (mi-kroh-SIS-tik uh-DEE-muh). *Pathologic condition.* Tiny fluid-filled globules present in the corneal epithelium in some corneal dystrophies. See also BULLAE, MICROCYSTIC DYSTROPHY.

microdermatoblepharopigmentation (mi-kroh-DUR-muh-toh-blef-uh-roh-pig-men-TAY-shun) **blepharopigmentation.** *Surgical procedure.* Application of tiny pigment granules under the skin ("tatoo") between the lashes or eyebrows for cosmetic purposes; results in "permanent eyeliner."

microkeratome (mi-kroh-KEHR-uh-tome). *Surgical instrument.* Used for shaving and reshaping a disc of cornea to change its refractive error. See also KERATOMILEUSIS, EPIKERATOPHAKIA.

micrometer (MI-kro-mee-tur), **micron (μ)**. *Measurement.* One-millionth of a meter; 1/1000 of a millimeter.

Micronase. *Drug.* Trade name of glyburide medication; for treating diabetes.

micronystagmus (mi-kroh-ni-stag-mus). *Function.* Extremely fine, involuntary, rhythmic side-to-side eye movements that are part of the normal fixation mechanism of the eyes. See also NYSTAGMUS.

microorganism. Animal or plant of microscopic size, such as a bacterium, virus, fungus or parasite.

microphakia (mi-kroh-FAY-kee-uh). *Congenital anomaly.* Abnormally small crystalline lens.

microphthalmia (mi-krahf-THAL-mee-uh), **microphthalmos.** *Congenital anomaly.* Abnormally small eyeball. See also COLOBOMA, CYSTIC MICROPHTHAL-MIA, NANOPHTHALMOS.

micropsia (mi-KRAHP-see-uh). *Symptom.* Disturbance of visual perception in which objects appear smaller than true size. See also MACROPSIA, META-MORPHOPSIA.

microsaccades (mi-kroh-suh-KAHDZ). *Function.* Extremely fine eye movements that hold the image of a viewed object on the most sensitive visual fibers (fovea).

microspherophakia (mi-kroh-SFIR-oh-FAY-kee-uh). *Congenital anomaly.* Abnormally small lens, having a spherical rather than biconvex form. Usually associated with weak lens zonules. May block pupil, causing glaucoma. See also WEILL-MARCHESANI SYNDROME.

microstrabismus (mi-kroh-struh-BIZ-mus), **microtropia, monofixation syndrome, small angle strabismus.** *Functional defect.* Eye misalignment with a small, usually inward, deviation and some fusion ability. Deviation usually increases with disruption of fusion (as with covering one eye). Affected eye may be amblyopic and/or anisometropic, usually with a small central suppression scotoma. See also FOUR-PRISM-DIOPTER TEST.

microtropia. See MICROSTRABISMUS.

Microvit (Premiere). *Surgical instrument.* Used for posterior microsurgery. Provides illumination and a needlelike cutting tool for vitrectomy. Optional attachments available for phacofragmentation and bipolar coagulation.

microvitreoretinal blade (MVR). *Surgical instrument.* Very sharp, small cutting tool that produces precisely-sized holes through the sclera and pars plana, to serve as entry ports for microsurgical instruments in vitreous and retinal surgery.

midbrain. *Anatomy.* Upper part of the brainstem above the pons. Contains the nuclei of the 3rd (oculomotor), 4th (trochlear), and 6th (abducens) cranial nerves and their interconnections, and control centers for pupil function and horizontal and vertical gazes.

mid-pupillary line, pupillary axis. Imaginary reference line passing from a fixation object through the center of the pupil.

midriasis. Incorrect spelling of MYDRIASIS.

migraine (MI-grayn). *Pathologic condition.* Vascular (blood vessel) disorder; spasm, then dilation, of blood vessels within the skull frequently results in a severe headache. Often one-sided and accompanied by nausea. May be preceded by an aura of taste or smell, "lightning flashes" or expanding circles of light (scintillating scotoma). When aura is visual, called an ophthalmic migraine.

> **retinal**: transient vision loss in one eye, usually followed by a headache on the same side.

> **ophthalmoplegic**: preceded by aura of lightning flashes and expanding circles of light, accompanied by temporary ocular motor nerve palsies. Caused by decreased blood flow (from blood vessel spasm) to part of the brain; headache and pain are caused by subsequent blood vessel dilation. Uncommon.

Mikulicz's syndrome (MIK-uh-lit-ziz). *Pathologic condition.* Chronic form of sarcoid in which there is cellular (lymphocyte) accumulation and enlargement of the tear and salivary glands.

milia (MIL-ee-uh). *Pathologic condition.* Small, round, white, slightly elevated cysts (dilated sweat glands) of superficial skin. May appear on eyelids.

Millard-Gubler syndrome (mee-LAR GU-blur). *Pathologic condition.* Paralysis of the 6th (abducens) cranial nerve and 7th (facial) cranial nerve on one side of the body and paralysis of the arm and leg on the opposite side.

miliary aneurisms (Leber's). See LEBER'S MILIARY ANEURISMS.

Miller Fisher syndrome. *Pathologic condition.* Painless rapid onset of bilateral external ophthalmoplegia (restricted eye movement due to extraocular muscle paralysis) and sometimes paralysis of the internal eye muscles (affecting pupils, eyelids and accommodation). Associated with absent or poor peripheral reflexes, unsteady gait, and bilateral weakness of facial muscles. Complete recovery usually occurs within three months. Variant of Guillain Barre syndrome. See also WERNICKE'S ENCEPHALOPATHY.

millijoule (mJ). *Measurement.* Unit of energy; 1/1000 of a joule. Used in comparing lasers or laser beams.

millimicron (mµ) (mih-lee-MI-krahn), **nanometer**. *Measurement.* Unit of wavelength of light equal to 10^{-9} meter. Nanometer is preferred term.

miner's nystagmus. *Functional defect.* Involuntary rhythmic eye movements that occur with prolonged exposure to darkness.

minima. 1. Plural of minimum. 2. In geometric optics, the troughs of wavelengths of light.

minimum perceptible acuity. *Measurement, function.* Degree to which a person can detect small dots, lines or patterns on a plain background.

minimum separable acuity. *Measurement, function.* Degree to which a person can distinguish two objects (dots, lines, patterns) that are just far enough apart to be seen as two, not one.

"ministroke." See TRANSIENT ISCHEMIC ATTACK.

minus cylinder, concave cylinder. *Optical device.* Toric lens that has maximum minus power in one meridian and no optical power in the meridian perpendicular to it. See also ASTIGMATISM.

minus cylinder grinding. *Optics.* Cylindrical lens with minus power ground on the lens surface closest to the eye.

minus lens, concave *(or)* **diverging lens**. *Optical device.* Lens that is thicker at the edges than in the center, increasing divergence of incoming light rays. Corrects nearsightedness (myopia).

Miocel (MI-oh-sel). *Drug.* Trade name of drug containing physostigmine and pilocarpine; for treating glaucoma.

Miochol, Miochol-E (MI-oh-kol). *Drug.* Trade name of rapid acting acetylcholine liquid that decreases size of pupil; for irrigating the anterior chamber during intraocular surgery.

miosis (mi-OH-sis). *Function.* State of pupillary constriction. Normal response to a bright light stimulus, focusing on a near object (accommodation), or instillation of certain drugs.

Miostat. *Drug.* Trade name of rapid acting carbachol liquid that decreases size of pupil; for irrigating anterior chamber during intraocular surgery.

miotic (mi-AH-tik). 1. *Description.* Refers to small pupils. 2. *Drug.* Cholinergic stimulating agent (parasympathomimetic drug) that mimics the actions of parasympathetic nerves by simulating acetylcholine chemically; causes small pupils (miosis), increases aqueous outflow, and opens the trabecular meshwork. Examples: carbachol, pilocarpine.

mires. *Optics.* Focusing guides on an optical instrument that aid in measurement (e.g., the circular targets in a keratometer or two half-circles in an applanation tonometer).

mitogen (MI-toh-jen). *Chemical.* Stimulates cellular division and growth.

mitomycin C (MMC). *Drug.* Anti-cancer drug that also retards wound healing. Used as eyedrops to prevent recurrence of a pterygium, or to prevent blebs from scarring over after glaucoma surgery.

Mittendorf's dot. *Anatomy.* Remnant of an embryonic hyaloid artery. Visible on slit lamp examination as a small dense floating opacity just behind the posterior lens capsule. Does not affect vision.

mixed astigmatism. *Refractive error.* Optical defect in which one focal line is in front of the retina (corrected by a minus cylinder lens) and the other focal line is behind the retina (corrected by a plus cylinder lens).

Mizuo's phenomenon. *Clinical sign.* In Oguchi's disease, a return to normal fundus coloration when retina is dark adapted, from an unusual golden color when light-adapted.

Möbius' (or Moebius) syndrome (MEE-bee-us or MOH-bee-us), **congenital bulbar paralysis *(or)* facial diplegia, von Graefe's syndrome**. *Congenital anomaly.* Bilateral malformation in the cranial nuclei of the 6th (abducens) and 7th (facial) nerves. Results in inability to move either eye outward past the midline or close the eyelids, a large inward eye deviation (esotropia), and an expressionless facial appearance.

Mohs' technique (mohz). *Surgical procedure.* Lengthy technique for removing a tumor in small stages, so as little normal tissue as possible is excised. Requires careful monitoring by a pathologist. Especially useful for eyelid tumors.

Moll glands. *Anatomy.* Sweat glands near the eyelash follicles on the eyelid margins. See also STYE.

molluscum contagiosum (muh-LUS-kum kun-tay-gee-OH-sum). *Pathologic condition.* Small, wart-like skin lesion with a pitted white center, found on or around the eyelids; caused by a virus. A cause of chronic conjunctivitis.

molluscum sebaceum (sih-BAY-shum), **keratoacanthoma**. *Pathologic condition.* Benign, fast-growing, cup-shaped skin lesion with a central crater that tends to form on the lids and face. Often regresses spontaneously.

Molteno implant. See MOLTENO VALVE.

Molteno valve (mahl-TEE-noh), **Molteno implant**. *Surgical device.* Implant tube used for controlling abnormally high intraocular pressure in glaucoma.

mongolism, Down's syndrome, trisomy 21. *Congenital defect.* Mental retardation associated with an extra chromosome (#21). Eye signs include lower eyelid margins that slant upward toward the lateral canthi (mongoloid slant), Brushfield spots in the iris, cataracts, inward deviation (esotropia), nearsightedness (myopia), blepharitis and keratoconus.

mongoloid slant. *Anatomy*. Eyelids whose outer corners (away from nose) are higher than the inner corners. See also ANTIMONGOLOID SLANT.

MONGOLOID SLANT

monochromacy (mon-oh-KROH-muh-see), **achromatopsia**. *Congenital defect*. Rare inability to distinguish colors. Nonprogressive; hereditary.

   cone (atypical): vision is relatively normal.

   rod (typical): vision is poor. Associated with light sensitivity (photophobia), involuntary eye oscillations (nystagmus) and absent or nonfunctioning retinal cones.

monochromat (mon-oh-KROH-mat). Individual who cannot distinguish colors; may have only one type of retinal cone (cone monochromat) or lack all cone function (rod monochromat).

monochromatic. *Optics*. Describes color produced by light waves of the same frequency.

monocular (mon-AHK-yu-lur). *Description*. Located in (or referring to) one eye.

monocular depth perception. *Function*. Appreciation of an object's distance through cues available to one eye, e.g., geometric pespective, motion parallax, overlap, relative size, shadow, aerial haze. See also BINOCULAR PARALLAX.

monocular diplopia (dih-PLOH-pee-uh), **polyopia**. *Symptom*. Multiple images seen with one eye. Commonly caused by early cataracts or irregular corneas.

monocyte. *Anatomy*. Type of white blood cell.

monofixation syndrome, microstrabismus, microtropia, small angle strabismus. *Functional defect*. Eye misalignment with small, usually inward, deviation and some fusion ability. Deviation usually increases with disruption of fusion (as with covering one eye). Affected eye may be amblyopic and/or anisometropic, usually with a small central suppression scotoma. See also FOUR-PRISM-DIOPTER TEST.

Mooren's ulcer (MOR-enz). *Pathologic condition*. Painful loss of corneal surface tissue caused by chronic, progressive inflammation, usually near the corneo-scleral junction (limbus). Difficult to control. Most common in the elderly.

Moraxella lacunata (mor-aks-EL-uh lah-ku-NAH-tuh). *Microorganism*. Gram-negative rod-shaped bacteria seen in pairs. Causes eye infection, e.g., chronic blepharoconjunctivitis.

Morgagnian cataract. *Pathologic condition*. Totally opaque lens that has begun to shrink and liquify; remaining hard nucleus floats within the lens capsule. Degraded lens protein molecules may leak into aqueous through the lens capsule and cause phacolytic glaucoma.

morning glory anomaly. *Congenital anomaly*. Optic disc that is large, distorted and bell-shaped (resembles morning glory flower), with blood vessels emerging from it like spokes on a wheel. Vision is poor. Rare, unilateral. Central nervous system malformations may be found. Variant of optic nerve coloboma. See also OPTIC NERVE HYPOPLASIA.

morning glory detachment. *Pathologic condition*. Advanced state of retinal separation from underlying pigment epithelium. Retina appears wrinkled and folded, resembling a bell-shaped morning glory flower.

Morquio-Brailsford syndrome (MOR-kee-oh). *Pathologic condition*. Hereditary form of mucopolysaccharoidosis (type IV), a deficiency of enzyme N-acetyl-alpha-D-glucosominidase. Characterized by severe skeletal abnormalities, heart problems, and moderate corneal clouding (only ocular abnormality).

mosaic degeneration, crocodile shagreen. *Pathologic condition*. Polygonal, light gray corneal opacities centrally located at Decemet's (posterior) or Bowman's (anterior) level. Represents a mild age-related degenerative change with little or no affect on vision.

motility (moh-TIL-ih-tee), **ocular motility**. *Function, test*. Study of extraocular muscles and their effect on eye movement. See also BINOCULARITY, STRABISMUS.

motion parallax. *Function.* Important monocular cue to depth perception. As the head or eye is moved from side to side, distant objects appear to move more slowly than closer objects. See also PARALLAX.

motor fusion. *Function.* Corrective eye movements (vergences) that enable the eyes to maintain single binocular vision of an approaching object. Occurs in response to double vision, which triggers corrective alignment movements to bring both images back onto the foveae. See also NORMAL RETINAL CORRESPONDENCE.

motor nerve, efferent nerve, output nerve. *Anatomy.* Nerve that carries impulses away from the central nervous system toward the body; e.g., 3rd (oculomotor) cranial nerve. See also SENSORY NERVE.

MRI (magnetic resonance imaging). *Test.* Type of imaging technique using high intensity magnets and computers; permits examination of soft tissues inside the body that cannot be seen with x-rays. Newer term for NMR (nuclear magnetic resonance). See also CT SCAN.

mucin (MYU-sin). *Anatomy.* Moist viscid secretions from small mucous glands, such as in the conjunctiva and linings of the mouth and nose. Serves as a protective lubricant.

mucocele (MYU-koh-seel). *Pathologic condition.* Enlarged cavity with accumulated mucous secretion, usually found around the nasal sinuses.

mucoid. *Description.* Mucus-like. Can refer to the inner mucinous layer of the tear film. See also MUCIN.

mucopolysaccharoidoses (MYU-koh-PAH-lee-SAK-uh-roy-DOH-sees). *Pathologic condition.* Group of connective tissue disorders involving mucopolysaccharide metabolism. Specific enzyme deficiencies result in varying degrees of skeletal and systemic abnormalities, mental retardation, and corneal clouding. See also HUNTER'S, HURLER'S, MAROTEAUX-LAMY, MORQUIO-BRAILSFORD AND SCHEIE SYNDROMES, SAN FILIPPO TYPE III.

mucormycosis (myu-kor-mi-KOH-sis). *Pathologic condition.* Rare fungus infection that originates in the nose and sinuses. Caused by *Mucor,* which invades the eye and brain structures through the arteries, causing blood vessel obstructions. Eye signs are lid swelling, bulging (proptosis), and restricted movements, with meningo-encephalitis. Associated with uncontrolled diabetes or renal acidosis. Often fatal.

Mueller cell. See MÜLLER CELL.

Mueller's muscle. See MÜLLER'S MUSCLE.

Müller cell (MYU-lur); also spelled Mueller. *Anatomy.* Retinal connective tissue cell that provides nutrients and forms internal structural support. See also B-WAVE.

Müller's muscle; also spelled Mueller's. *Anatomy.* 1. Smooth muscle sheets that provide "tone" for the upper and lower eyelids. Controlled by sympathetic nerves. 2. Circular muscle fibers at the innermost part of the ciliary muscle.

multifocal lens. *Optical device.* Eyeglass lens that incorporates several different optical powers, to permit focusing at different distances. See also ADD, BIFOCAL, PROGRESSIVE ADDITION LENS, TRIFOCAL.

multiple sclerosis (MS). *Pathologic condition.* Chronic central nervous system disorder in which there is loss of the protective myelin sheath surrounding nerve tissue (demyelination). Eye findings include optic nerve inflammation (especially retrobulbar neuritis) with reduced vision, double vision (caused by internuclear ophthalmoplegia), and involuntary eye oscillations (nystagmus). See also NEUROMYELITIS OPTICA.

Munchausen's syndrome. Feigning symptoms of a disease or injury in order to undergo diagnostic tests, hospitalization, or medical or surgical treatment.

Munsell scale (muhn-SEHL). Standardized scale of colored materials having variations in hue and saturation, for standardizing test targets used for color vision assessment.

Munson sign. *Clinical sign.* Bowing of the lower eyelid margin upon looking down. Caused by cone-shaped protrusion of the cornea in keratoconus.

mural cells. *Anatomy.* Cells found in retinal capillary walls.

Murine Plus. *Drug.* Trade name of tetrahydrozoline eyedrops; decongestant that "whitens" the eyes.

Murine Tears. *Drug.* Trade name of polyvinyl alcohol eyedrops or ointment; for treating dry eyes.

Murocel. *Drug.* Trade name of methylcellulose eyedrops for treating dry eyes.

Muro-128. *Drug.* Trade name of hypertonic sodium chloride eyedrops or ointment.

muscae volitantes (MUS-kee vol-ih-TAN-tuz). *Symptom.* Dark specks (floaters) seen when looking at a bright, overly illuminated field, such as the sky. Caused by minute residue of fetal vascular (hyaloid) system floating in the vitreous. See also FLOATERS.

muscle cone. *Anatomy.* Cone-shaped tissue behind the eyeball formed by intraocular muscles (medial rectus, lateral rectus, superior rectus, inferior rectus, superior oblique), their muscle sheaths and intermuscular membranes. Tip of cone is at the innermost point (apex) of the orbit.

muscle hook. *Surgical instrument.* Used for holding an extraocular muscle.

muscle of Riolan (ree-oh-LAN), **pars ciliaris.** *Anatomy.* Part of orbicularis oculi muscle, located in the eyelid behind the eyelash follicles. Helps inner (by nose) eyelid margin hug close against the eyeball

muscle-paretic nystagmus (puh-RET-ik ni-STAG-mus). *Functional defect.* Involuntary, rhythmic eye movements (nystagmus) that occur when stress is placed on a weak extraocular muscle. Example: when right lateral rectus is partially paralyzed, the right eye oscillates on right-gaze.

muscle sheath. *Anatomy.* Thin fibrous tissue that forms an enclosure for an extraocular muscle. See also INTERMUSCULAR MEMBRANE.

Mustarde flap (mus-TAR-day). *Surgical procedure.* Method of reconstructing all or the outer half of the lower eyelid. Skin tissue is dissected from the cheek, lined with a mucous membrane and cartilage graft, and rotated to form a new eyelid. Eliminates a large skin fold on either side of the nose (epicanthal fold). See also TENZEL FLAP.

"mutton fat" KPs (keratic precipitates). *Clinical sign.* Large clusters of inflammatory cells and white blood cells from the iris and ciliary body that enter the aqueous and adhere to the endothelium (innermost corneal surface). Sign of granulomatous inflammation. Occurs in various types of uveitis. Called "punctate" if KPs are smaller (nongranulomatous).

myasthenia gravis. *Pathologic condition.* Abnormality of the nerve-muscle junction, leading to excessive muscle fatigability. Eye signs include drooping eyelids (ptosis) and double vision, which appear or worsen as the day progresses. See also TENSILON.

Mydfrin. *Drug.* Trade name of phenylephrine; dilates the pupil by contracting the iris dilator.

Mydrapred (MID-ruh-pred). *Drug.* Trade name of eyedrop containing atropine and prednisone; for treating iritis.

Mydriacyl (mid-RI-uh-sil). *Drug.* Trade name of tropicamide eyedrops that dilate the pupils and paralyze accommodation; used in eye examinations.

mydriasis (mid-RI-uh-sis). *Function.* Increase in pupil size (dilation). Occurs normally in the dark or artificially with certain drugs.

mydriatic (mid-ree-AT-ik). *Drug.* Stimulates sympathetic nerve fibers, causing the iris dilator to contract (dilating the pupils), or blocking parasympathetic nerve fibers (paralyzing the iris sphincter muscle). Examples: Atropine, Cyclogyl, Mydriacyl, Neosynephrine. See also CYCLOPLEGIA.

mydriatic provocative test. For narrow angle glaucoma; glaucoma suspect is given 1 or 2 drops of a mild dilating drop, e.g., eucatropine, then intraocular pressure is checked after 1 hour. An increase of 8 mm or more is considered positive. See also DARKROOM PROVOCATIVE TEST.

myectomy (mi-EK-tuh-mee). *Surgical procedure*. Removing part of an extraocular muscle to decrease its action and help correct an eye deviation.

myelin (MI-uh-lin). *Anatomy*. Fatty sheath that covers some nerves, acting as an electrical insulator that speeds conduction of nerve impulses. See also MULTIPLE SCLEROSIS, MYELINATED NERVE FIBERS.

myelinated nerve fibers (MI-uh-lin-ay-tid), **meduated nerve fibers**. *Congenital anomaly*. Nerve fibers in the retina that are covered with patches of myelin. Non-progressive, asymptomatic. Requires no treatment.

myeloma (mi-uh-LOH-muh). *Pathologic condition*. Malignant plasma cell tumor.

myocardial infarction (MI), "coronary," heart attack. *Pathologic condition*. Sudden blockage of a blood vessel that supplies nutrients to the heart. Results in death (infarction) of some of the heart muscle.

myoclonus. *Function*. Abrupt, irregular, shock-like contractions of muscles.

myokymia (mi-oh-KI-mee-uh). *Functional defect*. Sporadic twitching of part of an eyelid muscle, often caused by fatigue.

myoneural junction, neuromuscular junction. *Anatomy*. Microscopic area where a motor nerve fiber comes in contact with a muscle fiber.

myopexy. *Surgical procedure*. Attaching muscle to tissue with a fixation suture.

myopia (mi-OH-pee-uh), **nearsightedness**. *Refractive error*. Focusing defect in which the eye is overpowered. Light rays coming from a distant object are brought to focus in front of the retina. Requires a minus lens correction to "weaken" the eye optically and permit clear distance vision.

> **axial**: caused by an eyeball that is too long for its optical power.

> **index**: type of REFRACTIVE (below). Caused by increase in the index of refraction of the crystalline lens. Usually associated with early cataract (resulting in "second sight") or diabetes mellitus.

> **refractive**: caused by overpowered optical elements in the eye, e.g., curvature of the cornea or lens and/or increased index of refraction of the lens (index myopia).

myopic (mi-AHP-ik). *Description*. Nearsighted.

myopic astigmatism. *Refractive error*. Optical defect in which light rays entering the eye are bent unequally in different meridians, preventing a sharp focus on the retina. The light rays form two focal lines perpendicular to each other. Corrected by a cylindrical (toric) eyeglass or contact lens.

> **simple**: one focal line forms on the retina; the other forms in the vitreous in front of the retina.

> **compound**: both focal lines form in front of the retina.

myopic crescent. *Anatomy*. Semilunar shaped depigmented zone on the optic disc in high myopes. See also MYOPIC DEGENERATION.

myopic degeneration, degenerative *(or)* malignant myopia. *Pathologic condition*. Uncommon form of nearsightedness (myopia) accompanied by progressive stretching changes and gradual damage to the retina, choroid, vitreous, sclera and optic nerve.

myositis (mi-uh-SI-tus). *Pathologic condition*. Inflammation of a muscle, usually causing discomfort or pain.

myotomy (mi-AH-tuh-mee). *Surgical procedure*. Method of cutting an extraocular muscle to reduce its pull.

MZM. *Drug*. Trade name of methazolamide; for treating glaucoma.

N

N, CN. Abbreviation for cranial nerve; used with nerve number (e.g., N II, CNII). Nerves involved with visual function are listed under CN.

Nadbath facial nerve block. *Surgical procedure*. Injection of an anesthetic drug behind the ear to decrease sensation from the 7th (facial) cranial nerve. See also ATKINSON, O'BRIEN, AND VAN LINT FACIAL NERVE BLOCK.

nadolol. *Drug*. Heart medication; for treating high blood pressure (hypertension). Trade name: Corgard. See also ATENOLOL, METAPROLOL, TIMOLOL.

Nagel anomaloscope (NAH-gul an-AHM-uh-luh-skohp), **anomaloscope**. *Instrument*. Used for sensitive color vision evaluation and diagnosis; patient mixes red and green in an attempt to match hue and brightness of a yellow standard.

nanometer (nm) (NAN-oh-mee-tur), **millimicron**. *Measurement*. Unit of wavelength of light equal to 10^{-9} meter. Nanometer is preferred term.

nanophthalmos (nan-ahf-THAL-mus). *Congenital anomaly*. Abnormally small eyeball, often two-thirds normal size, accompanied by proportionately small eye structures. See also COLOBOMA, CYSSTIC MICROPHTHALMIA.

naphazoline (nuh-FAZ-oh-leen). *Drug*. Sympathomimetic, decongestant eyedrop that constricts blood vessels. For "whitening" the eyes. Trade names: AK-Con, Albalon, Clear Eyes, Degest-2, Naphcon, Opcon, Vasoclear, Vasocon.

Naphcon (NAF-kon). *Drug*. Trade name of naphazoline eyedrops; for "whitening" the eyes.

Naphcon-A. *Drug*. Trade name of drug containing naphazoline (a decongestant) and pheniramine (an antihistamine); for treating allergic conjunctivitis.

narrow angle glaucoma (glaw-KOH-muh), **angle closure *(or)* acute angle closure *(or)* closed-angle glaucoma**. *Pathologic condition*. Sudden rise in intraocular pressure in patients with narrow anterior chamber angles. Aqueous behind the iris cannot pass through the pupil and pushes the iris forward, preventing aqueous drainage through the angle (pupillary block).

nasal. *Location*. 1. Inward (toward the nose). 2. The half of the eye or visual field from the vertical midline inward. See also TEMPORAL.

nasal sinuses. *Anatomy*. The ethmoid, frontal, maxillary and sphenoid sinuses.

nasal step. *Functional defect*. Step-like visual field defect located at the outer limit of the nasal field. Most commonly associated with retinal nerve fiber layer damage due to glaucoma.

nasociliary nerve (nay-zoh-SIL-ee-eh-ree). *Anatomy*. Branch of the ophthalmic division of the 5th (trigeminal) cranial nerve. Provides pain fibers to the globe and supplies sensory fibers to the iris, cornea, ciliary muscle, and skin at the tip of the nose. See also CILIARY NERVES.

nasolacrimal duct (NLD) (nay-zoh-LAK-rih-mul), **lacrimal duct, tear duct**. *Anatomy*. Tear drainage channel that extends from the lacrimal sac to an opening in the mucous membrane of the nose.

nasolacrimal duct obstruction. See BLOCKED TEAR DUCT.

nasolacrimal probing. *Surgical procedure*. Opening the tear drainage system by passing a thin metal rod through the passage and pressing gently to break any obstruction. See also DACRYOSTENOSIS.

Natacyn. *Drug*. Trade name for natamycin eyedrops; for treating fungal infections.

natamycin (naa-tuh-MI-sin). *Drug*. Suspension applied topically to the cornea for treating corneal fungal ulcers; formerly known as pimaricin. Trade name: Natacyn. See also AMPHOTERICIN B, CLOTRIMAZOLE, FLUCYTOSINE, KETOCONAZOLE, MICONAZOLE.

Nd:YAG laser. *Surgical instrument.* Laser that produces a short pulsed, high energy light beam to cut, perforate, or fragment tissue. Acronym: neodymium yttrium-aluminum-garnet. See also PHOTOCOAGULATION.

near point of accommodation (NPA), punctum proximum of accommodation. *Measurement.* Position closest to the eye where a small object (usually small print) can be kept in sharp focus by maximal accommodation. See also PRINCE'S RULE.

near point of convergence (NPC), punctum proximum of convergence. *Measurement.* Point where convergence and binocular single vision can no longer be maintained as an object approaches an eye.

nearsightedness, myopia. *Refractive error.* Focusing defect in which the eye is overpowered. Light rays coming from a distant object are brought to focus in front of the retina. Requires minus lens correction to "weaken" the eye optically and permit clear distance vision. Types listed under MYOPIA.

near vision. *Measurement.* Visual acuity measured with target at 16 in. (approximately 40 cm), corresponding to normal reading distance.

nebula (NEB-yu-luh). *Pathologic condition.* Least dense type of corneal opacity. See also LEUKOMA, MACULA.

necrosis. *Clinical sign.* Death of cells or tissue in a localized area. Caused by disease, injury, or insufficient blood supply.

necrotizing scleritis. *Pathologic condition.* Severe inflammation of the sclera that spreads and destroys involved tissue and produces pain and redness. Associated with systemic disease e.g., rheumatoid arthritis. Requires immediate treatment.

needle holder. *Surgical instrument.* Holds a suture needle.

needling. *Surgical procedure.* Puncturing the lens capsule to allow absorption of the lens substance, to aid in extraction of a congenital cataract. Obsolete.

Nefrin. *Drug.* Trade name for phenylephrine; "whitens" the eyes.

negative vertical vergence *(or)* divergence, left sursumvergence, right deosumvergence. *Function.* Downward movement of the left eye relative to the right, usually to maintain single binocular vision, e.g., when increasing amounts of base-up prism are placed in front of the left eye.

Neisseria catarrhalis (ni-SIR-ee-uh kat-uh-RAL-is). *Microorganism.* Gram-negative round bacteria. Rare cause of eye infections.

Neisseria gonorrhea. *Microorganism.* Gram-negative spherical bacteria. Causes severe eye infections, especially in newborn whose mothers have venereal disease.

Neisseria meningitidis (men-in-JIT-ih-dis). *Microorganism.* Gram-negative round bacteria. Can cause a severe infection of the membranes surrounding the brain.

Neo-Cortef (NEE-oh KOR-tef). *Drug.* Trade name of ointment containing neomycin and hydrocortisone; for treating keratitis and conjunctvitis.

neodymium:YAG laser. See ND:YAG LASER.

neomycin (nee-oh-MI-sin). *Drug.* Antibiotic used for mild external eye infections.

neoplasm. *Pathologic condition.* New abnormal growth of tissue that has no physiological function. Usually malignant.

Neosporin (nee-oh-SPOR-in). *Drug.* Trade name of ointment containing polymyxin B, bacitracin and neomycin; for treating conjunctivitis.

Neosynephrine (nee-oh-sin-EF-rin). *Drug.* Trade name of phenylephrine hydrochloride; used in low concentration to "whiten" the conjunctiva, or in stronger concentration to dilate the pupils.

neovascular glaucoma (nee-oh-VAS-kyu-lur glaw-KOH-muh), **hemorrhagic *(or)* rubeotic glaucoma.** *Pathologic condition.* Severe, hard-to-control form of glaucoma that leads to a painful eye with high intraocular pressure, corneal swelling, and "cell and flare" in the anterior chamber. Caused by abnormal new blood vessel formation (neovascularization) on the iris, that extends over trabecular meshwork causing closure of angle drainage structures. Associated with severe diabetic retinopathy and other problems that cause blockage of retinal blood vessels, especially veins. See also RUBEOSIS IRIDIS.

neovascularization (nee-oh-VAS-kyu-lur-ih-ZAY-shun). *Pathologic condition.* Abnormal formation of new blood vessels, usually in or under the retina or on the iris surface. May develop in diabetic retinopathy, blockage of the central retinal vein, or macular degeneration.

> **preretinal**: develops on the retinal surface, which tends to bleed. Complication of various blood vessel diseases, such as diabetes.

> **subretinal**: develops between (under) the retinal pigment epithelium and the choroid; may cause fluid leakage and bleeding under the retina with eventual destruction of function in the overlying retina. Occurs in some forms of macular degeneration.

nephropathic cystine storage disease (neh-froh-PATH-ik, SIS-teen). See LIGNAC-FANCONI'S SYNDROME.

Neptazane. *Drug.* Trade name of methazolamide tablets; for treating glaucoma.

nerve fiber bundle defect. *Functional defect.* Arc-shaped blind spot (scotoma) within the visual field caused by damage to the retinal nerve fiber layer near the optic nerve head. See also CENTROCECAL SCOTOMA.

nerve fiber layer (NFL). *Anatomy.* Innermost retinal layer (closest to vitreous). Contains axons from ganglion cells that follow a characteristic pattern toward the optic disc, where all fibers exit the eye as the optic nerve.

neuritis. *Pathologic condition.* Inflammation of a nerve.

> **optic**: Inflammation of the optic nerve. May accompany demyelinating disease (e.g., multiple sclerosis) or infections from the meninges, orbital tissues or paranasal sinuses. Characterized by rapid onset of decreased vision and, usually, discomfort with eye movement and a central visual field defect. See also PAPILLITIS, RETROBULBAR NEURITIS.

> **retrobulbar**: inflammation of the optic nerve behind the optic disc (within the orbit), which hides early disc changes. Visual acuity is markedly reduced. Frequently in patients with multiple sclerosis.

neuroblastoma. *Pathologic condition.* Highly malignant tumor of the sympathetic nervous system, found in children. Usually begins in the abdomen (adrenal medulla), then spreads by metastasis to the orbit (usually lateral orbital wall) and brain. Eye signs include orbital and lid bleeding ("black eye"), marked proptosis (bulging), and inflammation of the eyelids.

neurofibromatosis (NU-roh-fi-broh-muh-TOH-sis), **Recklinghausen's *(or)* von Recklinghausen's disease**. *Pathologic condition.* One of several hereditary disorders (called phakomatoses) characterized by small tumors under the skin and in the central nervous system, and bony defects in the orbital bones. Common sites include the upper eyelid, optic nerve, 8th (acoustic) cranial nerve, and spinal cord. See also LISCH NODULES.

neuromuscular junction, myoneural junction. *Anatomy.* Microscopic area where a motor nerve fiber comes in contact with a muscle fiber.

neuromyelitis optica (NU-roh-mi-uh-LI-tis AHP-tih-kuh), **Devic's disease**. *Pathologic condition.* Rare demyelinating central nervous system disorder characterized by paraplegia and inflammation of both optic nerves, causing marked loss of vision. Similar to multiple sclerosis.

neuroretinitis (NU-roh-ret-in-I-tus). *Pathologic condition.* Inflammation of the retina near the optic nerve.

neuroretinopathy (NU-roh-ret-in-AHP-uh-thee). *Pathologic condition.* Non-inflammatory retinal abnormality occurring near the optic nerve.

neuropathy (nur-AHP-uh-thee). *Pathologic condition.* Non-inflammatory nerve abnormality.

neurotrophic keratitis (nu-roh-TROH-fik kehr-uh-TI-tis). *Pathologic condition.* Corneal inflammation resulting from trauma or corneal exposure following damage to corneal nerves. Accompanied by loss of corneal sensitivity (corneal anesthesia).

neutral density filter. *Test instrument.* Gray transparent material placed before the eyes to differentiate organic amblyopia (irreversible; reduces vision) from functional amblyopia (reversible; improves or does not affect vision). Used also as sunglasses, to decrease amount of light entering the eye.

neutrality. *Optics.* In retinoscopy, endpoint for assessing a refractive error, when the light reflex seen through the retinoscope totally fills the pupil. See also "AGAINST" MOTION, "WITH" MOTION.

neutralize. *Function.* 1. To determine the optical error of an eye or power of an unknown lens by adding appropriate opposite-powered lenses. 2. In retinoscopy, to reach a condition where the pupil is totally filled with light from the retinoscope, signifying that the proper corrective lens is in front of the eye. 3. To determine misalignment of an eye by adding corrective prisms.

neutrophil (NU-troh-fihl), **polymorphonuclear leukocyte, poly.** *Anatomy.* Type of white blood cell important in combatting acute (especially bacterial) infections.

nevus (NEE-vus). *Anatomic defect.* Mole. Small, flat, usually pigmented benign tumor made up of specific cells called nevus cells; found in skin and eye tissues. Does not interfere with tissue function; very rarely undergoes transformation into a malignant melanoma.

nevus of Ota, oculodermal melanocytosis. *Congenital defect.* Pigmented area on cheek, eyelids, forehead or nose.

Newcastle's disease. *Pathologic condition.* Rare viral infection that causes conjunctivitis. Seen in poultry handlers who accidentally self-innoculate while immunizing chickens. No treatment; usually resolves in 1–2 weeks.

Nicolet system. *Test.* For contrast sensitivity, detecting subtle gradations in grayness between detail in the test target and the background.

nictitation. *Function.* Blinking or winking. Usually refers to animals that have a thin membrane (nictitating membrane) functioning as a third eyelid that sweeps laterally across the surface of the eye.

nidus (NI-dus). *Localized site.* 1. Place where something originates, develops, or is fostered. 2. Tissue where organisms causing a disease lodge and multiply. Plural: nidi.

Niemann-Pick disease (NEE-min), **sphingomyelin lipidosis.** *Pathologic condition.* Defect of fat metabolism caused by a deficiency of the enzyme sphingomyelinase. Fatty deposits accumulate in many organs, nerve tissue, and eyes. Retinal changes may include cherry red spots or grayish haze. Life span is about 20 years. Hereditary. See also SPHINGOLIPIDOSES.

nifedipine (nih-FED-ih-peen). *Drug.* Heart medication; acts as a calcium channel blocker for heart pain (angina) and high blood pressure (hypertension). Trade name: Procardia. See also VERAPAMIL.

night blindness, nyctalopia. *Functional defect.* Inefficient dark adaptation that results in markedly reduced vision in dim light. Usually indicates a defect in the (retinal) rods. May be progressive.

night vision, rod *(or)* **scotopic vision.** *Function.* Refers to visual acuity at low light levels; primarily a function of (retinal) rods. Maximum sensitivity usually occurs after 30 minutes in the dark. See also DARK ADAPTATION.

Nizoral. *Drug.* Trade name of ketoconazole; for treating fungal infections.

Nocardia asteroides (noh-KAHR-dee-uh as-tur-OY-deez). *Microorganism.* Gram-positive filamentous bacteria. May cause corneal ulcers.

nodal point, optical center. *Optics.* Reference point on the principal axis of an optical system though which incoming light rays are not bent by a lens or optical surface, so that incident and transmitted rays make equal angles with the optic axis. In the eye, lies on the optic axis near the rear surface of the lens.

non-accommodative esotropia. *Functional defect.* Excessive turning of an eye inward (toward nose) that is not influenced by the refractive correction of any hyperopia (farsightedness).

noncomitant strabismus (non-KAHM-ih-tunt struh-BIZ-mus), **incomitant strabismus.** *Functional defect.* Eye deviation that varies in amount in different positions of gaze.

non-contact tonometer, pneumotonometer, pneumatic *(or)* **"puff" to-nometer.** *Instrument.* Gas-pressurized device that measures intraocular pressure by blowing a puff of air against the cornea to flatten it slightly; does not come in contact with eye. See also TONOMETRY.

non-granulomatous uveitis (non-gran-yu-LOH-muh-tus yu-vee-I-tis). *Pathologic condition.* Uveal inflammation thought to be a hypersensitivity reaction. Characterized by blurred vision, ciliary flush, sensitivity to light, cells in the anterior chamber, and fine deposits on inner corneal surface. Usually acute, unilateral and self-limiting. See also PUNCTATE KERATIC PRECIPITATES.

non-optic reflex eye movements. *Function.* Eye movements initiated by the inner ear (vestibular system), head motion or head position, rather than by visual stimuli.

nonproliferative retinopathy (ret-in-AHP-uh-thee), **background retinopathy.** *Pathologic condition.* Retinal changes associated with early diabetic retinopathy. Common retinal findings include microaneurysms, "dot and blot" hemorrhages, hard exudates, and dilation of retinal veins. Specifically excludes presence of abnormal new blood vessels (neovascularization). See also PROLIFERATIVE RETINOPATHY.

non-steroid anti-inflammatory drugs. See NSAIDS.

norfloxacin. *Drug.* Antibiotic eyedrop used for treating ocular infections. Trade name: Chibroxin.

normal. *Optics.* Line perpendicular to the surface of a medium.

normal retinal correspondence (NRC). *Function.* Foveae of both eyes work together as corresponding retinal points, with resultant images blended (fused) in the occipital cortex of the brain, allowing single binocular vision. See also ANOMALOUS RETINAL CORRESPONDENCE.

Norman-Wood syndrome. *Congenital anomaly.* Form of amaurotic familial idiocy, a disorder characterized by nervous system and retinal disease. Eye signs include lesions in the area providing central vision (macula) and optic nerve degeneration.

normotensive. *Description.* Refers to normal arterial blood pressure readings.

Norrie's syndrome. *Congenital abnormality.* Blindness at birth, with bilateral retinal pseudotumor, retinal detachment, phthisis, deafness and mental retardation. Hereditary; X-linked (recessive).

no-stitch, one- *(or)* **two-stitch surgery.** *Surgical procedure.* Cataract extraction technique using minimal size incision into the eye, with lens fragmentation and removal by phacoemulsification. See also EXTRACAPSULAR CATARACT EXTRACTION.

Nothnagel's syndrome. *Pathologic condition.* Brainstem abnormality producing paralysis of eye muscles innervated by the 3rd (oculomotor) cranial nerve on the same side, and unsteady limb movement on the opposite side. See also BENEDIKT'S SYNDROME, WEBER'S SYNDROME.

Novocain. *Drug.* Trade name of procaine, an injectable anesthetic agent.

NSAIDs (non-steroid anti-inflammatory drugs). *Drug.* Class of prostaglandin-inhibiting drugs (e.g., aspirin, ibuprofen). Used as a substitute for steroids in controlling minimal inflammations.

nuclear (NU-klee-ur). *Description.* 1. Refers to an optically dense center of the eye's crystalline lens. 2. Refers to cranial nerve nuclei in the brain.

nuclear sclerosis (sklur-OH-sis). *Pathologic condition.* Type of early cataract characterized by increasing hardness or density at the center of the eye's crystalline lens. Usually results in a refractive change toward increasing myopia. Occurs with aging.

nucleus (NU-klee-us). *Anatomy.* 1. Key central element of a cell that contains hereditary material (DNA). 2. The optically dense center of the eye's crystalline lens. 3. Controlling neural elements in the brain, such as those that give rise to the 12 cranial nerves. Plural: nuclei.

nucleus of Perlia (PUR-lee-uh). *Anatomy.* Central portion of 3rd (oculomotor) cranial nerve nucleus in brainstem. Function not well understood, though probably related to accommodation and convergence mechanisms.

null point. Position of gaze where eye movements of congenital nystagmus are reduced or eliminated.

nummular. *Description.* Coin-shaped; circular or oval, e.g., nummular keratitis.

numo. Incorrect spelling of PNEUMO.

nutritional amblyopia (am-blee-OH-pee-uh). *Functional defect.* Vision loss accompanied by dense central visual field defects in both eyes. Caused by B vitamin deficiency, usually in patients who consume excessive tobacco and alcohol. See also AMBLYOPIA.

nyctalopia (nik-tuh-LOH-pee-uh). See NIGHT BLINDNESS.

nystagmoid (nih-STAG-moyd). *Functional defect.* Jerky, non-rhythmic oscillating eye movements. Usually associated with poor vision.

nystagmus (ni-STAG-mus), **jerk nystagmus**. *Functional defect.* Involuntary, rhythmic side-to-side or up and down (oscillating) eye movements that are faster in one direction than the other. See also NULL POINT.

> **caloric**: same as VESTIBULAR (below).
>
> **endpoint**: side-to-side movements that occur with effort to maintain extreme positions of gaze.
>
> **gaze paretic**: movements begin when gaze is attempted in a direction to which the eyes cannot move easily. Associated with drugs, multiple sclerosis, tumors, or circulatory problems.
>
> **labyrinthine**: same as VESTIBULAR (below).
>
> **latent**: movements occur in one eye when other eye is covered; may be more marked in one eye than the other.
>
> **muscle-paretic** (puh-RET-ik): occurs when stress is placed on a weak extraocular muscle, e.g., when the right lateral rectus is partially paralyzed, the right eye oscillates on right-gaze.
>
> **miner's**: caused by darkness.
>
> **optokinetic (OKN)**: produced by viewing a series of vertical bars or other patterned contours; slow following phase (pursuit) toward the side of target movement, with rapid jerk return (saccade) in the opposite direction. Normal. Also called "railroad" nystagmus.
>
> **pendular**: movements are approximately equal in each direction. Associated with congenital nystagmus or central vision loss before age 2.
>
> **"railroad"**: same as OPTOKINETIC (above).
>
> **rotary**: twitching movements in clockwise or counterclockwise rotation around the visual axis. Frequent in brain-damaged children.
>
> **sensory**: caused by severe visual loss in early childhood. See also ALBINISM, ANIRIDIA, CONGENITAL CATARACT.
>
> **vestibular**: occurs when inner ear labyrinths are irritated or diseased.

nystagmus blockage syndrome (ni-STAG-mus). *Functional defect.* Inward eye deviation (esotropia) caused by excessive convergence stimulation, which lessens or eliminates oscillating eye movements (nystagmus).

O

obicularis. Incorrect spelling of ORBICULARIS.

objective test. Examination that does not require answers or observations by the patient. See also SUBJECTIVE TEST.

object of regard, fixation object. *Test object.* Object used to control the patient's direction of attention during certain diagnostic tests.

obleek. Incorrect spelling of OBLIQUE.

obligatory suppression. *Functional defect.* Non-perception of image by a misaligned eye when both eyes are open; continues when straight eye is covered. Unconscious mechanism to avoid double vision (diplopia). Associated with amblyopia. See also FACULTATIVE SUPPRESSION.

oblique astigmatism (uh-STIG-muh-tizm). *Refractive error.* Astigmatic refractive error whose axis lies in a position that is neither vertical (90°) nor horizontal (180°).

O'Brien facial nerve block. *Surgical procedure.* Injection of an anesthetic drug in front of the ear to decrease sensation from the 7th (facial) cranial nerve. See also ATKINSON, NADBATH, VAN LINT FACIAL NERVE BLOCKS.

obstruction. *Pathologic condition.* Blockage; may be complete or partial.

obtunded. *Description.* Reduced in intensity or sensitivity; made dull.

occipital lobe. *Anatomy.* Rear part of each cerebral hemisphere in the brain. Responsible for vision and visual perception.

occluded pupil, occlusio pupillae. *Pathologic condition.* Covering of the pupillary opening by a membrane, usually after inflammation; blocks aqueous flow from the posterior to the anterior chamber.

occluder. *Instrument.* Used for covering one eye during testing or treatment (e.g., paddle, patch).

occlusio pupillae. See OCCLUDED PUPIL.

occlusion. 1. *Pathologic condition.* Blockage, as of a blood vessel. 2. *Treatment.* Covering one eye, as with a patch after surgery, injury, or in amblyopia. 3. *Test technique.* Covering one eye.

occlusion amblyopia (am-blee-OH-pee-uh). *Functional defect.* 1. Reduced visual acuity caused by prolonged patching of the better-seeing eye (which has no detectable anatomic damage to visual pathways) to promote use of the weaker eye; usually reversible. 2. Poor vision in an eye with an optical defect (e.g., cataract) that prevents formation of clear retinal image, resulting in inadequate sensory information to the brain. Unrelated to retinal or neurological disease.

Occucoat. *Drug.* Trade name of methylcellulose viscoelastic agent.

Octopus. *Instrument.* Trade name of computerized apparatus for detection and mapping of visual field defects. See also PERIMETER.

Ocu-Chlor. *Drug.* Trade name of chloramphenicol eyedrops or ointment.

Ocuclear. *Drug.* Trade name of oxymetazoline eyedrops; "whitens" the eye.

Ocufen. *Drug.* Trade name of flubiprofen, an anti-inflammatory, non-steroidal agent.

Ocuflox. *Drug.* Trade name of ofloxacin antibiotic eyedrops.

ocular adnexa (ad-NEKS-uh), **adnexa oculi, appendages of the eye**. *Anatomy.* Structures surrounding the eyeball; includes eyelids, eyebrows, tear drainage system, orbital walls and orbital contents.

ocular albinism (AL-bin-iz-um). *Congenital abnormality.* Lack of pigment (may be partial) in the iris and choroid. Results in reddish pupils and iris (from choroidal vessels seen through the overlying retina). Usually accompanied by poor vision, light sensitivity (photophobia), and involuntary oscillating eye movements (nystagmus). See also ALBINISM.

ocular biometry. *Test.* For measuring the distance between various ocular structures (e.g., axial length), usually with A-scan or B-scan ultrasound instruments.

ocular bobbing. *Clinical sign.* Disordered, spontaneous, fast downward jerk of both eyes followed by a slow return to the straight-ahead (primary) position. Related to advanced disease of the brainstem, usually in a comatose patient. See also REVERSE BOBBING.

ocular dysmetria (dis-MEE-tree-uh). *Clinical sign.* Uncoordinated eye movements, with "overshooting" of the eyes upon effort to view an object; small side-to-side eye movements occur until a stable end-point is reached. Sign of cerebellar system disease. See also OCULAR FLUTTER, OPSOCLONUS.

ocular flutter. *Clinical sign.* Brief, intermittent, spontaneous movements of both eyes in the straight-ahead position. Sign of cerebellar disease. See also DYSMETRIA, OPSOCLONUS.

ocular histoplasmosis (his-toh-plaz-MOH-sis), **presumed ocular histoplasmosis syndrome**. *Pathologic condition.* Chorioretinal disease characterized by fluid leakage, hemorrhage, and scarring of the macula (disciform degeneration), atrophy near the optic disc, and "punched out" choroidal lesions in the peripheral retina. Epidemiologically linked to histoplasmosis allergy. See also HISTO SPOTS.

ocular hypertensive (OHT) (hi-pur-TEN-siv), **glaucoma suspect**. Patient with intraocular pressure elevated above 21 mm of mercury, with no obvious optic nerve damage or visual field defects. Glaucoma may or may not develop with time.

ocularist (ahk-yu-LEHR-ist). *Vision care specialist.* Professional who designs and fits artificial eyes.

ocular media. *Anatomy.* Transparent optical surfaces and liquids within the eye through which light rays pass before reaching the retina; includes cornea, aqueous, lens and vitreous.

ocular motility, motility. *Science, function, test.* Deals with extraocular muscles and their effect on eye movements. See also BINOCULARITY, STRABISMUS.

ocular motor. *Description.* Refers to eye movements. Sometimes called oculomotor.

ocular motor palsies. See OCULOMOTOR PALSIES.

ocular myoclonus (mi-oh-KLOH-nus). *Clinical sign.* Quick bursts of parallel side-to-side eye movements. Associated with lesions in the pons or pretectal brainstem areas.

ocular pemphigus (PEM-fih-gus), **pemphigoid**. *Pathologic condition.* Chronic, progressive blistering and scarring of the eyes' mucous membranes, leading to adhesions between palpebral and bulbar conjunctiva. Causes severe drying and opacification of the cornea and may be devastating to vision. No known treatment. Occurs over age 60. See also SYMBLEPHARON.

ocular torticollis (tor-tih-KOL-is). *Functional defect.* Abnormal head turn or tilt that develops to compensate for a vertical extraocular muscle weakness.

Oculinum (ahk-yu-LI-num). *Drug.* Trade name for botulinum toxin; used as an alternative or in addition to surgery to correct eye misalignments.

oculist (AH-kyu-list). Obsolete term for ophthalmologist.

oculo-auriculo-vertebral dysplasia (AH-kyu-loh ah-RIK-yu-loh vur-TEE- brul dis-PLAY-zhuh), **Goldenhar's syndrome**. *Congenital anomaly.* Characterized by ear and spine deformities, small jaw, and sometimes deafness. Associated eye findings include unilateral conjunctival and corneal dermoids, eyelid colobomas, and Duane's retraction syndrome.

oculo-cardiac reflex. *Function.* Decrease in heart rate following manipulation of the eyes or extraocular muscles.

oculo-cephalic reflex (sef-AL-ik), **vestibulo-ocular reflex**. *Function*. Involuntary eye rotation in the opposite direction from head rotation to maintain fixation on a non-moving target. May be abnormal with some brainstem defects. See also DOLL'S HEAD PHENOMENON, OTOLITH APPARATUS, VESTIBULAR SYSTEM.

oculo-cerebro-renal syndrome, Lowe's syndrome. *Pathologic condition*. Characterized by mental retardation, renal problems, cataracts and congenital glaucoma. Rare. Hereditary, X-linked (affects males; female carriers have only cataracts).

oculodermal melanocytosis (MEH-lun-oh-si-TOH-sus), **Ota's nevus**. *Congenital defect*. Pigmented area on cheek, eyelids, forehead, or nose.

oculo-digital reflex. *Symptom*. Constant rubbing or pressing on the eyes with the fists or fingers. Common in blind children.

oculo-glandular syndrome, Parinaud's oculo-glandular conjunctivitis. *Pathologic condition*. Rare type of conjunctivitis characterized by conjunctival lesions surrounded by follicles, usually in one eye, with fever and malaise. Caused by various organisms.

oculogyric crisis. *Pathologic condition*. Involuntary spasmodic upward rotation of the eyes that occurs with basal ganglia disease, e.g., Parkinson's.

oculo-mandibulo-dyscephaly (dis-EF-uh-lee), **Francois** *(or)* **Hallermann-Streiff syndrome**. *Congenital anomaly*. Bone deformity of the skull and face. Characterized by a bird-like face with small jaw and "parrot-beak" nose, dwarfism, small eyes, congenital cataracts, and poor vision. Rare; hereditary. See also MANDIBULOFACIAL DYSOSTOSIS.

oculomotor. Name of the 3rd cranial nerve. Also used to refer to eye movements in general; in that case, the preferred term is ocular motor.

oculomotor apraxia (ay-PRAKS-ee-uh), **congenital** *(or)* **Cogan's congenital oculomotor apraxia**. *Congenital abnormality*. Inability to make voluntary eye movements. Results in head-thrusting movement to bring the eyes into desired gaze positions. Usually improves with age.

oculomotor decussation (dek-uh-SAY-shun). *Anatomy*. Crossing over of the nerve pathways that control horizontal gaze; occurs in the brainstem between the 3rd and 4th cranial nerve nuclei. Lesions below this level cause horizontal gaze deficits on same side; above, on opposite side.

oculomotor nerve. *Anatomy*. Third cranial nerve; primary motor nerve to the eye. Originates in front of the cerebral aqueduct in the midbrain area of the brainstem, runs through the cavernous sinus to enter the orbit through the superior orbital fissure, where it divides. Superior division sends branches to the superior rectus and eyelid levator muscles; inferior division sends branches to the medial rectus, inferior rectus and inferior oblique muscles, and carries parasympathetic fibers to the pupil sphincter and ciliary body muscles.

oculomotor palsies, ocular motor palsies. *Functional defect*. General term for eye deviations caused by a weakened 3rd (oculomotor), 4th (trochlear) and/or 6th (abducens) cranial nerve supplying the extraocular muscles. See also INCOMITANT STRABISMUS.

oculomotor palsy. *Functional defect*. Eye deviation caused by a weakened 3rd cranial nerve, which supplies four extraocular muscles.

oculoplastic surgery, ophthalmic plastic and reconstructive surgery. Subspecialty of ophthalmology that deals with diseases and reconstructive aspects of the eyelids, canthi, lacrimal system and orbit.

oculopressive device. *Instrument*. Used before surgery to press on the eye, to reduce intraocular pressure. See also HONAN CUFF.

oculo-respiratory reflex. *Function*. Temporary stoppage of breathing (apnea) during eye surgery induced by tugging extraocular muscles and surrounding orbital tissues.

Ocupress. *Drug*. Trade name of carteolol; for treating glaucoma.

Ocusert. *Drug*. Trade name of slowly dissolving membrane that is inserted in the lower conjunctival sac to provide continuous release of pilocarpine for seven days; for treating glaucoma.

Ocutome (AHK-yu-tohm). *Surgical instrument*. Needle-like cutting device. Used for cutting and removing vitreous or cataracts.

OD *(oculus dexter)*. Right eye.

oedema, edema. *Clinical sign*. Swelling of tissue from fluid accumulation.

oftamology, ofthamology. Incorrect spelling of OPHTHALMOLOGY.

Oguchi's disease (oh-GU-cheez). *Pathologic condition*. Form of night blindness. Hereditary; found almost exclusively in Japanese.

one and one-half syndrome. *Pathologic condition*. Brainstem lesion of the medial longitudinal fasciculus (MLF) and paramedian pontine reticular formation (PPRF). Produces a horizontal gaze palsy to the same side and an internuclear ophthalmoplegia (INO) during gaze to the opposite side. Result is a full outward eye movement on one side, with nystagmus, and no other horizontal movement.

one-snip *(or)* **two-snip operation**. *Surgical procedure*. Technique(s) for opening a constricted punctum leading to the lacrimal canaliculus.

one-stitch *(or)* **two-** *(or)* **no-stitch surgery**. *Surgical procedure*. Cataract extraction technique using minimal size incision into the eye, with lens fragmentation and removal by phacoemulsification. See also EXTRACAPSULAR CATARACT EXTRACTION.

onchoceriasis (ocular), river blindness. *Pathologic condition*. Infection caused by the microfilaral stage of a worm that invades the eye, primarily the cornea. Most common cause of blindness in Africa, Central and South America.

opacity. Condition of being opaque. Refers to anything that blocks normal transmission of light through a transparent medium.

opaque media. *Pathologic condition*. Cloudiness or opacification of the parts of the eye that are usually transparent (cornea, aqueous, lens, vitreous).

Opcon. *Drug*. Trade name of naphazoline eyedrops; "whitens" the eyes.

Opcon-A. *Drug*. Trade name of eyedrops containing pheniramine (an antihistamine) and naphazoline (a decongestant); for relief of itchy, red eyes.

open angle. *Description*. Iris that is not in contact with the corneal periphery, allowing adequate space for aqueous fluid to filter through the trabecular meshwork. Normal. See also ANGLE.

open angle glaucoma (OAG) (glaw-KOH-muh), **chronic** *(or)* **primary open angle glaucoma**. *Pathologic condition*. Most common type of glaucoma. Caused by gradual blockage of aqueous outflow from the eye despite an apparently open anterior chamber angle. If untreated, results in gradual, painless, irreversible loss of vision. Usually in both eyes.

"open sky" vitrectomy (vit-REK-toh-mee). *Surgical procedure*. Cutting and removal of vitreous using front access to inside of eye, by incising the corneal edge (limbus) for at least 180° or by removing a corneal button and extracting the lens.

operating microscope. *Instrument*. Modified microscope used for microsurgery on the eye. Has foot-operated focusing controls, observer eyepieces, and a beam splitter for a camera attachment. May be mounted on a stand or the ceiling.

operculum (oh-PUR-kyu-lum). *Pathologic condition*. Flap of torn retina; may be partially attached or totally free in the vitreous.

optamology, opthalmology, opthamology. Incorrect spelling of OPHTHALMOLOGY.

Ophthaine (AHF-thayn). *Drug*. Trade name of proparacaine anesthetic eyedrops.

ophthalmia neonatorum (ahf-THAL-mee-uh nee-oh-nuh-TOR-um). *Pathologic condition.* Severe eye infection (gonococcal) of newborn infants acquired from the birth canal. Also called gonorrheal ophthalmia. See also CREDE'S PROPHYAXIS.

ophthalmia nodosa. *Pathologic condition.* Nodular swelling of the conjunctiva due to penetration of ocular tissue by the hairs of certain insects (e.g., caterpillars) and vegetable matter.

ophthalmic artery (ahf-THAL-mik). *Anatomy.* First branch of internal carotid artery after it enters the cranial cavity. Supplies most of the blood vessels to the eye and orbit.

ophthalmic assistant. See OPHTHALMIC MEDICAL ASSISTANT.

ophthalmic insert. *Drug.* Slowly dissolving membrane containing medication that is inserted in the lower conjunctival sac (fornix) to provide continuous release of medication over several hours. Trade name: Ocusert.

ophthalmic medical assistant. *Vision care specialist.* Certified allied health person in ophthalmology trained to perform preliminary examinations and specialized ophthalmic tests. Three levels: ophthalmic assistant (COA), lowest; ophthalmic technician (COT); ophthalmic technologist (COMT), highest.

ophthalmic nerve. *Anatomy.* First of three divisions of the 5th (trigeminal) cranial nerve. Divides into three branches (lacrimal, frontal, nasociliary) just before entering the orbit through the superior orbital fissure.

ophthalmic technician. See OPHTHALMIC MEDICAL ASSISTANT.

ophthalmic technologist. See OPHTHALMIC MEDICAL ASSISTANT.

ophthalmodynamometer (ahf-THAL-moh-di-nuh-MAH-mih-tur). *Instrument.* Calibrated device applied to the eye. Used for measuring blood pressure in the ophthalmic artery. See also OPHTHALMODYNAMOMETRY.

ophthalmodynamometry (ODN) (ahf-THAL-moh-di-nuh-MAH-mih-tree). *Test.* Measurement of blood pressure in the ophthalmic artery with an instrument that increases intraocular pressure and induces pulsations in the central retinal artery at the disc margin. Useful in suspected carotid artery insufficiency.

ophthalmologist (ahf-thal-MAH-loh-jist). *Medical specialist.* Physician (MD) specializing in diagnosis and treatment of refractive, medical and surgical problems related to eye diseases and disorders.

ophthalmology (ahf-thal-MAH-loh-gee). *Medical specialty.* Deals with the eye, its function and diseases. Includes diagnosis and medical/surgical management.

ophthalmopathy. *Pathologic condition.* Any non-specific abnormality of the eyeball, e.g., endocrine (Graves'), external.

    Graves (endocrine): chronic inflammatory condition affecting the extraocular muscles and orbit, causing abnormal eye movements, lid retraction, and/or eye bulging (proptosis). Characteristic of thyroid eye disease.

ophthalmopathy. *Pathologic condition.* Chronic inflammatory condition affecting the extraocular muscles and orbit, causing abnormal eye movements and/or eye bulging (proptosis). Characteristic of thyroid eye disease.

ophthalmoplegia (ahf-thal-muh-PLEE-juh). *Pathologic condition.* Paralysis of more than one eye muscle, in one or both eyes.

    external: acquired paralysis of all extraocular muscles, causing restriction of eye movement, and the levator muscle, causing a droopy lid (ptosis). See also CHRONIC PROGRESSIVE EXTERNAL OPHTHALMOPLEGIA.

    internal: loss of muscle function inside the eye, with loss of accommodation, and a large pupil that does not constrict to light or to near stimuli. Caused by paralysis of parasympathetic nerve fibers affecting the iris sphincter and ciliary muscle.

painful: inflammatory condition characterized by severe pain and restricted eye movement due to palsies of the 3rd (oculomotor), 4th (trochlear), 5th (trigeminal) and 6th (abducens) cranial nerves; sympathetic nerve fibers and the optic nerve may be involved. No optic disc swelling (papilledema). Affects one eye; occurs during 4th or 5th decade of life. Also called Tolosa-Hunt syndrome. See also CAVERNOUS SINUS SYNDROME, ORBITAL APEX SYNDROME, SUPERIOR ORBITAL FISSURE SYNDROME.

total: combination of INTERNAL, EXTERNAL.

ophthalmoplegic exophthalmos (ahf-thal-moh-PLEE-gik ex-ahf-THAL-mus). *Anatomic defect.* Inability to rotate the eye because of abnormal bulging forward (proptosis) of the eyeball.

ophthalmoplegic migraine. *Pathologic condition.* Uncommon form of migraine headache preceded by an aura of lightning flashes and expanding circles of light, accompanied by temporary ocular motor nerve palsies. Caused by decreased blood flow (from blood vessel spasm) to part of brain; headache and pain caused by subsequent blood vessel dilation.

ophthalmoscope (ahf-THAL-muh-skohp). *Instrument.* Illuminated instrument for visualizing the interior of the eye (especially the fundus).

direct: provides a magnified (15x) upright view with a small (8°) field of view; consists of a bright light source and incorporated focusing lenses.

indirect: creates an inverted, magnified (3x) image of the fundus projected in front of the eye, with a wide (30°) field of view. Consists of a bright light source and a hand-held high-plus lens. Binocular model allows stereoscopic depth perception of the fundus.

ophthalmoscopy (ahf-thal-MAHS-kuh-pee). Use of an ophthalmoscope to examine the internal structures of the eye, especially the fundus (back of interior of eye).

Ophthetic (ahf-THET-ik). *Drug.* Trade name of proparacaine anesthetic eyedrops.

Ophthocort (AHF-thoh-kort). *Drug.* Trade name of antibiotic eyedrops containing chloramphenicol, polymyxin and hydrocortisone; for treating conjunctival and corneal infections.

opsin (AHP-sin). *Chemical.* Colorless protein found in rod and cone outer segments; carries specific photochemicals derived from vitamin A that are necessary to change light energy into electrical energy.

opsoclonus (ahp-soh-KLOH-nus). *Clinical sign.* Sequence of erratic, jerky movements of both eyes, usually in a horizontal direction. Sign of cerebellar disease. See also DYSMETRIA, OCULAR FLUTTER.

optamology, opthalmology, opthamology. Incorrect spelling of OPHTHALMOLOGY.

optical axis, lens *(or)* principal axis. *Optics.* Imaginary line that passes through the optical centers of both surfaces of any lens.

optical center, nodal point. *Optics.* Reference point on an optical system's principal axis though which incoming light rays are not bent by the lens or optical surface, so that incident and transmitted rays make equal angles with the optic axis. In the eye, lies on the optic axis near the rear surface of the lens.

optical zone. *Optics.* Central, optical portion of the cornea or a contact lens.

optic atrophy (AT-roh-fee). *Pathologic condition.* Optic nerve degeneration characterized by optic disc paleness. Usually results in irreversible loss of vision.

optic axis, geometric axis. *Optics.* Imaginary line that passes through the centers of curvature of the cornea and lens.

optic canal. *Anatomy.* Passage in the skull connecting the orbit with the intracranial cavity. Transmits the optic nerve.

optic chiasm (KI-azm), **chiasm**. *Anatomy.* Important X-shaped part of the retina-to-brain nerve chain, where retinal nerve fibers from the nasal portion of both eyes cross to the opposite side and optic nerves from the two eyes join and form the optic tracts. Located at the base of the brain just above the pituitary gland. See also OPTIC TRACT.

optic cup. 1. *Anatomy.* White depression in the center of optic disc; usually occupies one-third or less of the total disc diameter. 2. *Embryology.* Early stage in a developing eye; outpouching from the primitive brain.

optic disc, disc, optic nerve head. *Anatomy.* Ocular end of the optic nerve. Denotes the exit of retinal nerve fibers from the eye and entrance of blood vessels to the eye.

optic foramen (for-AY-min). *Anatomy.* Opening in the sphenoid bone at the back of the orbit through which pass the ophthalmic artery, optic nerve, and sympathetic nerves.

optic glioma (glee-OH-muh). See OPTIC NERVE GLIOMA.

optician (ahp-TISH-un), **dispensing optician.** *Vision care specialist.* Professional who makes and adjusts optical aids, e.g., eyeglass lenses, from refraction prescriptions supplied by an ophthalmologist or optometrist.

optic nerve. *Anatomy.* Second cranial nerve. Largest sensory nerve of the eye; carries impulses for sight from the retina to the brain. Composed of retinal nerve fibers that exit the eyeball through the optic disc and exit the orbit through the optic foramen.

optic nerve coloboma. *Congenital anomaly.* Defect in the optic nerve, often including the optic disc, usually the lower segment. Results from incomplete fusion of fetal fissure during gestation. See also MORNING GLORY SYN-DROME, PAPILLEDEMA.

optic nerve glioma (glee-OH-muh). *Pathologic condition.* Slow-growing (over years), non-malignant congenital tumor of the optic nerve or optic chiasm composed of glial supportive cells. Often presents with eye protrusion (proptosis), enlarged optic foramen and decreased vision. Often seen with neurofibromatosis. See also HAMARTOMA.

optic nerve head. See OPTIC DISC.

optic nerve hypoplasia (hi-poh-PLAY-zhuh). *Congenital abnormality.* Small optic disc; sometimes surrounded by a double ring (scleral halo) and often a pigment epithelium halo. Vision may or may not be reduced.

optic nerve pit. *Congenital defect.* Incomplete coloboma of the optic disc, sometimes associated with fluid leakage under the retina that simulates central serous choroidopathy.

optic nerve sheath decompression (ONSD). *Surgical procedure.* Cutting a rectangular window in the sheath surrounding the optic nerve to reduce pressure on the nerve.

optic neuritis. *Pathologic condition.* Inflammation of the optic nerve. May accompany demyelinating disease (e.g., multiple sclerosis) or infections from the meninges, orbital tissues or paranasal sinuses. Characterized by rapid onset of decreased vision and, usually, discomfort with eye movement and a central visual field defect. See also PAPILLITIS, RETROBULBAR NEURITIS.

optic neuropathy. *Pathologic condition.* Non-inflammatory abnormality or degeneration of the optic nerve.

optic radiations, geniculo-calcarine tract. *Anatomy.* Visual nerve pathway between the lateral geniculate body and the calcarine fissure of the occipital visual cortex in the brain. Consists of crossed nasal retinal fibers from one eye and uncrossed temporal retinal fibers from the other eye.

Opticrom. *Drug.* Trade name of cromolyn; for treating allergic conjunctivitis.

optics. *Science.* Branch of physics that deals with the properties and behavior of light, e.g., its refraction and reflection by lenses, prisms, mirrors and the eye. See also LENS, PHYSIOLOGIC OPTICS, PRISM.

optic tract. *Anatomy.* Visual nerve pathway between the optic chiasm and the lateral geniculate body. Consists of nasal retinal fibers from the eye on the opposite side (contralateral eye) and uncrossed temporal retinal fibers from the eye on the same side (ipsilateral eye).

optic vesicle (VES-uh-kul). *Anatomy.* Embryologic outgrowth of neural ecto-derm from each side of the primitive forebrain, appearing in the 3-week-old fetus as a hollow ball of cells. Eventually forms the retina, retinal pig-ment epithelium, ciliary body epithelium and iris epithelium.

Optimyd (AHP-tih-mihd). *Drug.* Trade name of prednisolone eyedrops, anti-inflammatory steroid used for treating infections inside the eye.

Optipranolol. Trade name of metipranolol; for treating glaucoma.

optokinetic nystagmus (OKN) (ahp-toh-kin-ET-ik ni-STAG-mus), **"railroad" nystagmus**. *Function.* Involuntary rhythmic eye movements produced by viewing a series of vertical bars or other patterned contours while the in-dividual or target is moving; slow following phase (pursuit) is in the direc-tion of target movement, with rapid jerk return (saccade) in the opposite direction. Normal.

optometer (ahp-TAHM-ih-tur). *Instrument.* Measures accommodation exerted by an eye as it views an object.

optometric technician (ahp-toh-MET-rik). *Vision care specialist.* Paraprofes-sional who performs vision tests for an optometrist.

optometrist (ahp-TAHM-uh-trist). *Vision care specialist.* Doctor of optometry (OD) specializing in vision problems, treating vision conditions with specta-cles, contact lenses, low vision aids and vision therapy, and prescribing medications for certain eye diseases.

optometry (ahp-TAHM-uh-tree). *Vision care specialty.* Deals with function and disorders of the eye. Includes detection of disease and some types of management.

optomotor reflexes (ahp-toh-MOH-tur), **pursuit mechanism**. *Function.* Slow, involuntary parallel movement of both eyes that allows following of moving objects. Also seen in slow phase of optokinetic nystagmus response and doll's head phenomenon.

optotype (AHP-toh-tipe). *Test instrument.* Letter, number, or symbol used in testing vision. See also CROWDING PHENOMENON.

oral. *Method.* Route of medication delivery: by mouth. See also PARENTERAL.

ora serrata (OR-uh seh-RAH-tuh). *Anatomy.* Front edge of the retina, located about 6.5 mm behind the corneo-scleral junction (limbus). Has a tooth-like appearance.

Oratol (OR-uh-tol). *Drug.* Trade name of dichlorophenamide, oral drug used for treating glaucoma. See also CARBONIC ANHYDRASE INHIBITOR.

orbicularis oculi (or-bik-yu-LEHR-is AHK-yu-li). *Anatomy.* Elliptical muscle sheet surrounding the eye that closes the eyelids (gently by palpebral portion, as in blinking, or tightly by orbital portion, as in crying or sneezing). Innervated by the 7th (facial) cranial nerve.

orbit. *Anatomy.* Pyramid-shaped cavity in the skull (apex toward back of head), about 2 inches deep and lined by the orbital bones (ethmoid, frontal, lacri-mal, maxillary, nasal, palatine, sphenoid). Contains the eyeball, its muscles, blood supply, nerve supply and fat.

orbital apex. *Anatomy.* Narrow innermost part of pyramid-shaped bony orbit, near the optic foramen and superior orbital fissure.

orbital apex syndrome. *Pathologic condition.* Disorder in the muscle cone at the rear of the orbit; causes limitation of eye movement, bulging eye (proptosis), and decreased corneal and eyelid sensation. Optic nerve in-volvement causes decreased vision and visual field loss, distinguishing it from superior orbital fissure syndrome. See also CAVERNOUS SINUS SYNDROME, TOLOSA-HUNT SYNDROME.

orbital cellulitis (sel-yu-LI-tis). *Pathologic condition.* Infection of the orbital contents, often caused by streptococci or staphylococci. Produces swelling and redness of eyelids, bulging eye (proptosis), limitation of eye movement, and swelling of orbital tissues. Usually spreads from an infected ethmoid, sphenoid, maxillary or frontal sinus into the orbit (bony cavity containing eyeball). See also PRESEPTAL CELLULITIS.

orbital decompression. *Surgical procedure.* Removal of any part of the bony orbital wall to permit enlarged orbital contents to expand without pushing the eye forward.

   lateral: removal of the side of the orbital wall to permit enlarged orbital contents (as in Grave's disease) to expand laterally. Also called Krönlein procedure.

orbital fascia (FASH-uh). *Anatomy.* Protective, supportive tissue surrounding the eyeball; includes check ligaments, intermuscular membrane, muscle sheaths, orbital septum, periorbita and Tenon's capsule.

orbital fat pads. *Anatomy.* Four lobes of fat located between each of the rectus muscles and the tissue lining the bony orbital walls.

orbital fissures. *Anatomy.* Slit-like openings in the bones that form the back and floor of the orbit; passageway for blood vessels and nerves to and from the brain.

   inferior: opening at the junction of the sphenoid and maxillary bones, through which pass the infraorbital and zygomatic nerves and the infraorbital artery.

   superior: opening between the lesser and greater wings of the sphenoid bone. Site of entry to the orbit for the 3rd (oculomotor), 4th (trochlear), and 6th (abducens) cranial nerves, and site of exit for the superior ophthalmic vein.

orbital fissure syndrome, superior orbital fissure syndrome. *Pathologic condition.* Characterized by a droopy eyelid, decreased corneal and eyelid sensation, numbness, and the eye positioned downward and outward. Disease involvement of structures passing through the superior orbital fissure cause a large pupil, paralysis of the 3rd (oculomotor), 4th (trochlear), ophthalmic division of 5th (trigeminal), and 6th (abducens) cranial nerves and sympathetic nerves, with no engorged veins. See also CAVERNOUS SINUS SYNDROME, ORBITAL APEX SYNDROME, TOLOSA-HUNT SYNDROME.

orbital floor fracture. *Injury.* Break in bony orbital floor caused by blunt trauma to the eye or orbit. See also BLOWOUT FRACTURE.

orbital implant. Plastic or glass sphere placed in the eye socket after surgical removal of an eyeball. Buried under Tenon's capsule and conjunctiva. See also ENUCLEATION, PROSTHESIS.

orbital periosteum (per-ee-AHS-tee-um), **periorbita**. *Anatomy.* Tight connective tissue sheet that lines the orbital bones.

orbital pseudotumor (SU-doh-tu-mur). *Pathologic condition.* Inflammation in the orbit that mimics a tumor mass.

orbital septum, palpebral fascia, septum orbitale. *Anatomy.* Sheet-like fibrous membrane that forms a protective barrier between the eyelid and the bony orbit; located between orbital rim of bone and the tarsal plate of the lid. Supports eyelid structures, prevents orbital fat from bulging into the lids, and prevents lid inflammations from entering the orbit.

orbitonometer (or-bit-uh-NAHM-ih-tur). *Instrument.* Used for measuring resistance to compression of the orbital contents.

orbitotomy (or-bit-AHT-uh-mee). *Surgical procedure.* Opening made into the orbital space, for biopsy, abscess drainage, or tumor mass or foreign body removal.

organic amblyopia (am-blee-OH-pee-uh), **irreversible amblyopia**. *Func-*

tional defect. Poor vision in one or both eyes caused by non-apparent damage to the visual system. Therapy is ineffective. See also AMBLYOPIA, NEUTRAL DENSITY FILTER.

organic visual loss. *Pathologic condition*. Decreased vision that has a pathological cause.

organized vitreous (VIT-ree-us). *Pathologic condition*. Formation of opaque fibrous vitreous strands within the normal jelly-like vitreous. Occurs with resolution of inflammation, hemorrhage or trauma.

Orinase. *Drug*. Trade name of tolbutamide medication; for treating diabetes.

Orthofusor (OR-thoh-fyu-zur). Booklet of stereoscopic pictures for viewing through Polaroid glasses, for eye muscle imbalances. Concentrating on different aspects of the pictures improves convergence and divergence .

orthokeratology (or-thoh-kehr-uh-TAH-luh-jee). *Treatment*. A system of treating myopia and astigmatism with a sequential series of flatter-than-normal contact lenses that gradually flatten the cornea. Controversial.

orthopnea (or-THAHP-nee-uh). *Pathologic condition*. Difficulty breathing when lying down.

orthophoria (or-thoh-FOR-ee-uh). *Function*. Absence of eye deviation (or tendency toward deviation); no ocular movement is elicited by covering an eye while the other eye views a target. See also COVER TEST.

orthoposition. Intersection of both primary lines of sight at the fixation object.

orthoptics. *Science*. Discipline dealing with the diagnosis and treatment of defective eye coordination, binocular vision, and functional amblyopia by non-medical and non-surgical methods, e.g., glasses, prisms, exercises.

orthoptist (or-THAHP-tist). *Vision care specialist*. Certified allied health person in ophthalmology who analyzes and treats patients with dysfunctions of binocularity and/or ocular motility.

Ortho-rater. *Instrument*. Trade name of device for testing visual acuity, binocularity, color vision and stereo acuity; incorporates viewing tubes and polarizing materials. Often used for vision testing by Department of Motor Vehicles.

OS *(oculus sinister)*. Left eye.

oscillopsia (ahs-sil-AHP-see-uh). *Optical illusion*. Illusion of object movement; accompanies acquired nystagmus.

Osmitrol. *Drug*. Trade name of mannitol; intravenous treatment for an acute glaucoma attack.

Osmoglyn (AHZ-moh-glin). *Drug*. Trade name of glycerin solution oral medication; for treating an acute glaucoma attack.

osmotic agent (ahz-MAH-tik). *Drug*. Lowers intraocular pressure by temporarily increasing osmotic pressure of blood so that fluid is drawn from the eye. Used for breaking an acute glaucoma attack. Examples: glycerin, isosorbide, mannitol, sodium ascorbate.

osteogenesis imperfecta (AHS-tee-oh-JEN-uh-sis im-pur-FEK-tuh), **van der Hoeve's syndrome**. *Pathologic condition*. Characterized by blue scleras, deafness and fragile bones. Congenital; hereditary.

Ota's nevus (OH-tuz NEE-vus), **oculodermal melanocytosis**. *Congenital defect*. Pigmented area on cheek, eyelids, forehead, or nose.

otolith apparatus (OH-toh-lith). *Anatomy*. Non-visual reflex system that keeps the eyes fixed in position with respect to gravity despite a change in head position; depends on normal function of the utricle in the inner ear. See also VESTIBULAR SYSTEM.

OU *(oculus uterque)*. *Anatomy*. Denoting both eyes used together. Term incorrectly used for denoting each of two eyes separately.

outer canthus (KAN-thus), **lateral canthus**. *Anatomy*. Angle formed by the outer (away from nose) junction of the upper and lower eyelids.

outer limiting membrane, external limiting membrane. *Anatomy.* Layer of retina between the visual cells (rods and cones) and their nuclei.

outer nuclear layer. *Anatomy.* Retinal layer that contains rod and cone nuclei. See also INNER NUCLEAR LAYER.

outer plexiform layer. *Anatomy.* Retinal layer containing intercellular connections, where rod and cone axons synapse with bipolar and amacrine dendrites.

outer retina. *Anatomy.* Refers to visual cells and retinal pigment epithelium (pigment cell layer just outside retina that nourishes retinal visual cells).

outer segment (of rods and cones). *Anatomy.* Tiny, outermost part of visual cells in the retina; photosensitive column of double membrane protein-lipid discs that contain visual pigments. See also IODOPSIN, RHODOPSIN.

outflow (aqueous). *Function.* Passage of aqueous fluid from the eye through the anterior chamber angle structures.

outflow facility. *Measurement.* Ease with which aqueous fluid exits the eye through the trabecular meshwork into the canal of Schlemm and out through the episcleral veins.

output nerve, efferent *(or)* **motor nerve**. *Anatomy.* Nerve that carries impulses from the central nervous system toward the body; e.g., the 3rd (oculomotor) cranial nerve. See also INPUT NERVE.

overlap. Monocular cue to depth perception: an object that appears to cover a portion of another object must be in front of it, and thus closer. See also MONOCULAR DEPTH PERCEPTION.

over-refraction. 1. *Test.* Determination of the best optical correction using the patient's own eyeglasses as a baseline for adding new optical power. 2. *Optical device.* Soft contact lens or eyeglasses worn to improve vision after cataract surgery, when an intraocular lens has been implanted.

overwear syndrome (OWS). *Pathologic condition.* Corneal swelling and epithelial erosion following prolonged contact lens wear (usually over 10 hrs./day). Symptoms are pain and sensitivity to light. See also CORNEAL BEDEWING.

oxymetazoline. *Drug.* Weak sympathomimetic eyedrops that constrict blood vessels to "whiten" the eye. Trade name: Ocuclear.

P

pachometer (pak-AHM-ih-tur), **pachymeter** (pak-IM-ih-tur). *Instrument.* Used for measuring corneal thickness or anterior chamber depth, using the optical principle of split images. Usually a slit lamp attachment.

pachometry (pak-AHM-ih-tree), **pachymetry** (pak-IM-ih-tree). *Test.* For measuring corneal thickness. See also PACHOMETER.

paddy keratitis (kehr-uh-TI-tis). *Pathologic condition.* Corneal inflammation found in rice field workers. Cause unknown.

Paget's disease (PAA-jets). *Pathologic condition.* Systemic disease characterized by abnormal bone thickening and thinning, primarily of the skull. Sometimes associated with reddish-brown subretinal streaks resembling blood vessels (angioid streaks) that can lead to macular degeneration.

palatine (PAL-uh-teen). *Anatomy.* Bone that forms part of the medial floor of the orbit (eye socket). Smallest of the seven bones forming the orbit.

palinopsia (pal-in-AHP-see-uh), **visual perseveration**. *Functional defect.* Recurrence of visual sensations following removal of a viewed object. May be mistaken for monocular double vision.

pallor of disc. *Clinical sign.* Paleness of optic nerve head, suggesting optic nerve damage and reduced function. See also OPTIC ATROPHY.

palpate. To examine by touch.

palpebral (pal-PEE-brul). *Description.* Refers to the eyelid.

palpebral conjunctiva (kahn-junk-TI-vuh). *Anatomy.* Mucous membrane lining the inner surfaces of the upper and lower eyelids.

palpebral fascia (FAA-shuh), **orbital septum, septum orbitale**. *Anatomy.* Sheet-like fibrous membrane that forms a protective barrier between the eyelid and the bony orbit. Located between the orbital rim of the bone and the tarsal plate of the lid. Supports eyelid structures, prevents orbital fat from bulging into the lids, and prevents lid inflammations from entering the orbit.

palpebral fissure, palpebral opening. *Anatomy.* Elliptical opening between the upper and lower eyelids that exposes the eyeball. Measured (in mm) while the eye is open and in primary position.

palpebral fissure length. *Measurement.* Distance between the inner (nasal) and outer (temporal) canthi of the eyelids.

palpebral fissure width *(or)* **height, fissure width** *(or)* **height**. *Measurement.* Distance from the center of lower eyelid margin to the center of the upper eyelid margin, measured when the eye is open.

palpebral opening. See PALPEBRAL FISSURE.

palsy, paralysis. *Functional defect.* Complete or partial loss of muscle function, usually due to nerve damage Plural: palsies.

pancytopenia (pan-si-tuh-PEE-nee-uh). *Pathologic condition.* Marked decrease in the number of all types of circulating blood cells (red, white, platelets), resulting in decreased hematocrit and hemoglobin levels.

pannus (PAN-us). *Pathologic condition.* Infiltration of the cornea (just under the surface) by abnormal blood vessels and fibrous tissue.

panophthalmitis (pan-ahf-thal-MI-tis). *Pathologic condition.* Infection or inflammation of all structures of the eyeball.

panretinal photocoagulation. See PRP.

pantoscopic tilt (pan-tuh-SKAH-pik). Angle of an eyeglass lens with respect to the vertical plane. Tilting the lower edge closer to the cheek permits the fixation line to pass perpendicular to the lens surface on down-gaze.

Panum's fusion area (PAN-umz). Zone immediately to the front and back of a fixation object, where single binocular vision with depth perception is possible. Outside this area, diplopia occurs. See also HOROPTER.

panuveitis (pan-yu-vee-I-tis). *Pathologic condition.* Inflammation of the entire uveal layer of the eye. See also ANTERIOR UVEITIS, POSTERIOR UVEITIS.

papilla (puh-PIH-luh). *Anatomy.* Small elevation. Plural: papillae.

> **Bergmeister's**: small mass of fetal glial tissue that remains on the surface of the disc after birth. Congenital remnant; not harmful.

> **optic**: incorrect (but commonly used) term for optic nerve head.

> **lacrimal**: slight elevation on eyelid margin near the nose; pierced by the opening to the tear drainage system (punctum).

papilledema (pap-il-uh-DEE-muh), **choked disc.** *Clinical sign.* Swelling of the optic disc with engorged blood vessels, associated with elevated pressure within the skull. Characterized by blurred optic disc edges, flame-shaped nerve fiber layer hemorrhages next to the disc, and an enlarged physiologic blind spot. Vision is normal.

papillae (pap-IH-lee). *Pathologic condition.* Tiny elevations of palpebral conjunctiva that contain the central tufts of blood vessels. Found in many types of conjunctivitis but most prominent in allergic conjunctivitis.

papillitis (pap-ih-LI-tis). *Pathologic condition.* Optic disc swelling caused by local inflammation. Usually acute and associated with moderate-to-severe vision loss. See also OPTIC NEURITIS.

papillomacular bundle (PAP-ih-loh-MAK-yu-lur). *Anatomy.* Densely packed group of retinal nerve fibers that extend from the macula to the optic disc in an ovoid pattern. See also CENTROCECAL SCOTOMA.

paracentesis (pehr-uh-sen-TEE-sis), **anterior chamber tap, keratocentesis**. *Surgical procedure.* Corneal puncture with removal of some anterior chamber fluid (aqueous) for analysis or to reduce eye pressure quickly and temporarily.

paracentral scotoma (pehr-uh-SEN-trul skuh-TOH-muh). *Functional defect.* Non-seeing area in the visual field, located within 20° above, below, nasal, or temporal to fixation, but not involving the central 5°.

paradoxic diplopia (dih-PLOH-pee-uh). *Functional defect.* Double vision, with unexpected spatial localization of images relative to the actual position of the eyes. Usually found after strabismus surgery; caused by abnormal retinal correspondence.

paradoxic pupil. *Functional defect.* Any unexpected pupillary reaction, e.g., when the pupil is expected to contract with light stimulation, it dilates, and vice versa. Seen with optic nerve hypoplasia, achromatopsia, congenital stationary night blindness.

parafovea (pehr-uh-FOH-vee-uh). *Anatomy.* Area immediately surrounding the foveal area of the retina. Extends out to 5° from fixation, but excludes the central 2°.

parafoveal fixation. *Functional defect.* Fixation by a non-foveal retinal point located between 2° and 5° from fixation. Found in amblyopia.

parallax. *Optics.* Change in relative position of objects visualized from different positions. See also PHI PHENOMENON.

> **binocular p**: binocular cue to depth pereption. Each eye views an object from a slightly different position, so the images are slightly different; fusion of the two images in the brain creates perception of depth.

> **motion p**: important monocular cue to depth perception. As the head or an eye is moved from side to side, distant objects appear to move more slowly than closer objects.

paralysis, palsy. *Functional defect.* Complete or partial loss of muscle function, usually due to nerve damage.

paralytic ectropion. *Functional defect*. Lower eyelid that sags away from normal contact with the eyeball due to 7th (facial) cranial nerve weakness.

paramacular fixation (pehr-uh-MAK-yu-lur). *Functional defect*. Fixation by a non-macular retinal point located in the retinal zone outside the macula. The paramacula is a poorly defined area somewhat larger than the para-foveal zone but is usually used synonymously.

paramedian pontine reticular formation (PPRF) (pon-TEEN reh-TIK-yu-lur), **horizontal** *(or)* **pontine gaze center**. *Anatomy*. Region near the center of the brainstem (in the pons) at the level of the 6th (abducens) cranial nerve nucleus. Believed to organize and integrate fast horizontal parallel movements (saccades) of both eyes.

parasellar syndrome (pehr-uh-SEL-ur), **cavernous sinus syndrome**. *Pathologic condition*. Characterized by restricted eye movement, venous blood congestion, and swelling and engorgement of eyelids, conjunctiva and orbital tissues, making the eye bulge forward (proptosis). Caused by blood clot, tumor, or infection in the cavernous sinus (intracranial space behind orbit), producing weakness of the 3rd (oculomotor), 4th (trochlear), 5th (trigeminal), and 6th (abducens) cranial nerves. See also ORBITAL APEX S., SUPERIOR ORBITAL FISSURE S., TOLOSA-HUNT S.

parastriate area (pehr-uh-STRI-ayt), **Brodmann area 18**. *Anatomy*. Area in the occipital lobe of the brain surrounding Brodmann area 17 (primary visual cortex). Serves as visual association area, helping to interpret visual messages from area 17. See also BRODMAN AREA 19, OCCIPITAL CORTEX.

parasympathetic nervous system. *Anatomy*. Part of the autonomic nervous system. Nerve fibers to the eye travel within the 3rd cranial (oculomotor) nerve and provide innervation to the ciliary body, for accommodation and aqueous production, and iris sphincter, to decrease pupil size (miosis). Controlled by acetylcholine, a chemical that allows nerve transmission, aided by the enzyme cholinesterase.

parasympatholytic (pehr-uh-sim-path-oh-LIT-ik). *Description*. Refers to chemicals that block the action of acetylcholine in nerve transmission, thus reducing the effect of the parasympathetic nerves.

parasympatholytic drug, cholinergic blocking agent. *Drug*. Blocks parasympathetic nerve fibers by inhibiting the action of acetylcholine in nerve transmission. Causes enlarged pupils (mydriasis) and ciliary muscle paralysis (cycloplegia), resulting in loss of focusing ability at near (accommodation). Used for cycloplegic refraction and for treating uveitis. Examples: atropine, cyclopentolate, tropicamide.

parasympathomimetic (pehr-uh-sim-path-oh-mim-ET-ik). *Description*. Refers to chemicals that enhance the action of acetylcholine in nerve transmission, making the parasympathetic nerves more effective.

parasympathomimetic drug, cholinergic stimulating agent. *Drug*. Mimics action of parasympathetic nerve fibers, causing small pupils (miosis), dilating blood vessels and increasing accommodation. Works by (1) simulating acetylcholine chemically (miotics), which increases aqueous outflow and opens trabecular meshwork to treat glaucoma; examples: carbachol, pilocarpine; (2) inactivating cholinesterase (anti-cholinesterase), for treating accommodative esotropia and myasthenia gravis; examples: diisopropyl fluorophosphate, echothiophate iodide, edrophonium chloride, pyridostigmine bromide.

Paredrine (PEHR-uh-dreen). *Drug*. Trade name for hydroxyamphetamine eyedrops that cause mild pupillary dilation. No longer available.

parenteral (puh-REN-tuh-rul). *Method*. Introduction of medication, etc., by any route but the mouth, usually by injection.

paresis. *Pathologic condition*. Incomplete or partial paralysis.

paresthesia (pehr-iz-THEE-zhuh). *Symptom.* Unusual sensation (e.g., tingling) usually associated with irritation or injury of a nerve.

paretic muscle (pehr-ET-ik). *Functional defect.* Extraocular muscle weakened by damaged nerve supply, which needs more than usual innervation to perform its normal function.

parietal lobe (puh-RI-uh-tul). *Anatomy.* Upper mid-part of each cerebral hemisphere in the brain. Responsible for body sensations. See also FRONTAL LOBE, OCCIPITAL LOBE, TEMPORAL LOBE.

Parinaud's oculo-glandular conjunctivitis (PEHR-in-ohdz), **oculoglandular syndrome**. *Pathologic conditon.* Rare type of conjunctivitis characterized by conjunctival lesions surrounded by follicles, usually in one eye, with fever and malaise. Caused by various organisms.

Parinaud's syndrome, dorsal midbrain *(or)* pretectal *(or)* Sylvian aqueduct *(or)* tectal midbrain syndrome. *Pathologic condition.* Decreased ability to move the eyes up or down; attributed to brainstem lesion near vertical gaze center. Sometimes associated with inability to converge and poor pupil responses to light. See also ARGYLL-ROBERTSON PUPILS.

Parlodel. *Drug.* Trade name of bromocriptine, anti-cancer medication.; used for shrinking pituitary tumors.

pars ciliaris (parz sil-ee-EHR-is), **muscle of Riolan**. *Anatomy.* Part of orbicularis oculi muscle, located in the eyelid behind the eyelash follicles. Helps inner eyelid margin hug close to the eyeball.

pars plana ciliaris (PLAY-nuh). *Anatomy.* Flattened back portion of the ciliary body; located about 4 mm behind the corneo-scleral junction (limbus), between the ciliary processes and the ora serrata. See also PARS PLICATA.

pars plana incision. *Surgical procedure.* Surgical cut into the eyeball that passes through the sclera and the pars plana area of the ciliary body, between the pars plicata and the ora serrata. Entrance site for instruments commonly used for vitrectomy procedures.

pars plana vitrectomy (vih-TREK-tuh-mee). *Surgical procedure.* Removal of vitreous, blood, and/or membranes from the eye, entering through the pars plana with a needle-like rotary cutter that has fluid injection and suction capabilities.

pars planitis (pluh-NI-tis), **peripheral uveitis**. *Pathologic condition.* Chronic inflammation of the ciliary body (pars plana zone) that leads to coalescence of debris in the lower part of the vitreous and the appearance of a "snowbank" overlying the pars plana.

pars plicata ciliaris (plih-CAH-tuh, sil-ee-EHR-is). *Anatomy.* Anterior (front) portion of ciliary body that includes ciliary processes. See also PARS PLANA.

partial excimer trabeculectomy (EKS-ih-mur truh-bek-yu-LEK-tuh-mee). *Surgical procedure.* Removing the top of Schlemm's canal with an excimer laser, then placing a conjunctival flap over the opening to form a filtering bleb. Decreases outflow resistance for glaucoma control.

partially seeing child. *Legal description.* Child whose best corrected vision is lower than 20/70 in the better eye; eligible for instruction by teacher of visually handicapped.

partial myectomy (mi-EK-toh-mee). *Surgical procedure.* Removal of a portion of extraocular muscle to decrease its effective action and help correct an eye deviation.

partial-thickness graft, lamellar graft *(or)* keratoplasty. *Surgical procedure.* Removal of outer corneal layers (lamellae) and replacement with normal corneal tissue from a donor. See also CORNEAL TRANSPLANT, PENETRATING KERATOPLASTY.

partial thromboplastin time. See PTT.

passive forced duction test, forced duction *(or)* traction test. Forcibly moving the eyeball into different positions by grasping the anesthetized conjunctiva and episclera with forceps at the corneo-scleral junction (limbus). For determining any mechanical restrictions to movement.

past pointing. *Functional defect*. Misjudgment of an object's location; occurs with recent onset of a palsied extraocular muscle or eccentric fixation.

Patau's syndrome (pat-OHZ), **D trisomy** *(or)* **trisomy 13 syndrome**. *Congenital anomaly*. Multiple defects in the brain, face and eyes, caused by an extra chromosome. Fatal.

patch corneal graft. *Surgical procedure*. Replacement of a diseased or ulcerated section of cornea with healthy donor cornea tissue.

patching. *Treatment*. Covering an amblyopic patient's preferred eye by occlusion, to improve vision in the other eye.

patent (PAY-tunt). *Description*. Open, as a channel.

pathogenesis. *Process*. Mechanism or course of events in the development of an abnormal condition or disease.

pathognomonic (PATH-ug-nuh-MAHN-ik). *Description*. Sign or symptom that is so often associated with a particular disease or condition that a diagnosis can be made from its presence.

pathologic, pathological. *Description*. Altered or caused by a disease or abnormal function. See also PHYSIOLOGIC.

pathologic diplopia. *Functional defect*. Double vision caused by misalignment of one eye. Temporary in children; permanent in adults.

pathway (visual). *Anatomy*. Complete course of nerve fibers originating from the retinal visual cells as they travel to the occipital cortex in the brain. Consists of retinal photoreceptors (rods and cones), retinal nerve fiber layer, optic nerve, optic tract and optic radiations. Divided into anterior and posterior pathways.

Paton's lines. *Clinical sign*. Circumferential retina folds around the optic disc in established papilledema.

paving stone degeneration, cobblestone *(or)* **peripheral chorioretinal degeneration**. *Degenerative change*. Flat yellowish round areas of retinal thinning and loss of pigment near the ora serrata, through which underlying choroid can be seen. No affect on vision. Occurs with advancing age.

peaked pupil, ectopic *(or)* **up-drawn pupil**. *Abnormal condition*. Pupil that is displaced from its normal position. May occur from a congenital defect, ocular surgery, or trauma.

peau d'orange (poh-doh-RAHNJ). *Description*. Rippled orange peel-like appearance of pigmentary retinal mottling, seen with angioid streaks.

pedicle flap, transposition flap. *Surgical procedure*. Tongue-shaped section of skin and its subcutaneous tissue that has been cut to maintain its blood supply. Used for covering a defect (from trauma or surgical removal of a tumor or scar). Variation of the rotation flap.

pellagra (peh-LEG-ruh). *Pathologic condition*. Caused by a deficiency of B_2 vitamin complex. Characterized by skin disease, diarrhea, mental disturbances and optic nerve degeneration.

Pelli-Robson charts. *Test*. For contrast sensitivity, detecting subtle gradations in grayness between a test target and the background.

pemphigoid (PEM-fuh-goyd), **ocular pemphigus**. *Pathologic condition*. Chronic progressive blistering and scarring of the eyes' mucous membranes, leading to adhesions between palpebral and bulbar conjunctiva. Causes severe drying and opacification of the cornea and may be devastating to vision. No known treatment. Occurs over age 60. See also SYMBLEPHARON.

pemphigus. See PEMPHIGOID.

penalization (peh-nul-ih-ZAY-shun). *Treatment*. Treatment of amblyopia with atropine, miotics or special glasses, to handicap one eye in order to force the use of the amblyopic eye. See also PATCHING.

pendular nystagmus (ni-STAG-mus). *Functional defect.* Involuntary, rhythmic eye movements in which both eyes move together at about the same speed and amount in each direction. Associated with congenital nystagmus or central vision loss before age 2.

penicillin. *Drug.* Antibiotic agent used for treating eye infections.

penetrating keratoplasty (PKP) (KEHR-uh-toh-plas-tee). *Surgical procedure.* Removal of full thickness of cornea and replacement with donor cornea. See also CORNEAL TRANSPLANT, LAMELLAR KERATOPLASTY.

perfluoropropane, C_3F_8. *Gas.* Injected into the eye to produce a nontoxic, expansive gas bubble to tamponade (push) dislocated parts into place. See also PNEUMATIC RETINOPEXY, SULPHUR HEXAFLUORIDE.

perfusion (pur-FYU-zhun). *Technique.* Causing a liquid (usually nuitrient fluid or blood) to flow over or through an organ.

periarteritis nodosa (PAN) (pehr-ee-ahr-tur-I-tis), **polyarteritis.** *Pathologic condition.* One of the connective tissue (collagen) diseases. Associated with inflammatory and degenerative changes in the blood vessels, most often affecting the middle-aged. Characterized by fever, weight loss, abdominal pain, and kidney, heart and lung disease. Eye signs include decreased vision, double vision, conjunctival swelling, corneal and scleral degeneration, restricted eye movements, swollen optic nerve heads (papilledema), and retinal cotton-wool spots.

peribulbar (pehr-ee-BUHL-bahr). *Location.* Close to or surrounding the eyeball.

peribulbar injection, periocular injection. *Technique.* Injection of drugs through the skin or conjunctiva to surround the eyeball.

pericentral scotoma (skuh-TOH-muh). *Functional defect.* Blind patch of visual field located within 20° of fixation, not including the central 5°.

perichiasmal (pehr-ee-ki-AZ-mul). *Location.* Refers to the area surrounding the optic chiasm.

perifovea (pehr-ee-FOH-vee-uh). *Anatomy.* Retinal area within 10° of fixation, not including the central fovea.

perimeter (pur-IM-ih-tur). *Instrument.* For plotting the central or peripheral field of vision. See also PERIMETRY.

> **arc**: for plotting peripheral field; obsolete.

> **automated**: stationary (static) luminous stimuli are presented in pre-arranged locations and plotted by computer. Trade names: Dicon, Humphrey Analyzer, Octopus, Squid.

> **manual**: luminous stationary (static) and moving (kinetic) targets of various sizes and intensities are projected onto standardized background illumination. Not computerized. Trade names: Goldmann, Marco, Topcon.

perimetry (puh-RIM-ih-tree). *Test.* Method of charting extent of a stationary eye's field of vision with test objects of various sizes and light intensities. Aids in detection of damage to sensory visual pathways. See also CONFRONTATION FIELDS.

> **kinetic**: stimuli are moved from a non-seeing area until first perceived.

> **static**: stimuli are not moved but are gradually increased in intensity until first perceived.

> **suprathreshold static**: uses static targets to identify minimum target threshold intensity that can be seen just within a kinetic isopter.

periocular (pehr-ee-AHK-yu-lur). *Location.* Area surrounding the eyeball.

periorbita (pehr-ee-OR-bit-uh), **orbital periosteum.** *Anatomy.* Tight layer of connective tissue that lines the orbital bones.

periosteum (peh-ree-AHS-tee-um). *Anatomy.* Fibrous membrane that tightly covers the surfaces of bones.

peripapillary (pehr-ee-PAP-ih-lehr-ee). *Location.* Area surrounding the optic nerve head.

peripapillary atrophy. *Pathologic condition.* Loss of pigment epithelium and choroid, exposing a white ring of sclera around the optic disc.

peripheral anterior synechia (PAS) (sin-EE-kee-uh), **goniosynechiae**. *Pathologic condition.* Abnormal adhesion that binds the front surface of the peripheral iris to the back surface of the cornea, usually near the anterior chamber angle. Sign of previous iris inflammation. May cause glaucoma by blocking aqueous outflow through the anterior chamber angle. See also ANTERIOR SYNECHIA, POSTERIOR SYNECHIA.

peripheral chorioretinal degeneration. See PAVING STONE DEGENERATION.

peripheral curve. *Optics.* One of a series of curves at the edge of a contact lens, flattened to conform to the shape of the cornea.

peripheral fusion. *Function.* Blending (in brain) of similar images from the peripheral areas of both eyes into one image; some stereopsis may result. See also CENTRAL FUSION, MONOFIXATION SYNDROME.

peripheral iridectomy (PI) (ir-ih-DEK-tuh-mee). *Surgical procedure.* Removal of a full-thickness wedge of iris tissue at the iris base (near the corneal limbus), usually between the 10 and 2 o'clock meridians. Permits aqueous to flow more easily from the posterior to anterior chamber. See also SECTOR IRIDECTOMY.

peripheral vision. *Function.* Side vision; vision elicited by stimuli falling on retinal areas distant from the macula.

periphlebitis (pehr-ee-fluh-BI-tis). *Pathologic condition.* Inflammation of the tissues closely surrounding a vein.

perivasculitis (pehr-ee-vas-kyu-LI-tis). *Pathologic condition.* Inflammation of blood vessel walls and surrounding tissue. In the retina, produces clusters of exudates that lie along vessel paths. Associated with intraocular eye inflammations, e.g., in sarcoid. See also CANDLEWAX DRIPPINGS.

peroxisomal disorder (pehr-ahks-ih-SOH-mul). *Pathologic condition.* Group of hereditary retinal dystrophies that result in marked vision loss. Caused by increased levels of long chain fatty acids and a lack of peroxisomes needed to break down these acids. See also REFSUM'S DISEASE.

persistent hyperplasia of the primary vitreous, persistent hyperplastic primary vitreous. See PHPV.

persistent pupillary membrane. *Congenital anomaly.* Fine strands of unabsorbed fetal iris stroma bridging across the pupil. Clinically unimportant.

petechia (puh-TEE-kee-yuh). *Clinical sign.* Purplish-red pinpoint spots caused by tiny hemorrhages in the skin.

Peter's anomaly, anterior chamber cleavage syndrome, mesodermal dysgenesis of cornea. *Congenital anomaly.* Central cornea malformation characterized by adherence of the iris to Descemet's membrane and the endothelium (innermost corneal layer). May be associated with iridocorneal angle abnormalities and cataract.

Petizaeus-Merzbacker syndrome. *Pathologic condition.* One of the leukodystrophies; characterized by mental retardation, uncoordinated movements (ataxia), abnormal reflexes, and paralysis. Eye signs include nystagmus, optic atrophy, pigmentary retinal degeneration. Onset in infancy or childhood. Hereditary; X-linked (recessive).

pH. Measure of the acidity or alkalinity of a solution; indicator of hydrogen ion concentration. Scale ranges from 0 (acidic) to 14 (alkaline); 7 is neutral.

phaco-, phako- (FAY-koh). Prefix: refers to the eye's natural crystalline lens.

phaco-anaphylactic uveitis (an-uh-fih-LAK-tik yu-vee-I-tis). *Pathologic condition.* Hypersensitivity reaction to an individual's own natural lens protein after the capsule is torn (from cataract extraction or trauma). Occurs as inflammation, with cells (KPs) that adhere to the corneal endothelium.

phacodonesis (fay-koh-doh-NEE-sis). *Functional defect.* Lens that wobbles with eye movement. Caused by broken suspensory (zonular) lens attachments.

phacoemulsification (fay-koh-ee-mul-sih-fih-KAY-shun). *Surgical procedure.* Use of ultrasonic vibration (from irrigation-aspiration instrument) to shatter and break up a cataract, making it easier to remove. See also EXTRACAPSULAR CATARACT EXTRACTION.

phacolytic glaucoma (fay-koh-LIT-ik glaw-KOH-muh), **lens-induced glaucoma**. *Pathologic condition.* Increased intraocular pressure caused by mechanical blockage of the eye's drainage channels (trabecular meshwork) by cells carrying lens protein. Associated with advanced (hypermature) cataract or lens trauma.

phagocyte (FAG-oh-site). *Anatomy.* Cell that scavenges, removing microorganisms, debris, dead tissue, and foreign proteins from body tissues.

phakic (FAY-kik). *Description.* Refers to an eye that possesses its natural lens.

phako-. See PHACO-.

phakoma. *Pathologic condition.* Small grayish-white tumor in the retina.

phakomatoses (fay-koh-muh-TOH-sees). *Pathologic condition.* Group of hereditary diseases and syndromes characterized by spots, tumors and cysts in various parts of the body. Those with ocular findings include tuberous sclerosis; von Hippel-Lindau, von Recklinghausen and Bourneville diseases; Louis-Bar, Sturge Weber and Wyburn Mason syndromes.

phase. *Optics.* Portion of a wavelength cycle.

Phenergan (FEN-ur-gan). *Drug.* Trade name for type of phenothiazine, a tranquilizing agent used also to prevent vomiting.

phenothiazine (feen-oh-THI-uh-zeen). *Drug.* Class of drugs used as tranquilizing agents and to prevent vomiting. Trade names: Compazine, Phenergan, Thorazine.

phenylephrine (fen-il-EF-rin). *Drug.* 1. Stimulates sympathetic nerve fibers, causing pupil to enlarge, for eye examination, breaking iris-to-lens adhesions (posterior synechiae), treating iritis, and preventing iris cyst formation caused by phospholine iodide. Trade names: AK-Dilate, AK-Mydfrin, Mydfrin, Neosynephrine. 2. Weak sympathomimetic eyedrops that constrict blood vessels to "whiten" eye. Trade names: AK-Nefrin, IsoptoFrin, Nefrin.

phenylketonuria (PKU) (feen-il-kee-tohn-YU-ree-uh). *Pathologic condition.* Genetic metabolic disorder caused by absence of enzyme phenylalanine hydroxylase in the liver. Characterized by mental retardation, epilepsy, restlessness, tendon reflex, hyperactivity tremors, light colored irides, and increased light sensitivity (photophobia). Affects children under age 5.

pheochromocytoma. *Pathologic condition.* A tumor derived from chromaffin cells in the adrenal gland, usually associated with paroxysmal or sustained hypertension. Plural: pheochromocytomas, pheochromocytomata.

phi phenomenon. *Function.* Apparent movement of an object that occurs between rapid sequential presentations of still images, e.g., in motion pictures or when eyes that are misaligned are alternately covered.

phlebitis (fluh-BI-tus), **thrombophlebitis**. *Pathologic condition.* Inflammation of a vein.

phlyctenular keratoconjunctivitis (flik-TEN-yu-lur KEHR-uh-toh-kon-junk-tih-VI-tis). *Pathologic condition.* Inflammation of the conjunctiva and cornea associated with small nodular lesions (phlyctenules) at the corneal edge; may promote abnormal new blood vessel growth (neovascularization). Suspected cause is hypersensitivity to bacterial proteins, particularly tuberculoprotein or staphylococcal protein.

phlyctenule (flik-TEN-yool). *Anatomic defect.* Wedge-shaped nodular lesion (lymphocytic infiltration) at the corneal edge. May promote abnormal new blood vessel growth (neovascularization). See also PHLYCTENULAR KERATOCONJUNCTIVITIS.

phoria (FOR-ee-uh), **heterophoria**. *Functional defect.* Latent tendency of eyes to deviate that is prevented by fusion. Thus a deviation occurs only when a cover is placed over an eye; when uncovered, the eye straightens. See also ESOPHORIA, EXOPHORIA, HYPERPHORIA, HYPOPHORIA, ORTHOPHORIA.

phoropter (FOR-ahp-tur or for-AHP-tur). *Instrument.* Refraction device for determining an eye's optical correction. Incorporates spherical and cylindrical lenses, prisms, occluders and pinholes.

phosphene (FAHS-feen). See PHOTOPSIA.

Phospholine iodide (PI) (FAHS-fuh-leen I-uh-dide). *Drug.* Trade name of echothiophate iodide; for treating open angle glaucoma and accommodative esotropia.

photism (FOH-tizm). *Function.* Sensation of vision.

photoablation (foh-toh-uh-BLAY-shun). *Surgical procedure.* Destruction of tissue with light or laser energy.

photochemistry. *Function.* Chemical change brought about by light stimulation, e.g., in the retinal rods and cones. See also IODOPSIN, RHODOPSIN.

photochromic lenses (foh-toh-KROHM-ik). *Optical device.* Eyeglass lenses that darken when exposed to sunlight and lighten to almost clarity when not in the sun.

photocoagulation (foh-toh-koh-ag-yu-LAY-shun). *Surgical procedure.* Application of a laser beam to burn or destroy selected intraocular structures, e.g., abnormal blood vessels or tumors, or to create new fluid passages. See also PHOTOABLATION, PHOTODISRUPTION.

photodisruption (foh-toh-dis-RUP-shun). *Surgical procedure.* Fragmenting tissue with light energy. Usually refers to a YAG laser used for obliterating a small area of tissue, as to form an optical opening in an opaque membrane, e.g., an opacified posterior capsule (after-cataract).

photokeratoscope (foh-toh-KEHR-uh-tuh-scohp). *Instrument.* Used for photographing the front surface contour of the cornea.

photokeratoscopy (foh-toh-kehr-uh-TAHS-kuh-pee). *Test.* Creating image patterns of reflected light rings from the cornea, which provides an accurate reconstruction of the shape of the anterior corneal surface. Used for calculation of corneal dioptric power. See also CORNEAL TOPOGRAPHY, PLACIDO DISK, VIDEOKERATOSCOPY.

photometry (foh-TAHM-uh-tree). *Science.* Deals with measurement of light intensity. See also DARK ADAPTATION, LIGHT ADAPTATION, WEBER'S LAW.

photon. *Optics.* The basic unit (quantum) of visible light energy.

photophobia (foh-toh-FOH-bee-uh). *Symptom.* Abnormal sensitivity to, and discomfort from, light. May be associated with excessive tearing. Often due to inflammation of the iris or cornea.

photopic vision (foh-TAHP-ik). *Function.* Eyesight under daylight conditions. Involves the cone photoreceptors, which function for sharp resolution of detail and color discrimination. See also LIGHT ADAPTATION, MESOPIC VISION, SCOTOPIC VISION.

photopsia (foh-TAHP-see-uh), **phosphene**. *Symptom.* Sensation of light or light flashes from mechanical or electrical irritation of the retina, neural pathways or brain, not from a light stimulus. See also ENTOPIC PHENOMENON.

photoreceptors (foh-toh-ree-SEP-turz), **retinal elements** *(or)* **visual cells, sensory receptors**. *Anatomy.* Rods and cones; retinal cells that convert light into electrical impulses for transmission of messages to brain.

photorefractive keratectomy (PRK), laser keratorefractive surgery, photorefractive surgery. *Surgical procedure.* Use of high intensity laser light (e.g., an excimer laser) to reshape the corneal curvature; for correcting refractive errors. Includes laser sculpting, LASIK.

photorefractive surgery. See PHOTOREFRACTIVE KERATECTOMY.

photostress test. For early macular degeneration; measures visual acuity rate of recovery (with a vision chart) after patient looks at a bright light to bleach the macula.

phototherapeutic keratectomy (PTK). *Surgical procedure*. Use of an excimer laser to remove corneal scars and smooth an irregular corneal surface.

photovaporization. *Surgical procedure*. Type of photocoagulation using an infrared carbon dioxide laser for cutting tissue through heat absorption. See also LASER.

PHPV (persistent hyperplasia of the primary vitreous, persistent hyperplastic primary vitreous). *Congenital anomaly*. Embryologic malformation caused by failure of normal regression of primary vitreous and hyaloid vascular system. Affected eye is usually slightly small (microphthalmic) with elongated ciliary processes, a shallow anterior chamber, cataract, and a white fibrovascular tract extending from the disc into the vitreous. See also HYALOID CANAL.

phthisical eye. See PHTHISIS BULBI.

phthisis bulbi (TI-sis BUL-bi), **phthisical eye**. *Pathologic condition*. Diseased or damaged eyeball that has lost function and shrunk. Associated with low intraocular pressure because the ciliary body stops producing aqueous fluid.

physiologic. *Description*. Normal condition or function. See also PATHOLOGIC.

physiologic blind spot (of Mariotte), blind spot. *Function*. Sightless area within the visual field of a normal eye. Caused by absence of light sensitive photoreceptors where the optic nerve enters the eye.

physiologic diplopia (dih-PLOH-pee-uh). *Function*. Binocular phenomenon of seeing double. Affects objects not directly fixated by both eyes, resulting in doubling of distant objects when near object is viewed, and vice versa. Normal. See also DIPLOPIA.

physiologic nystagmus (ni-STAG-mus). *Function*. Involuntary, rhythmic side-to-side eye movements (of small degree) that occur during normal fixation. Eye is never completely stationary.

physiologic optics. *Science*. Study of fundamental phenomena of vision, light and seeing; includes optics of the eye, and eyeglass and contact lens correction for vision improvement.

physiologic position of rest, dissociated *(or)* **fusion-free** *(or)* **heterophoric position**. *Function*. Position assumed by the eyes, relative to each other, when one eye is covered or its vision obstructed. See also PHORIA.

physostigmine (fi-zoh-STIG-meen), **eserine**. *Drug*. Early ophthalmic drug for treating glaucoma. Indirectly stimulates parasympathetic nerves; prolonged use causes conjunctival irritation. Rarely used today. See also MIOCEL.

phytanic acid storage disease (fi-TAN-ik), **heredopathia atactica polyneuritiformis, Refsum's disease**. *Pathologic condition*. Enzymatic blockage of phytanic acid decomposition. Characterized by fatty acid accumulation, drop foot, increased cerebrospinal fluid, cerebral degeneration, inability to sleep, electrocardiogram changes, retinal pigment epithelium degeneration (causing defective dark adaptation and constricted visual fields), nystagmus, ptosis (droopy eyelids), and small pupils. Hereditary. See also RETINITIS PIGMENTOSA.

picosecond (PEE-coh-sek-und). *Unit of measure*. One-trillionth of a second.

"pie in the sky" defect, superior quadrantanopia. *Functional defect*. Upper quadrant visual field defect on the same side of each eye. Caused by damage to inferior fibers of the optic radiations in the temporal lobe of the brain (in Meyer's temporal loop).

Pierre Robin syndrome. *Congenital anomaly*. Multiple deformities resulting from incomplete development of the maxilla and mandible bones, e.g., small jaw, cleft palate, low-set ears, abnormal tongue position. Characteristic eye findings include congenital cataracts and glaucoma, large corneas, and retinal degeneration that often leads to retinal detachment.

piggyback lens. *Optical device.* Hard contact lens worn over a soft contact lens. Used when hard lenses are not tolerated, e.g., in severe keratoconus.

pigment clumping. *Anatomic defect.* Irregularly shaped patches of pigment deposits under the retina. Usually found where there has been previous irritation of the retinal pigment epithelium, such as at the site of a vitreous tug or retinal tear, or at the healed site of minimal inflammation.

pigment dropout. *Anatomic defect.* Atrophy of the retinal pigment epithelium. Appears as "windows" when visualized with fluorescein angiography. The causes are similar to pigment clumping (above), but damage is greater.

pigment epitheliitis (ep-ih-thee-lee-I-tis), **retinal pigment epitheliopathy**. *Pathologic condition.* Damage to the pigment epithelium with cellular loss and, later, pigment clumping and pigment dropout, usually in the macular area. Probably viral in origin. Sudden onset; gradual recovery of normal vision within 3 months.

pigment epithelium (PE) (ep-ih-THEE-lee-um), **retinal pigment epithelium**. *Anatomy.* Pigment cell layer (hexagonal cells densely packed with pigment granules) just outside the retina that nourishes retinal visual cells. Firmly attached to underlying choroid and overlying retinal visual cells.

pigmentary dispersion glaucoma (glaw-KOH-muh). *Pathological condition.* Type of open angle glaucoma caused by pigment granules gradually breaking free from the iris and ciliary epithelium, deposited on the back corneal surface, lens and zonules, and plugging the trabecular meshwork (which increases intraocular pressure). See also KRUKENBERG'S SPINDLE.

pilo (PI-loh). *Drug.* Slang for pilocarpine.

Pilocar (PI-loh-kahr). *Drug.* Trade name of pilocarpine eyedrops; for treating glaucoma.

pilocarpine (pi-loh-KAHR-peen). *Drug.* Stimulates parasympathetic nerve receptors, producing small pupils (miosis), increased accommodation and increased aqueous outflow. For treating glaucoma. Trade names: Adsorbocarpine, Isopto Carpine, Pilocar, PIlocar, Pilocel, P.V. Carpine. See also PARASYMPATHOMIMETIC DRUGS.

Pilocel (PI-loh-sel). *Drug.* Trade name of pilocarpine eyedrops; for treating glaucoma.

pimaricin (pih-MEHR-uh-sin). *Drug.* Antibiotic drug suspension applied topically to the cornea for treating fungal ulcers. Now known as NATAMYCIN.

pincushion distortion. *Optics.* Type of optical distortion especially apparent in a high-plus spectacle lens. Produced when peripheral zones of a lens have greater magnification than the central zone.

pinealoma (pi-nee-uh-LOH-muh). *Pathologic condition.* Pineal body tumor that may impinge on the roof of the midbrain, producing defective pupil function and/or reduced ability to move the eyes vertically.

pinguecula (pin-GWEK-yu-luh). *Anatomic defect.* Yellowish-brown subconjunctival elevation composed of degenerated elastic tissue; may occur on either side of the cornea. Benign. Plural: pingueculae. See also PTERYGIUM.

pingueculum. Incorrect word; correct word is PINGUECULA.

pinhole (ph). *Test instrument.* Opaque disc with one or more holes ranging from 0.5 to 2 mm in diameter. Looking through the hole with one eye (other eye covered) will improve vision if reduced vision is caused by an optical defect or refractive error. See also DILATED PINHOLE TEST.

"pink eye," conjunctivitis. *Pathologic condition.* Inflammation of the conjunctiva (mucous membrane covering white of eye and inner eyelid surfaces). Characterized by discharge, grittiness, redness and swelling. Usually viral in origin; may be contagious.

pisciform (PI-sih-form). *Description.* Shaped like a fishtail. Describes deposits found in flavimacular retinopathy.

pit, optic nerve pit. *Congenital defect.* Incomplete coloboma of the optic disc, sometimes associated with fluid leakage under the retina that simulates central serous choroidopathy.

pituitary ablation. *Surgical procedure.* Destruction of the pituitary gland.

pituitary apoplexy. *Pathologic condition.* Catastrophic expansion and destruction of the pituitary gland by a pituitary tumor. Causes severe headaches and double vision. May result in sudden profound loss of vision in one or both eyes.

pituitary gland, pituitary body, hypophysis. *Anatomy.* Master gland of the body that controls the activity of other glands; makes several hormones. Hangs sac-like from base of brain, between and behind the orbits and below the optic chiasm. See also SELLA TURCICA.

pituitary tumor (pih-TU-ih-tehr-ee). *Pathologic condition.* Abnormal tissue growth within or near the pituitary gland; may exert pressure on the optic nerves and chiasm, causing decreased vision, bitemporal visual field defects, and optic nerve degeneration. Most common types are chromophobe adenoma, acidophilic adenoma and basophilic adenoma. See also BITEMPORAL HEMIANOPSIA, CRANIOPHARYNGIOMA.

Placido disk (pluh-SEE-doh). *Test instrument.* Simplified type of keratoscope that permits evaluation of the smoothness and regularity of the corneal surface, for detecting corneal distortion or high astigmatism. Composed of alternating black and white rings and a central hole; reflected onto corneal surface as examiner views the cornea through the central hole.

plano (PLAY-noh). *Optics.* Lens that has no focusing power, neither plus nor minus.

> **plano concave**: minus-powered lens, flat on one side, curved inward on other side.

> **plano convex**: plus-powered lens, flat on one side, curved outward on the other side.

plaque (plak). *Pathologic condition.* Small differentiated area on the surface of the body or a blood vessel, e.g., fatty and calcium deposits (atheroma) in an artery in atherosclerosis.

Plaquenil (PLAK-wuh-nil). *Drug.* Trade name of hydroxychloroquine; for treating malaria, lupus erythematosus or rheumatoid arthritis.

plasma-lecithin deficiency (LES-ih-thin). *Pathologic condition.* Characterized by inability to metabolize fats (lipids), anemia, and grayish deposits in the corneal periphery.

plastic iritis. *Pathologic condition.* Iris and ciliary body inflammation characterized by presence of large amount of protein and fibrin, thus markedly slowing aqueous flow in the anterior chamber; sometimes forms a clot.

plateau iris. *Anatomic variant.* Configuration of the iris in which there is a prominent peripheral roll that may occlude the trabecular meshwork and cause acute angle closure glaucoma when the pupil is dilated, but does not have the typical pupillary block mechanism.

platybasia. *Pathologic condition.* An upward bulge into the posterior fossa of the base of the skull around the foramen magnum.

pleomorphism. See POLYMORPHISM.

pleoptics (plee-AHP-tiks). *Treatment.* Systematic method for analyzing and treating decreased vision from eccentric fixation, by reestablishing foveal fixation. See also EUTHYSCOPE, PROJECTOSCOPE.

plexus. *Anatomy.* Network, such as of interlacing blood vessels or nerves.

plica lacrimalis (PLEE-kuh lak-rih-MAA-lis), **Hasner's valve**. *Anatomy.* Mucous membrane fold at lower end of the nasolacrimal duct. Acts as a valve in preventing air from entering the lacrimal sac when the nose is blown.

plica semilunaris (sem-ee-lu-NEH-ris), **semilunar fold**. *Anatomy* Crescent-shaped, fleshy mound of conjunctival tissue at the inside (nasal) corner of each eye.

plus cylinder. *Optical device.* Lens with no optical power in one meridian (axis) and maximum plus-power in the perpendicular direction.

PLUS disease. *Congenital anomaly.* Dilated tortuous retinal blood vessels in conjunction with retinopathy of prematurity. Prognosis for vision is poor.

plus lens, converging lens, convex lens. *Optical device.* Lens that is thicker in the center than at the edges, adding optical power to incoming light rays. Corrects farsightedness (hyperopia).

PMMA (polymethylmethacrylate). *Chemical.* Plastic polymer used in making hard contact lenses.

pneumatic retinopexy. *Surgical technique.* For retinal detachment repair; intraocular injection of an inert gas bubble to press on the retina and seal the retinal break. See PERFLUOROPROPANE, SULPHUR HEXAFLUORIDE.

pneumatic tonometer. See PNEUMOTONOMETER.

pneumo (NU-moh), **Streptococcus pneumoniae**. *Microorganism.* One of the most common gram-positive bacteria that causes eye infections, especially corneal ulcers. Bacteria grow in pairs. See also PSEUDOMONAS AERUGINOSA, STAPHYLOCOCCUS AUREUS.

pneumotonometer (nu-moh-tuh-NAH-mih-tur), **non-contact *(or)* pneumatic *(or)* "puff" tonometer**. *Instrument.* Gas-pressurized device that measures intraocular pressure by blowing a puff of air against the cornea to flatten it slightly; does not come in contact with eye. See also TONOMETRY.

polarization. *Process.* A change in light effected by certain crystals or materials whereby light is separated into beams that vibrate in one plane only, instead of in all planes as does ordinary light. See also POLAROID.

Polaroid. Trade name for transparent material that allows vibrations of light to occur in one plane only, instead of in all planes as ordinary (unpolarized) light. See also VECTOGRAPH.

Polaroid vectograph slide. *Test chart.* Visual acuity master slide that is viewed with polarized glasses, allowing each eye to see letters or figures that are invisible to the other. Used for measuring stereo acuity and for testing visual acuity in monofixators and malingerers.

poliosis (poh-lee-OH-sis). *Clinical sign.* Absence of eyelash pigment (lashes are whitened). Associated with sympathetic ophthalmia, syphilis and Vogt-Koyanagi-Harada syndrome.

poly. See POLYMORPHONUCLEAR LEUKOCYTE.

polyarteritis (pah-lee-ahr-tur-I-tis), **periarteritis nodosa**. *Pathologic condition.* One of the connective tissue (collagen) diseases. Associated with inflammatory and degenerative changes in blood vessels, most often affecting the middle-aged. Characterized by fever, weight loss, abdominal pain, and kidney, heart and lung disease. Eye signs include decreased vision, double vision, conjunctival swelling, corneal and scleral degeneration, restricted eye movements, swollen optic nerve heads (papilledema), and retinal cotton-wool spots.

polycoria (pah-lee-KOR-ee-uh). *Pathologic condition.* More than one pupillary opening in the iris. May be congenital or result from iris disease.

polycythemia (pol-ee-si-THEE-mee-uh). *Clinical sign.* Increased number of red blood cells.

polymegethism. *Pathologic condition.* Significant increase in size variation of corneal endothelial cells as measured by specular microscopy (e.g., after long-term contact lens wear).

polymethylmethacrylate (PAH-lee-METH-il-meth-AK-rih-layt). See PMMA.

polymorphism, pleomorphism. *Description.* The state or quality of having or assuming many forms.

polymorphonuclear leukocyte (PMN) (PAH-lee-MOR-foh-NU-klee-ur LU-koh-site), **poly, neutrophil**. *Anatomy.* Type of white blood cell important in combatting acute (especially bacterial) infections.

polymyalgia rheumatica (PAH-lee-mi-AL-juh ru-MAA-tih-kuh). *Pathologic condition.* Stiffness and pain in many muscles, especially in the shoulder, associated with weight loss and temporal arteritis. Thought to be an auto-immune disease.

polymyxin B. *Drug.* Antibiotic agent used for treating eye infections.

polyopia (pah-lee-OH-pee-uh), **monocular diplopia**. *Symptom.* Multiple images seen with one eye. Commonly caused by early cataracts or irregular corneas.

polyostotic fibrous dysplasia (pah-lee-oh-STAH-tik, dis-PLAY-zhuh), **Albright's disease**. *Pathologic condition.* Characterized by pigmented skin lesions, early puberty, and bone abnormalities. Eye findings include eye protrusion (proptosis) and visual field defects resulting from optic nerve compression.

polys. See POLYMORPHONUCLEAR LEUKOCYTE.

Polysporin (pah-lee-SPOR-in). *Drug.* Trade name of antibiotic ointment containing polymyxin B and bacitracin; for treating corneal and conjunctival infections.

polytomography, tomography. *Clinical test.* X-ray imaging technique that utilizes moving film plate and an x-ray tube. Displays thin "slices" of tissue (structures in front and behind are blurred out and do not show).

polyvinyl alcohol. *Chemical.* Artificial tears solution or ointment used as a lubricant or wetting agent. Combined with ophthalmic drugs to prolong contact with the cornea. Trade names: AKWA Tears, Hypotears, Just Tears, Liquifilm Forte, Liquifilm Tears, Murine Tears, Puralube, Refresh, Tears Plus. See also METHYLCELLULOSE, TEAR FILM BREAKUP TIME.

Pompe's disease (pahm-PAYZ), **generalized gangliosidosis**. *Pathologic condition.* Genetic defect in enzyme B-galactosidase metabolism. Characterized by early and progressive brain degeneration, a macular cherry red spot, and death within 2 years. See also GANGLIOSIDOSIS, SPHINGOLIPIDOSES.

pons. *Anatomy.* Part of the brainstem; connects the midbrain with the medulla. Contains 6th (abducens) cranial nerve nucleus and horizontal gaze center.

pontine gaze center (PGC), horizontal gaze center, paramedian pontine reticular formation. *Anatomy.* Region near center of brainstem (in the pons) at the level of the 6th (abducens) cranial nerve nucleus; believed to organize and integrate fast, horizontal, parallel movements (saccades) of both eyes.

pontine lesion. *Pathologic condition.* Tumor in pons area of the brainstem. Affects other nearby areas, sometimes producing 6th (abducens) cranial nerve palsy, lack of corneal sensation (from involvement of 5th, trigeminal, cranial nerve), difficulty in making parallel eye movements (versions), or involuntary, rhythmic side-to-side eye movements (nystagmus).

Pontocaine (PAHN-tuh-kayn). *Drug.* Trade name of tetracaine anesthetic eyedrops.

popping (eye). 1. Self-inflicted finger pressure against upper and lower eyelid fold to push an eye partly out of its socket. May cause optic nerve compression. 2. *Test.* In an infant, spontaneously opening the eyelids in response to dimming room lights; provides evidence of visual function.

positive Seidel (si-DEL). *Test.* Bright green fluid flow seen after fluorescein is applied to the cornea; indicates wound leak of aqueous from the anterior chamber to the outside of the eye. See also SEIDEL SIGN.

positive vertical vergence *(or)* **divergence, right sursumvergence, left deorsumvergence**. *Function.* Upward movement of the right eye relative to the left, usually to maintain single binocular vision, e.g., when increasing amounts of base-down prism are placed in front of the right eye.

Posner-Schlossman syndrome, glaucomato-cyclitic crisis. *Pathologic condition.* Uveal inflammation resulting in acute increase in intraocular pressure. Characterized by corneal swelling, decreased aqueous outflow, and an open anterior chamber angle. Usually in one eye. See also SECONDARY GLAUCOMA.

post-chiasmal (ki-AZ-mul). *Location.* Refers to optic nerve fibers between the chiasm and the brain. Includes optic tract and optic radiations. See also PRE-CHIASMAL.

posterior. *Location.* On or near the back of an organ or of the body. See also ANTERIOR.

posterior capsule. *Anatomy.* Rear of the capsule enveloping the crystalline lens; lies against the anterior hyaloid membrane of the vitreous. See also ANTERIOR CAPSULE.

posterior capsulotomy (kap-sul-AH-tuh-mee). *Surgical procedure.* Opening in the rear lens capsule when it has become opacified after previous cataract surgery; usually made with a YAG laser. See also ANTERIOR CAPSULOTOMY, CAPSULE, CAPSULORHEXIS.

posterior chamber (PC). *Anatomy.* Space between the back of the iris and the front face of the vitreous; filled with aqueous fluid. See also ANTERIOR CHAMBER.

posterior chamber intraocular lens (PCIOL). *Optical device.* Plastic lens surgically implanted into the posterior chamber (behind the iris) to replace the eye's natural lens after cataract extraction. See also ANTERIOR CHAMBER INTRAOCULAR LENS.

posterior ciliary arteries (SIL-ee-ehr-ee). *Anatomy.* Six to 20 *short* ciliary arteries that supply blood to the optic nerve head, choroid and choriocapillaris, and two *long* ciliary arteries that join the anterior ciliary arteries to form the major arterial circle of the iris. Enter the eye around the optic nerve. See also ANTERIOR CILIARY ARTERIES, OPHTHALMIC ARTERY.

posterior fixation suture, Faden procedure, retroequatorial myopexy. *Surgical procedure.* Method of weakening a rectus muscle (medial, lateral, superior or inferior) by attaching it to the sclera 10-16 mm behind its insertion, thus restricting its action.

posterior hyaloid membrane (PHM) (HI-uh-loyd). *Anatomy.* Condensed tissue layer that attaches the vitreous firmly to the internal surface of the retina (limiting membrane).

posterior lip sclerectomy (skler-EK-toh-mee). *Surgical procedure.* Removal of a small section of sclera at the corneoscleral junction (limbus). Usually includes excision of a wide section of iris (iridectomy). Treatment for advanced glaucoma.

posterior pole. *Anatomy.* Back (posterior) curvature of the eyeball; usually refers to the retina between the optic nerve and the macular area. See also ANTERIOR POLE, GEOMETRIC AXIS.

posterior polymorphous dystrophy (PAH-lee-MOR-fus DIS-truh-fee). *Pathologic condition.* Development of calcium crystal plaques on innermost (endothelial) corneal surface. Does not usually affect vision. Hereditary (dominant); appears in early childhood.

posterior sclerectomy (skler-EK-tuh-mee). *Surgical procedure.* Removal of a small segment of sclera from the rear of the eyeball (globe).

posterior sclerotomy (skler-AHT-uh-mee). *Surgical procedure.* Incision into or through the sclera; usually with perforation of the choroid to drain subretinal fluid, as part of a retinal detachment repair.

posterior segment. *Anatomy.* Rear two-thirds of eyeball (behind the lens); includes the vitreous, retina, optic disc, choroid, pars plana, and most of the sclera. See also ANTERIOR SEGMENT.

posterior subcapsular cataract (PSC), cupuliform cataract. *Pathologic condition.* Opacity of the rear surface of the lens. Common; one type of "senile cataract" affecting the elderly but may occur at any age after chronic intraocular inflammations or prolonged use of steroid drugs.

posterior synechia (sin-EE-kee-uh). *Pathologic condition.* Adhesion(s) binding the pupillary margin and back surface of the iris to the front surface of the lens. See also ANTERIOR SYNECHIA, PERIPHERAL ANTERIOR SYNECHIA, PUPILLARY BLOCK.

posterior uveitis (yu-vee-I-tis). *Pathologic condition.* Choroidal or ciliary body inflammation; may produce cellular debris in vitreous and exudative retinal opacities.

posterior vitreous detachment (PVD), vitreous detachment. *Pathologic condition.* Separation of vitreous gel from the retinal surface. Frequently occurs with aging as the vitreous liquifies or in some disease states e.g. diabetes and high myopia. Usually innocuous, but can cause retinal tears, which may lead to retinal detachment.

postprandial. *Description.* After a meal.

potassium hydroxide (KOH). *Chemical.* Breaks cells apart to expose fungi for microscopic examination; placed on a slide with sample of corneal or conjunctival tissue to test for presence of fungi.

potential acuity meter (PAM). *Instrument.* Helps predict visual acuity potential in the presence of an opacity (e.g., cataract). Projects brightly illuminated Snellen chart through the least dense areas of an opacity onto the retina. See also LASER INTERFEROMETER.

power. *Optics.* Measure (in diopters) of the capability of a lens to converge (plus lens) or diverge (minus lens) light rays.

power density. *Measurement.* Amount of energy (as by laser) delivered into a unit area, e.g., joules per square centimeter.

PPD (purified protein derivative), tuberculin skin test. *Chemical.* Used as a skin test for tuberculosis.

pre-auricular nodes. *Anatomy.* Lymph nodes in front of the ears; enlarge with viral eye infections.

pre-chiasmal (ki-AZ-mul). *Location.* Refers to the optic nerve fiber pathway between the eyeball and the chiasm. See also POST-CHIASMAL.

pre-corneal tear film (KOR-nee-ul), **tear film**. *Anatomy.* Liquid that bathes the cornea and conjunctiva. Composed of three layers: outer oily layer secreted by meibomian glands, aqueous layer secreted by the lacrimal glands, inner mucin layer produced by the conjunctival goblet cells.

Pred Forte (pred FOR-tay). *Drug.* Trade name of prednisone eyedrops; anti-inflammatory steroid.

prednisolone (pred-NIS-uh-lohn). *Drug.* Steroid used in treatment of ocular inflammation. Trade names: Ak-Pred, Econopred, Infamase, Pred Forte.

prednisone (PRED-nih-sohn). *Drug.* Steroid used for treating conjunctival and corneal inflammation.

preferential looking technique (PLT). *Test.* Subjective vision evaluation for preverbal children; a patterned stimulus is presented in one of two possible locations. See also FIXATION PREFERENCE, FORCED PREFERENTIAL LOOKING.

Premiere. *Surgical instrument.* Used for anterior microsurgery. Provides a needlelike cutting tool for vitreous surgery, irrigation and aspiration. Optional attachments available for phacoemulsification.

Premiere Microvit. *Surgical instrument.* Used for posterior microsurgery. Provides illumination and a needlelike cutting tool for vitrectomy. Optional attachments available for phacofragmentation and bipolar coagulation.

Prentice's rule, formula for prismatic effect by lens. *Optics*. Equation for prismatic effect induced at any point in a lens. Prism diopters = decentration (in cm) x lens power (in diopters). See also PRISMATIC EFFECT BY LENS.

pre-placed sutures. *Surgical technique*. Stitches sewn into the cornea or sclera before cutting into an eye. Used during cataract surgery to allow rapid closure of the wound.

preretinal (pree-RET-ih-nul). *Anatomy*. Area immediately in front of the retina and behind the posterior vitreous face.

preretinal membrane. *Pathologic condition*. Abnormal tissue lining the inner retinal surface, tending to wrinkle it. May be thin and transparent, or thick, fibrous and opaque. See also MACULAR PUCKER.

preretinal neovascularization (nee-oh-vas-kyu-lur-ih-ZAY-shun). *Pathologic condition*. Abnormal formation of fragile new blood vessels on the retinal surface, which tend to bleed. Complication of various blood vessel diseases, such as diabetes. See also SUBRETINAL NEOVASCULARIZATION.

presbyopia (prez-bee-OH-pee-uh). *Functional defect*. Refractive condition in which there is a diminished power of accommodation arising from loss of elasticity of the crystalline lens, as occurs with aging. Usually becomes significant after age 45.

pre-septal cellulitis, lid cellulitis. *Pathologic condition*. Swelling or infection of eyelid tissue in front of the orbital septum. Does not affect the eyeball. See also ORBITAL CELLULITIS.

"press-on," Fresnel lens *(or)* **prism**. *Optical device*. Flexible plastic lens or prism that has an adhesive side for adhering to eyeglass lenses. Used for correcting eye deviations or refractive errors. See also FRESNEL PRINCIPLE.

presumed ocular histoplasmosis syndrome (POHS) (his-toh-plaz-MOH-sus), **ocular histoplasmosis**. *Pathologic condition*. Chorioretinal disease characterized by fluid leakage, hemorrhage and scarring in the macula (disciform degeneration), atrophy near the optic disc, and "punched-out" choroidal lesions in the peripheral retina. Epidemiologically and immunologically linked to histoplasmosis allergy. See also HISTO SPOTS.

pretectal area (pree-TEK-tul). *Anatomy*. Junctional zone on the top of the midbrain that contains the centers for pupillary reactions, vergence movements and vertical gaze.

pretectal syndrome, dorsal *(or)* **tectal midbrain syndrome, Parinaud's** *(or)* **Sylvian aqueduct syndrome**. *Pathologic condition*. Decreased ability to move the eyes up or down; attributed to brainstem lesion near the vertical gaze center. Sometimes associated with an inability to converge and poor pupil responses to light. See also ARGYLL-ROBERTSON PUPILS.

primary deviation. *Measurement*. Amount of eye deviation caused by a paralyzed muscle, measured when the normal eye is fixating. See also SECONDARY DEVIATION.

primary focal point. *Optics*. Object point on a lens axis that is imaged at infinity so that light rays refracted by the lens emerge in parallel bundles. See also SECONDARY FOCAL POINT.

primary line of sight, line of fixation, principal line of direction, visual axis *(or)* **line**. Imaginary line connecting a viewed object and the fovea.

primary mover, agonist. *Function*. Extraocular muscle mainly responsible for moving an eye into the desired position.

primary open angle glaucoma (POAG) (glaw-KOH-muh), **open angle** *(or)* **chronic open angle glaucoma**. *Pathologic condition*. Most common type of glaucoma. Caused by gradual blockage of aqueous outflow from the eye despite an apparently open anterior chamber angle. If untreated, results in gradual, painless, irreversible loss of vision. Usually in both eyes.

primary perivasculitis of the retina (pehr-ee-vas-kyu-LI-tis), **angiopathia**

retinae juvenilis, Eales' disease, periphlebitis retinae. *Pathologic condition.* Characterized by inflammation and possible blockage of retinal blood vessels, abnormal growth of new blood vessels (neovascularization), and recurrent retinal and vitreal hemorrhages. Found in young men. Cause unknown.

primary position. Straight-ahead position of both eyes when the head is also directed straight ahead.

primary visual cortex (KOR-teks), **Brodmann area 17, striate area**. *Anatomy.* Area in occipital lobes of the brain (cerebral end of sensory visual pathways that begin at the retina), where initial conscious registration of visual information takes place. See also OCCIPITAL CORTEX.

primary vitreous (VIT-ree-us). *Anatomy.* Earliest part of the vitreous to develop. Originates from mesodermal tissue during the 1st month of fetal life and regresses to form zonules and the hyaloid canal. See also PHPV, SECONDARY VITREOUS, TERTIARY VITREOUS.

Prince rule. *Instrument.* Scale ruler (marked in cm and/or diopters) used for measuring near-point of accommodation. Test card is moved along scale toward the eye until letters blur.

principal axis, lens *(or)* **optical axis**. *Optics.* Imaginary line that passes through the optical centers of both surfaces of any lens.

principal line of direction. See PRIMARY LINE OF SIGHT.

principal planes. *Optics.* Two imaginary planes that can theoretically replace all refracting surfaces in a complex lens system, to simplify calculations and measurements.

principal points. *Optics.* Two imaginary points of intersection, where the two principal planes cross the optical axis of a lens system.

principal visual direction (PVD). *Function.* Straight-ahead localization of images received on the fovea.

Priscoline (PRIS-koh-leen). *Drug.* Trade name of tolazoline; injection for dilating a blocked central retinal artery.

prism. *Optical device.* Wedge-shaped, transparent medium that bends light rays toward its base. Does not focus. See also PRISM DIOPTER.

prism adaptation test (PAT). Fresnel prisms are placed over eyeglass lenses in an attempt to gain binocular control of an eye misalignment.

prism + alternate cover test, alternate prism *(or)* **screen + cover test**. For measuring inward, outward, upward or downward eye deviations. As a target is viewed, a prism is placed over one eye and a cover over the other eye; the cover is moved from eye to eye. Eye movement is noted as prism power is changed. The power used when movement stops is the deviation measurement. See also SIMULTANEOUS PRISM AND ALTERNATE COVER TEST.

prismatic effect by lens. *Optics.* Light passing through a lens at a point other than its optical center is bent as though it were passing through a prism. See also PRISM.

  formula (Prentice's rule): equation for prismatic effect induced at any point in a lens. Prism diopters = decentration (in cm) x lens power (in diopters).

prism ballast. *Optical device.* Weight added to the edge of a contact lens to prevent lens rotation. Permits the lens to maintain a given orientation in order to correct astigmatism.

prism bar. *Test instrument.* Plastic holder with a series of prisms in increasing strengths; used in testing fusional vergence ability or measuring eye misalignments.

prism diopter (di-AHP-tur) (Δ). *Unit of measure.* 1. Prism strength: 1^Δ indicates deflection of a light ray by 1 cm at a distance of 1 m. 2. Eye deviation: 1 arc degree of deviation = 1.7^Δ (approx.).

PRK (photorefractive keratectomy), laser keratorefractive surgery, photo-

refractive surgery. *Surgical procedure*. Use of high intensity laser light (e.g., an excimer laser) to reshape the corneal curvature; for correcting refractive errors. Includes laser sculpting, LASIK.

probing, nasolacrimal probing. *Surgical procedure*. Opening tear drainge system by passing a thin rod through the passageway and pressing gently to break any obstruction. See also DACRYOSTENOSIS.

Procan. *Drug*. Trade name of procainamide; heart medication.

procaine. *Drug*. Injectable anesthetic agent used for eye surgery. Trade name: Novocain. See also BUPIVACAINE, LIDOCAINE, MEPIVACAINE, PROPARACAINE, XYLOCAINE.

procainamide. *Drug*. Heart medication; for treating irregular heartbeat. Trade names: Procan, Pronestyl. See also PROPANOLOL, QUININE.

Procardia. *Drug*. Trade name of nifedipine; heart medication.

prodrome (PRO-drohm). Earliest clinical symptoms of a developing medical condition.

profile analyzer. *Instrument*. Used for examining the smoothness of contact lens edges.

progressive addition lens. *Optical device*. Type of near-vision eyeglass lens designed so that power for near increases gradually from zero (in center) to maximum add (lower portion) with no telltale bifocal demarcation line.

progressive external ophthalmoplegia (PEO) (ahf-thal-muh-PLEE-juh), **chronic progressive external ophthalmoplegia**. *Pathologic condition*. Degenerative disease characterized by droopy eyelids (ptosis) and gradual paralysis of all extraocular muscles, with eventual loss of all eye movement; often associated with paralysis of other body muscle groups. Usually affects the elderly. See also EXTERNAL OPHTHALMOPLEGIA.

progressive myopic degeneration (mi-AH-pik), **degenerative *(or)* malignant myopia**. *Pathologic condition*. Nearsightedness associated with stretching of eye structures, with thinning and tearing of sclera, choroid, retinal pigment epithelium and retina, especially in the macular area and around the optic nerve, with "lacquer cracks" in Bruch's membrane. See also FUCHS' SPOT.

progressive supranuclear palsy (PSP). *Pathologic condition*. Progressive limitation of eye movement in the elderly. Begins with loss of downgaze; saccades and pursuit systems are involved, with smooth eye movements becoming jerky (cogwheeling). Body movements become rigid, speech articulation suffers, and mental deterioration sets in. Death occurs in a few years.

projector. *Instrument*. Used for projecting illuminated visual acuity and astigmatic charts onto screens, walls or mirrors, to aid in refraction.

projectoscope (proh-JEK-tuh-skohp). *Instrument*. Modified ophthalmoscope. Used for determining the retinal area used for fixation or stimulating the fovea during pleoptic treatment for eccentric fixation.

prolapse (PROH-laps). *Pathologic condition*. Slipping of tissue or an organ out of its normal position.

proliferative (diabetic) retinopathy (PDR) (ret-in-AHP-uh-thee), **retinitis proliferans**. *Pathologic condition*. Severe retinal blood vessel disease that may accompany advanced diabetes or other retinal blood vessel diseases (e.g., retinal vein occlusion, sickle cell disease). Findings include formation of abnormal new blood vessels (neovascularization) and/or fibrous tissue growing on retinal surface, later extending into the vitreous. Leads to vitreous hemorrhage, retinal detachment, and visual loss. See also BACKGROUND RETINOPATHY, PRERETINAL NEOVASCULARIZATION.

proliferative vitreoretinopathy (PVR) (VIT-ree-oh-ret-in-AHP-uh-thee). *Pathologic condition*. Development of fixed retinal folds from taut vitreal and preretinal fibrous membranes. Distorts retina; often results in a complicated retinal detachment. Repair requires vitrectomy, membrane peeling, and injection of gas or silicone oil. Previously known as MPP, MPR and MVR. See also MACULA PUCKER, NEOVASCULARIZATION.

Pronestyl. *Drug.* Trade name of procainamide; heart medication.

propanolol. *Drug.* Heart medication; for treating irregular heart beat, congestive heart failure and hypertension (high blood pressure.) Trade name: Inderal. See also PROCAINAMIDE.

proparacaine. *Drug.* Rapid, short-acting anesthetic eyedrop. Trade names: Alcaine, Ophthaine, Ophthetic, AK-Taine.

Propine. *Drug.* Trade name of dipivefrin; for treating glaucoma.

propositus. Family member first studied who becomes the starting point for a genealogical chart.

proptosis (prahp-TOH-sis), **exophthalmos**. *Anatomic defect.* Abnormal protrusion or bulging forward of the eyeball.

prosthesis (prahs-THEE-sis), **shell**. Cosmetic "false eye" replacement for a removed (enucleated) eye. Plexiglas shell painted to resemble a natural eye fits into conjunctival sac under the eyelids and over a buried implant.

protanomaly (proh-tuh-NAHM-uh-lee). *Functional defect.* Mild color vision defect (type of anomalous trichromatism); deficiency of red retinal receptors results in poor red-green discrimination. Congenital; hereditary (X-linked; present in 1% of males). See also DEUTERANOMALY, ERYTHROLABE, TRITANOMALY.

protanopia (proh-tuh-NOH-pee-uh). *Functional defect.* Severe type of color vision defect (form of dichromatism in which red appears dark); caused by total absence of red retinal receptors. Congenital; hereditary (X-linked; present in 1% of males).

prothrombin time. See PT.

provocative test. Any test that can reproduce signs of a suspected disease, to help confirm a diagnosis (e.g., water-drinking test for angle closure glaucoma).

proximal (PRAHKS-uh-mul). *Location.* Closer to a point of reference or to the midline of the body. See also DISTAL.

proximal convergence. *Function.* Portion of the total amount of available convergence, stimulated by the awareness of an object's nearness.

PRP (**panretinal photocoagulation**). *Surgical procedure.* Use of high intensity light or laser beam to create hundreds of tiny retinal burns. Produces regression of abnormal blood vessels (neovascularization) in patients who have proliferative retinopathy, usually from diabetes or retinal vein occlusion.

pseudoexfoliation. *Pathologic condition.* Deposits of unknown composition and origin appearing on lens surfaces, ciliary processes, zonules, inner iris surfaces, anterior chamber and trabecular meshwork. May be associated with high intraocular pressure and cataracts. See also TRUE EXFOLIATION.

pseudofacility (SU-doh-fuh-sil-ih-tee). Component of tonographic outflow facility that is an artifact. Results from suppression of aqueous secretion by the weight of the tonometer. May account for about 20% of the total outflow facility in normal eyes.

pseudo-isochromatic chart. *Test chart.* Composed of colored dots, differing in shade and hue, that form numbers and patterns that are not visible with color vision defects. See also HARDY-RAND-RITTLER PLATES, ISHIHARA TEST PLATES.

Pseudomonas aeruginosa (su-duh-MOH-nus eh-ru-jin-OH-suh). *Microorganism.* Long, slender, gram-negative rod bacteria frequently found in contaminated fluorescein solutions, saline, sulfonamides and contact lens solutions. Can cause severe eye infections, with corneal "melting" and loss of the eye within days. Most virulent of common bacterial causes of corneal ulcers. See also STAPHYLOCOCCUS AUREUS, STREPTOCOCCUS PNEUMONIAE.

pseudomyopia (mi-OH-pee-uh), **"school myopia."** *Functional defect.* Temporary blurring of distance vision brought about by ciliary muscle spasm (causing increased lens convexity, providing too much optical power). Occurs after prolonged near work or with emotional disturbance. See also ACCOMMODATIVE SPASM.

pseudo-papilledema (pap-il-uh-DEE-muh). *Anatomic defect.* Optic nerve head elevation that resembles optic nerve congestion caused by increased intracranial pressure. See also PAPILLEDEMA.

pseudophakia (SU-doh-FAY-kee-uh). *Anatomic change.* State of having an intraocular lens implant taking the place of the eye's natural lens. See also APHAKIA.

pseudophakodonesis (SU-doh-fay-koh-doh-NEE-sis). *Clinical sign.* Intraocular lens (IOL) movement within the eye that results from normal eye movement.

pseudophakos (su-doh-FAY-kus), **implant, intraocular lens, IOL**. *Optical device.* Plastic lens that is surgically implanted to replace the eye's natural lens.

pseudostrabismus (su-doh-struh-BIZ-mus). Erroneous appearance of eye misalignment. Caused by epicanthal folds or a visual axis not centered in the pupil. See also EPICANTHUS.

pseudotumor cerebri (SU-doh-tu-mur SEHR-uh-bri). *Pathologic condition.* Intracranial inflammation that resembles a brain tumor. Causes intracranial hypertension and can result in optic nerve head swelling (papilledema), headaches, protrusion of the eyeball (proptosis), and transient loss or reduction of vision. Tends to occur in obese females in their 30s.

pseudo-von Graefe's sign (GRAY-feez). *Clinical sign.* Inappropriate elevation of the upper eyelid on attempted down-gaze. Caused by misdirected (aberrant) nerve fiber regeneration following 3rd (oculomotor) cranial nerve palsy. See also ABERRANT REGENERATION, VON GRAEFFE'S SIGN.

pseudoxanthoma elasticum (PXE) (su-soh-zan-THOH-muh), **Gronblad Strandberg syndrome**. *Pathologic condition.* Elastic connective tissue disorder that gives skin a leathery quality and causes damage to major arteries. Eye findings include a network of pigmented lines (angioid streaks) under the retina due to defects in Bruch's membrane, and macular hemorrhages and scarring. Hereditary.

psychophysics. *Science.* Deals with the relationship between physical stimuli and an individual's subjective response, e.g., light and vision, sound and hearing.

psychoplegia, psychoplegic. Incorrect spelling of CYCLOPLEGIA, CYCLOPLEGIC.

PT (prothrombin time). *Lab test.* Blood test for helping evaluate many types of blood clotting disorders.

pterygium (tur-I-jee-um). *Pathologic condition.* Abnormal wedge-shaped growth on the bulbar conjunctiva. May gradually advance onto the cornea and require surgical removal. Probably related to sun irritation. Plural: pterygia. See also PINGUECULA, STOCKER LINE.

pterygoid-levator synkinesis (external) (TUR-ih-ghoyd leh-VAY-tur sin-kin-EE-sis), **Gunn** *(or)* **jaw winking** *(or)* **Marcus-Gunn jaw winking syndrome**. *Congenital defect.* Droopy eyelid (ptosis) that opens widely upon chewing, sucking or moving mouth to opposite side. Caused by abnormal innervation of levator muscle by 5th (trigeminal) cranial nerve.

ptosis (TOH-sis), **blepharoptosis**. *Functional defect.* Drooping of upper eyelid. May be congenital or caused by paralysis or weakness (paresis) of the 3rd (oculomotor) cranial nerve or sympathetic nerves, or by excessive weight of the upper lids. See also CONGENITAL DYSTROPHIC PTOSIS.

ptotic (TAH-tik). Refers to a droopy eyelid. See PTOSIS.

PTT (partial thromboplastin time). *Lab test.* Blood test for clotting disorders.

"puff" tonometer, pneumotonometer, non-contact *(or)* **pneumatic tonometer**. *Instrument.* Gas-pressurized device that measures intraocular pressure by blowing a puff of air against the cornea to flatten it slightly. Does not come in contact with eye. See also TONOMETRY.

Pulfrich phenomenon. *Function*. Illusion of stereopsis from nerve conduction delay between eye and brain that is greater on one side than the other. May be caused by reducing illumination to one eye with neutral density filter or by nerve disease (e.g., multiple sclerosis).

pulsating exophthalmos (eks-ahf-THAL-mus). *Pathologic condition*. Protrusion of the eyeball that is coincident with the heartbeat. Accompanies carotid-cavernous fistula.

Puralube. *Drug*. Trade name of polyvinyl alcohol drops; for treating dry eyes.

purulent (PYUR-yuh-lunt). *Description*. Containing or consisting of pus.

pulseless disease, idiopathic arteritis of Takayasu, Takayasu's disease. *Pathologic condition*. Inflammatory disorder of large arteries caused by obstruction. Characterized by insufficient blood flow reaching brain, upper extremities and eyes. Most frequently affects children and young people.

"punched-out" lesion. *Pathologic condition*. White, sharply defined area of one or more choroidal clearings or scars. Results from prior inflammation in the choroid, especially in the peripheral fundus. Occurs in presumed ocular histoplasmosis.

punctal ectopion. *Functional defect*. Lower eyelid whose inner side (closest to nose) sags away from normal contact with the eyeball.

punctal occlusion. *Surgical procedure*. Heat cautery or diathermy applied to the lacrimal punctum in the eyelid to seal it. Can reduce tear drainage in patients who have insufficient tears or dry eyes.

punctal plug. *Surgical device*. Plastic materials (polyhydroxethyl methacrylate or silicone) inserted into the punctum to prevent normal tear drainage, to preserve tears for helping keep the cornea and conjunctiva moist.

punctate keratitis (kehr-uh-TI-tus), **superficial** *(or)* **Thygeson's superficial punctate keratitis**. *Pathologic condition*. Corneal disease of unknown cause, characterized by small superficial corneal lesions. Other symptoms include foreign body sensation and sensitivity to bright light. Sometimes recurs after spontaneous remissions.

punctum (PUNK-tum). *Anatomy*. Tiny skin opening of the lacrimal canaliculus of each upper and lower eyelid, near the nose. Entrance to the tear drainage (lacrimal) system. Plural: puncta.
> **inferior**: opening in the papilla (elevation) of the lower eyelid margin). Lower entrance to the tear drainage system. Also called lower punctum.
> **superior**: opening in the papilla (elevation) of the upper eyelid margin. Upper entrance to the eye's tear drainage system. Also called upper punctum. See also SUPERIOR CANALICULUS.

punctum proximum of accommodation (PPA), near-point of accommodation. *Measurement*. Closest point to the eye where small print can be kept in clear focus. See also PRINCE RULE.

punctum proximum of convergence (PP), near-point of convergence. *Measurement*. Closest point to the eye where convergence and binocular single vision can be maintained as an object approaches.

pupil. *Anatomy*. Variable-sized black circular opening in the center of the iris that regulates the amount of light that enters the eye.

pupil dilator, dilator muscle *(or)* **pupillae, iris dilator**. *Anatomy*. Smooth iris muscle that contracts to enlarge the pupillary opening. Extends like wheel spokes from the pupillary margin to iris periphery. Innervated by sympathetic nerves.

pupillary axis, midpupillary line. Imaginary reference line passing from a fixation object through the center of the pupil.

pupillary block. *Functional defect*. Blockage of aqueous flow through the pupil, from the posterior chamber into the anterior chamber, caused by tight contact between the pupillary margin of the iris and the lens or vitreous face. See also IRIS BOMBE.

   aphakic: type of angle-closure glaucoma that occurs at some time after cataract extraction.

pupillary distance (PD), interpupillary distance. *Measurement.* Distance from the center of one pupil to the center of other pupil. Used for proper positioning of eyeglass lenses.

pupillary membrane. 1. *Anatomy.* Embryonic mesodermal tissue in the center of the iris that normally begins to disappear in a fetus's 8th month. Sometimes small traces remain. 2. *Abnormal growth.* Membrane covering the pupil. Usually caused by trauma or inflammation.

pupillary reflex. *Function.* Decrease in pupil size (constriction) that occurs with direct light stimulation to eye.

pupillometer. *Instrument.* 1. Used for measuring the distance from the center of the pupil to the center of the bridge of the nose (monocular interpupillary distance), for fitting spectacles. 2. Laboratory instrument for measuring size (diameter) of the pupil.

pupillotonia (pyu-pil-uh-TOH-nee-uh). See ADIE'S PUPIL.

purified protein derivative. See PPD.

Purkinje entoptic test. Self-evaluation of retinal function by visualizing one's own retinal blood vessels while a bright point-source of light (as from a penlight) enters the eye from the side or through a closed eyelid.

Purkinje images (pur-KIN-jee). *Optics.* Four sets of reflected images from the front and rear surfaces of the cornea and the front and rear surfaces of the lens; these surfaces act as mirrors, two convex and two concave. The brightest image is from front surface of cornea and is useful for taking K-readings for contact lens fitting or for measuring eye deviations.

Purkinje shift. *Optics.* Normal shift in wavelength to which eye is maximally light sensitive, from 555 nanometers (nm) when light-adapted to 507 nm when dark-adapted. Indicates the presence of the two types of retinal photoreceptors (rods and cones).

pursuit mechanism, optomotor reflexes. *Function.* Slow, involuntary parallel movement of both eyes that allows following of moving objects. Also seen in slow phase of optokinetic nystagmus response and doll's head phenomenon.

Purtscher's retinopathy (PUR-churz). *Pathologic condition.* Multiple retinal white patches, cotton-wool spots, hemorrhages, and swelling following severe chest trauma that causes a sudden increase in venous blood pressure. Temporary, with signs lasting only a few days.

"push plus." *Refraction technique.* Method for suppressing accommodation, to allow the maximum amount of plus optical power to be used for correcting a refractive error. See also ACCOMMODATIVE ESOTROPIA.

PVCarpine (KAR-peen). *Drug.* Trade name of pilocarpine eyedrops; for treating glaucoma.

pyogenic. *Description.* Producing pus.

pyrexia (pi-REK-see-uh). *Pathologic condition.* Fever.

pyridostigmine. *Drug.* Long-lasting anticholinesterase agent for treating myasthenia gravis. Trade name: Mestinon. See also EDROPHONIUM CHLORIDE.

pyrogenic. *Description.* Producing temperature elevation; causing fever.

Q

quadrantanopia (kwah-dran-tuh-NOH-pee- uh), **quadrantanopsia.** *Functional defect.* Visual field defect affecting one comparable (homonymous) quadrant in each eye (e.g., superior temporal in left eye, superior nasal in the right). Homonymous inferior, considered pathognomonic of parietal lobe involvement; homonymous superior, a lesion of temporal loop of the optic radiations.

    superior: upper quadrant visual field defect on the same side in each eye. Caused by damage to the inferior fibers of the optic radiations in the temporal lobe of the brain (in Meyer's temporal loop). Also called "pie in the sky" defect.

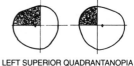

LEFT SUPERIOR QUADRANTANOPIA

quadrantanopsia (kwah-dran-tuh-NAHP-see-uh). See QUADRANTANOPIA.

quadrantic defect (kwah-DRAN-tik). *Functional defect.* Visual field defect limited to one quadrant.

Questran. *Drug.* Trade name of cholystyramine; for lowering cholesterol levels.

Quickert 3-suture operation, lid-bracing sutures. *Surgical procedure.* For repair of an inturned lower eyelid (ectropion). Three horizontal stitches are placed just below the tarsal edge of the lower lid at its inner, central, and outer portions. See also SENILE ENTROPION.

Quinidex. *Drug.* Trade name of quinidine, a heart medicaiton.

quinidine. *Drug.* Heart medication used for irregular heartbeat.

R

racemose (RAY-seh-mohs). *Description.* Resembling a bunch of grapes.

radial astigmatism. An image aberration created by light that hits a refractive surface obliquely. Not a refractive error.

radial keratotomy (RK) (keh-ruh-TAH-tuh-mee). *Surgical procedure.* Series of spoke-like (radial) cuts (usually 4–8) made in the corneal periphery to allow the central cornea to flatten, reducing its optical power and thereby correcting nearsightedness.

radiations (optic), geniculo-calcarine tract. *Anatomy.* Visual nerve pathway that travels back from the lateral geniculate body and ends in the calcarine fissure of the occipital visual cortex (in the brain). Consists of crossed nasal retinal fibers from one eye and uncrossed temporal retinal fibers from the other eye.

radiometry. *Measurement.* Detection and measurement of radiation.

radio-opaque, radiopaque. *Description.* Refers to a substance that is opaque to x-rays, and therefore visible on x-ray film. Radiopaque dye is useful diagnostically for outlining tube-like structures.

radiuscope (RAY-dee-uh-skohp), **contacto gauge.** *Instrument.* For measuring the back surface curvature (base curve) of a contact lens.

Raeder's syndrome (RAY-durz), **Raeder's paratrigeminal neuralgia.** *Pathologic condition.* Small pupil and droopy eyelid (ptosis). Associated with severe headaches and 5th (trigeminal) cranial nerve abnormalities. Sometimes called a painful Horner's syndrome.

"railroad" nystagmus, optokinetic nystagmus. *Function.* Involuntary, rhythmic eye movements produced by viewing a series of vertical bars or other patterned contours while the individual or the target is moving. Slow following phase (pursuit) is toward target movement, with rapid jerk return (saccade) in opposite direction.

Randot stereo test (RAN-daht). *Test chart.* For evaluating binocular depth perception; random-looking dot patterns become identifiable geometric figures when the patient wears eyeglasses with polarized filters. See also TITMUS CHART, TNO TEST.

range of accommodation. *Measurement.* Distance (from eye) between the nearest and farthest points at which clear vision can be maintained. See also AMPLITUDE OF ACCOMMODATION, FAR-POINT OF ACCOMMODATION, NEAR-POINT OF ACCOMMODATION.

raphe (ruh-FAY). *Anatomy.* Demarcation line between two halves of an organ or structure. In the eye, refers to the horizontal line (horizontal raphe) separating upper from lower temporal retinal nerve fiber layer patterns.

rapid eye movements (REM). *Function.* Bursts (about 1 min. each) of fast eye movements that occur periodically during sleep. Associated with dreams. See also SACCADES.

Rathke's pouch tumor (RATH-keez), **craniopharyngioma.** *Pathologic condition.* Congenital tumor that grows in cyst form into the 3rd ventricle of the brain, compressing visual fibers at the back of the chiasm. Eye signs are vision loss, swollen optic nerve heads (papilledema), and inferior temporal visual field loss (bitemporal hemianopsia). Usually apparent by age 10.

real image. *Optics.* Image formed by refracted converging light rays. Can be projected onto a screen. See also VIRTUAL IMAGE.

receptor amblyopia (am-blee-OH-pee-uh). *Functional defect.* Visual acuity deficiency (one or both eyes) caused by faulty positioning of the rods and cones (retinal receptors).

recession. *Surgical procedure*. Weakening an overactive extraocular muscle to correct an eye deviation. Muscle is removed from its insertion and repositioned farther back on the eyeball (globe). See also RESECTION.

recess-resect (R & R). *Surgical procedure*. For correcting an eye deviation; one extraocular muscle is repositioned farther back on eyeball to weaken it and its opposing muscle in the same eye (direct antagonist) is shortened, to strengthen it.

reciprocal innervation, Sherrington's Law. *Function*. As one extraocular muscle receives a nerve impulse to contract, its opposing muscle (direct antagonist) in the same eye simultaneously receives a nerve impulse to relax. See also HERING'S LAW, H_2S.

Recklinghausen's disease (REK-ling-how-zinz), **neurofibromatosis, von Recklinghausen's disease**. *Pathologic condition*. One of several hereditary disorders called phakomatoses. Characterized by small tumors under the skin and in the central nervous system, and bony defects in the orbital bones. Common tumor sites include upper eyelid, optic nerve, 8th (acoustic) cranial nerve, and spinal cord.

rectus. *Anatomy*. Four of the six muscles that move the eyeball: the inferior r., lateral r., medial r., and superior r. Plural: recti.

recurrent corneal erosion. *Pathologic condition*. Episodic, periodic loss of the outer layer of cornea (epithelium) due to its failure to adhere properly to Bowman's membrane; extremely painful. May follow minor scratch-type injury.

red eye. *Pathologic condition*. Lay term for any condition (e.g., conjunctivitis, uveitis) with dilation of conjunctival or ciliary blood vessels. See also CILIARY INJECTION, CONJUNCTIVITIS.

redoch phenomenon. *Incorrect spelling of* RIDDOCH PHENOMENON.

red reflex. *Function*. Normal red glow emerging from the pupil when the interior of the eye is illuminated.

reduced eye, Gullstrand's reduced eye. *Optics*. Simplified geometrical drawing of the eye that serves as a model for teaching optical concepts. See also SCHEMATIC EYE.

refixation. *Function*. Fast, voluntary movements as the eye shifts from one object to another or as it follows an object that is moving too fast to follow steadily.

reflection. 1. *Optics*. Bouncing back of light rays by a mirror-like surface. 2. *Surgical technique*. Folding back of tissue that has been cut but not severed.

reflection densitometry, densitometry. Laboratory measurement technique to determine amounts of various retinal photopigments in visual cells.

reflex. 1. *Function*. Involuntary response to a stimulus. 2. *Optics*. Slang for reflection.

> **corneal**: 1. Neurologic response: blink caused by touching the cornea. 2. Mirror-like reflection of a bright light from the corneal surface.

> **oculo-cardiac**: decrease in heart rate following manipulation of the eyes or extraocular muscles.

> **oculo-cephalic** (sef-AL-ik): involuntary eye rotation in the opposite direction from head rotation to maintain fixation on a non-moving target. May be abnormal with some brainstem defects.

> **oculo-digital**: constant rubbing or pressing on the eyes with the fists or fingers; common in blind children.

> **pupillary**: decrease in pupil size (constriction) that occurs with direct light stimulation to eye.

> **vestibulo-ocular**: same as OCULO-CEPHALIC (above).

reflex tearing. *Function*. Tears produced by the lacrimal glands in response to a corneal or conjunctival surface irritant. See also BASAL TEARING, SCHIRMER TEST.

reflux. To cause to flow back or spill out, or the material that flows back.

refraction. 1. *Optics*. Bending of light rays as they travel from a clear medium of one density to another of different density. See also VERGENCE POWER. 2. *Test*. Determination of an eye's refractive error and the best corrective lenses to be prescribed; series of lenses in graded powers are presented to determine which provide sharpest, clearest vision. 3. Prescription for eyeglasses or contact lenses resulting from this test. See also REFRACTOMETRY.

    cycloplegic: test performed after lens accommodation has been paralyzed with cycloplegic eyedrops. Eliminates variability in optical power caused by a contracting lens.

    manifest: test performed without using cycloplegic eyedrops.

refractive amblyopia (am-blee-OH-pee-uh), **ametropic amblyopia**. *Functional defect*. Vision loss associated with significant uncorrected refractive error. Vision may improve after eyeglass or contact lens correction is worn for several months. See also ANISOMETRIC AMBLYOPIA.

refractive error. *Functional defect*. Optical defect in an unaccommodating eye; parallel light rays are not brought to a sharp focus precisely on the retina, producing a blurred retinal image. Can be corrected by eyeglasses or contact lenses. See also AMETROPIA.

refractive index, index of refraction. *Measurement*. Ratio of the speed of light in air to the speed of light traveling through a particular substance. The greater the index, the more optical effect a substance produces.

refractive keratoplasty (KEHR-uh-toh-plas-tee). *Surgical procedure*. Any surgery on the cornea to change the optical power of the eye, e.g., epikeratophakia, keratomileusis, LASIK.

refractive media. *Optics*. The transparent parts of the eye's optical system through which light travels before being focused on the retina; includes tear film, cornea, lens, aqueous and vitreous.

refractive surgery, keratorefractive surgery. *Surgical procedure*. Various procedures that alter the shape of the cornea and thus how it bends light, in order to change the eye's refractive error. Can reduce or eliminate the need for spectacle or contact lens correction. Procedures include arcuate keratotomy, epikeratophakia, keratomileusis, keratophakia, laser sculpting, LASIK, photorefractive surgery, radial keratotomy, refractive keratoplasty, thermoplasty, transverse keratotomy.

refractometry. *Test*. Objective testing to determine the combination of spheres and cylinders that will optically correct an eye without determining what prescription a patient will accept subjectively.

Refresh. *Drug*. Trade name of polyvinyl alcohol eyedrops or ointment; for treating dry eyes.

Refresh Plus. *Drug*. Trade name of methylcellulose eyedrops; for treating dry eyes.

Refsum's disease (REF-sumz), **heredopathia atactica polyneuritiformis, phytanic acid storage disease**. *Pathologic condition*. Enzymatic blockage of phytanic acid decomposition. Characterized by fatty acid accumulation, drop foot, increased cerebrospinal fluid, cerebral degeneration, inability to sleep, electrocardiogram changes, retinal pigment epithelium degeneration (causing defective dark adaptation and constricted visual fields), involuntary rhythmic eye movements (nystagmus), droopy eyelids (ptosis), and small pupils. Hereditary. See also RETINITIS PIGMENTOSA.

Reis-Buckler's dystrophy (rice BU-klurz DIS-troh-fee). *Pathologic condition*. Corneal disease of the outer stroma (Bowman's membrane) leading to recurrent superficial erosions and conjunctival redness. Recurrent attacks lead to gradual corneal cloudiness with surface irregularities. Hereditary; starts in childhood.

Reiter's syndrome (RI-turz). *Pathologic condition.* Arthritis, urethritis, and conjunctivitis or iritis. Unknown cause.

relative afferent pupillary defect (RAPD) (AF-ur-unt), **afferent pupillary defect, Gunn** *(or)* **Marcus-Gunn pupil.** *Functional defect.* Diminished pupil reaction to light caused by slowed conduction in the optic nerve fibers, usually secondary to optic nerve disease. In dim illumination, a sudden bright light stimulus to the normal eye will result in both pupils contracting briskly. When the light stimulus is shifted to the defective eye, they contract less well, making them appear to be enlarged. See also SWINGING FLASHLIGHT TEST.

relative amblyopia (am-blee-OH-pee-uh). *Functional defect.* Co-existence of a visual acuity deficiency that is partly functional (reversible) and partly organic (irreversible).

relative convergence, relative fusional convergence. *Function.* Amount of base-out prism power that can be overcome while single clear binocular vision is maintained.

relative divergence, relative fusional divergence. *Function.* Amount of base-in prism power that can be overcome while single clear binocular vision is maintained.

relative scotoma. *Functional defect.* Area of reduced sensitivity within the visual field; can be detected only with smaller or dimmer test objects. See also ABSOLUTE SCOTOMA.

relative size. Monocular cue to depth perception; a familiar object's size helps in judging its distance. See also MONOCULAR DEPTH PERCEPTION.

relaxing incisions. *Surgical technique.* For reducing excessive traction. In the cornea, corneal astigmatism is decreased by flattening the curvature in a corneal meridian that has been steepened from trauma or sutures (from prior corneal surgery). See also RADIAL KERATOTOMY, REFRACTIVE KERATOPLASTY.

remission. Lessening of the signs and symptoms of a disease. See also EXACERBATION.

Remy separator (REE-mee). *Instrument.* Hand-held bar with a septum separating two targets, one seen by each eye. For divergence training at home.

reposit. *Surgical procedure.* To return displaced tissue to its normal position.

resection (ree-SEK-shun). *Surgical procedure.* Strengthening a weak extraocular muscle to correct an eye deviation. A section of muscle is removed at its insertion site on the eyeball, then the muscle is reattached to its original position. See also RECESSION.

residual astigmatism. Amount of astigmatism that remains after best refractive error correction with contact lenses.

restrictive syndrome. *Anatomic defect.* Eye deviation caused by mechanical obstruction in the orbit involving extraocular muscles; prevents free eyeball movement. See also BLOWOUT FRACTURE, BROWN'S SYNDROME, DUANE'S SYNDROME, FORCED GENERATION TEST, GRAVES' DISEASE, TRACTION TEST.

rete mirabile (REE-tee mih-RAB-ih-lee). *Pathologic condition.* Delicate web-like network of abnormal newly formed blood vessels (neovascularization) on or near the retinal surface. Form of proliferative retinopathy.

reticle (REH-tuh-kul), **reticule, graticule**. *Measuring device.* Grid or scale in the eyepiece of some optical instruments (e.g., microscope, lensometer) that aids in focusing, measuring or counting.

reticule. See RETICLE.

reticulum cell sarcoma. Obsolete term for HISTIOCYTIC LYMPHOMA.

reticular. *Description.* Netlike; resembling or forming a net.

retina (RET-ih-nuh), **tunica nervosa oculi**. *Anatomy.* Part of the eye (embryologically part of brain) that converts images from the eye's optical system into electrical impulses that are sent along the optic nerve for transmission to the brain. Forms a thin membranous lining of the rear two-thirds of the globe. Consists of layers that include rods and cones; bipolar, amacrine, ganglion, horizontal and Müller cells; and all interconnecting nerve fibers. See also EXTERNAL LIMITING MEMBRANE, INNER NUCLEAR LAYER, INNER PLEXIFORM LAYER, INTERNAL LIMITING MEMBRANE, NERVE FIBER BUNDLE LAYER, OUTER NUCLEAR LAYER, OUTER PLEXIFORM LAYER.

    inner: retinal layers that lie nearest the vitreous.

    outer: refers to visual cells and retinal pigment epithelium (pigment cell layer just outside the retina that nourishes retinal visual cells).

retinal. 1. (RET-in-ul). *Description.* Refers to the retina. 2. (ret-in-AL). *Chemical.* Older term for retinaldehyde.

retinal apoplexy (RET-in-ul AP-oh-plek-see). Obsolete term for central retinal vein occlusion.

retinal break. See RETINAL HOLE.

retinal correspondence. *Function.* Inherent relationship between paired retinal visual cells in the two eyes. Images from an object stimulate both cells, which transmit the information to the brain, permitting a single visual impression localized in the same direction in space.

    abnormal: binocular sensory adaptation to compensate for a long-standing eye deviation; fovea of the straight (non-deviated) eye and a non-foveal retinal point of the deviated eye work together, sometimes permitting single binocular vision despite the misalignment. Also called anomalous.

    normal: binocular condition in which both foveae work together as corresponding retinal points, with resultant images blended (fused) in the occipital cortex of the brain.

retinal cryopexy (KRI-oh-pek-see), **cryoretinopexy**. *Surgical procedure.* Use of intense cold to seal a retinal hole by creating a chorioretinal cold-burn and scar. Part of retinal detachment repair.

retinaldehyde (reh-tin-AL-duh-hide). *Chemical.* Aldehyde of vitamin A. Part of the photosensitive pigment found in the rod and cone outer segments. Necessary for chemical conversion of light energy to electrical energy.

retinal detachment (RD), retinal separation. *Pathologic condition.* Separation of sensory retina from the underlying retinal pigment epithelium. Disrupts visual cell structure and thus markedly disturbs vision. Almost always caused by a retinal tear; often requires immediate surgical repair. See also CHOROIDAL DETACHMENT, CRYORETINOPEXY, DIALYSIS, GIANT TEAR, HORSESHOE TEAR, MORNING GLORY DETACHMENT, RHEGMATOGENOUS RETINAL DETACHMENT, SCLERAL BUCKLE.

retinal dialysis. *Pathologic condition.* Tear in the peripheral retina at the ora serrata. Usually caused by blunt ocular trauma that loosens the vitreous base.

retinal elements. See RETINAL VISUAL CELLS.

retinal hole, retinal break *(or)* **tear**. *Pathologic condition.* Hole in retinal tissue. Usually caused by tug or traction on the vitreous; may be created deliberately during vitrectomy surgery.

retinal ischemia (iss-KEE-mee-uh). *Pathologic condition.* Abnormal reduction of the retinal blood supply from varying degrees of blood vessel blockage. May result in retinal edema, cotton-wool spots, microaneurysms, venous engorgement, and neovascularization.

retinal migraine (MI-grayn). *Pathologic condition.* Transient vision loss in one eye, usually followed by a headache on the same side. See also MIGRAINE.

retinal pigment epithelial detachment (RPED). *Pathologic condition.* Blisterlike elevation of the retinal pigment epithelium. May occur as part of macular degeneration, but is usually self-limited, reversible, and not significant.

retinal pigment epitheliopathy (ep-ih-thee-lee-AHP-uh-thee), **pigment epitheliitis**. *Pathologic condition.* Damage to the pigment epithelium with cellular loss and, later, pigment clumping and pigment dropout, usually in the macular area. Probably viral in origin. Sudden onset; gradual recovery of normal vision within three months.

retinal pigment epithelium (RPE) (ep-ih-THEE-lee-um), **pigment epithelium**. *Anatomy.* Pigment cell layer (hexagonal cells densely packed with pigment granules) just outside the retina that nourishes retinal visual cells. Firmly attached to underlying choroid and overlying retinal visual cells.

retinal tear. See RETINAL HOLE.

retinal rivalry. *Function.* Simultaneous transmission of incompatible images from corresponding retinal areas of the two eyes. Produces a peculiar sensation of patchy visibility with variable portions of both images seen at any one time.

retinal telangectasia, Leber's miliary aneurisms. *Pathologic condition.* Malformed, irregularly dilated retinal blood vessels in one eye that leak proteineaceous fatty exudates into and under the retina. Congenital; early stage of Coats' disease. Affects mostly males, with leakage occurring in late youth.

retinal visual cells, photoreceptors, retinal elements, sensory receptors. *Anatomy.* Rods and cones; retinal cells that convert light into electrical impulses for transmission of messages to the brain.

retinene. *Chemical.* Obsolete term for retinaldehyde.

retinitis (reh-tin-I-tis). *Pathologic condition.* Inflammation of the retina.

CMV (cytomegalovirus) r: virus infection that causes retinitis and vasculitis, with lesions that produce widespread destruction of retinal and choroidal structures. Occurs in infants and immunosuppressed adults, as in AIDS. See also ACUTE RETINAL NECROSIS, TOXOPLASMOSIS.

exudative r: chronic, progressive retinal disorder characterized by massive white exudates into and under the retina with eventual detachment. Associated with malformed, tortuous, dilated retinal blood vessels. Affects one eye; tends to occur in males. Also called Coats' disease. See also RETINITIS PROLIFERANS.

metastatic r: infection (purulent or septic) of the retina caused by microorganisms that reach it (as emboli) through the bloodstream.

neuroretinitis (NU-roh-ret-in-I-tus): inflammation of the retina near the optic nerve.

r. pigmentosa (RP): progressive retinal degeneration in both eyes. Night blindness, usually in childhood, is followed by loss of peripheral vision (initially as ring-shaped defect), progressing over many years to tunnel vision and finally blindness. Hereditary. See also LAURENCE-MOON-BIEDL SYNDROME, REFSUM'S DISEASE.

r. proliferans: severe retinal blood vessel disease that may accompany advanced diabetes or other retinal blood vessel diseases (e.g., retinal vein occlusion, sickle cell disease). Findings include formation of abnormal new vessels (neovascularization) and/or fibrous tissue growing on the retinal surface, later extending into the vitreous. Leads to vitreous hemorrhage, retinal detachment, and visual loss. Also called proliferative retinopathy. See also BACKGROUND RETINOPATHY, PRERETINAL NEOVASCULARIZATION.

r. punctata albescens (punk-TAH-tuh al-BES-enz): characterized by progressive night blindness, tiny white dots in the retina, constricted visual fields, and decreased central vision. Hereditary.

purulent r: infectious, with pus, as in METASTATIC (above).

r. sclopetaria: severe contusion lesion of the retina from shock wave generated from a shotgun pellet or BB striking the orbit or eyelid.

secondary r: follows uveal inflammation.

septic r: same as PURULENT (above).

retinoblastoma (ret-in-noh-blas-TOH-muh). *Pathologic condition.* Malignant intraocular tumor that develops from retinal visual cells. If untreated, seedling nodules produce secondary tumors that gradually fill the eye and extend along the optic nerve to the brain, ending in death. Most common childhood ocular malignancy. Hereditary.

retino-choroiditis. *Pathologic condition.* Inflammation of the retina and the choroid, e.g., toxoplasmosis.

retinocryopexy (ret-in-oh-CRI-oh-pex-ee), **cryo, cryopexy, cryoretinopexy**. *Surgical procedure.* Use of intense cold to seal a retinal hole by creating a chorioretinal cold-burn and scar to close a retinal tear or tack down a detached retina.

retinol (RET-ih-nol), **vitamin A**. *Chemical.* Vitamin A alcohol. Stored in the liver and perhaps the retinal pigment epithelium. Ultimately modified and used by rods and cones as the photosensitive pigment that initiates the visual process.

retinopathy (ret-in-AHP-uh-thee). *Pathologic condition.* Non-inflammatory degenerative disease of the retina.

cellophane r: retinal wrinkling in the macular area caused by contraction of the transparent membrane lying on the retinal surface. Distorts vision. Also called cellophane maculopathy, epiretinal membrane, epiretinal proliferation, macular pucker.

central serous r. (CSR): smooth blister-like elevation of the sensory retina in the area of central vision (macula), with localized detachment from the pigment epithelium. Results in reduction and/or distortion of vision, which usually recovers within a few months. Also called central serous chorioretinopathy, central serous choroidopathy.

chloroquin r: drug-induced bull's-eye maculopathy, frequently accompanied by impaired vision; may be reversible if drug is stopped in the early stages.

circinate r: ring-shaped deposit of exudates within the retina, usually around the macular area (area of central vision) from retinal vascular leakage. Many causes, especially diabetes.

diabetic r: retinal changes accompanying long-standing diabetes mellitus. Background retinopathy (non-proliferative) is the early stage; may advance to the proliferative stage, which includes the growth of abnormal new blood vessels (neovascularization) and accompanying fibrous tissue.

drug abuse r: various types of retinal pathology caused by long-term intravenous drug abuse.

familial exudative vitreal r. (FEVR): characterized by fluid leakage from the retina, and vitreo-retinal membrane formation with new blood vessels. Affects both eyes. Resembles retinopathy of prematurity but lacks history of prematurity. Rare; hereditary.

flavimacular r. (flah-vee-MAK-yu-lur): characterized by irregular, yellow flecked, deep retinal or pigment epithelial lesions. Often associated with a discrete macular abnormality. Vision may be affected. Rare; hereditary. Also called fundus flavimaculatus. See also STARGARDT'S DISEASE.

hemorrhagic r: massive intraretinal and nerve fiber layer hemorrhages with dilated and engorged veins (also swollen optic disc margins and retinal thickening). Caused by blockage of blood flow through the central retinal vein. Results in markedly decreased vision that rarely improves. May cause secondary glaucoma. Patients usually elderly. See also NEOVASCULAR GLAUCOMA, RUBEOSIS IRIDIS.

hypertensive r: retinal changes accompanying high blood pressure;

may include narrow arterioles, dull light reflections from blood vessel surfaces ("copper wiring"), vein irregularities, nicking where arteries cross veins, flame-shaped retinal hemorrhages, cotton-wool spots, and optic disc swelling when the process is advanced.

neuroretinopathy: non-inflammatory retinal abnormality that occurs near the optic nerve.

r. of prematurity (ROP): series of destructive retinal changes that may develop after prolonged life-sustaining oxygen therapy is given to premature infants. In the active stage, findings include dilated, tortuous peripheral blood vessels, retinal hemorrhages and abnormal newly formed blood vessels (neovascularization). Sometimes regresses; other times a peripheral fibrotic scar forms that detaches the retina. Can result in vision loss or blindness. Other possible complications: glaucoma, cataracts, myopia (nearsightedness), sunken eyes, eye misalignment. Previously called retrolental fibroplasia. See also ECTOPIC MACULA.

proliferative r: fibrous vascular membrane forms around abnormal, newly formed blood vessels (neovascularization), later extending into the vitreous. Associated with diabetes, sickle cell disease, and central vein occlusion. Also called retinitis proliferans.

Purtscher's r. (PUR-churz): multiple retinal white patches, cotton-wool spots, hemorrhages and swelling following severe chest trauma that causes a sudden increase in venous blood pressure. Temporary, with signs lasting only a few days.

solar r: macular damage from staring at the sun without proper protective filters, usually during a solar eclipse. A dazzling light sensation soon changes to a central blind spot (scotoma), usually with some permanent reduction in central vision caused by intense radiant energy absorbed in the retina and pigment epithelium. Also called eclipse blindness or solar maculopathy.

tapetoretinopathy (tuh-PEE-toh-): general term for a group of hereditary degenerations of the retinal pigment epithelium and sensory retina.

venous stasis r: characterized by engorged retinal veins, splinter hemorrhages in the nerve fiber layer, and optic disc swelling. Caused by occlusion or partial occlusion of the central retinal vein. Retinal findings are less severe and less extensive than in hemorrhagic retinopathy. Vision usually improves over months unless retinal swelling causes irreversible macular changes. Patients often middle-age or younger. See also AMAUROSIS FUGAX, CYSTOID MACULAR EDEMA.

retinopexy (RET-in-oh-pek-see). *Surgical procedure*. Use of diathermy or cold to repair a detached retina.

retinoschisis (ret-in-oh-SKEE-sis), **schisis**. *Degenerative change*. Abnormal splitting of the retinal sensory layers, usually in the outer plexiform layer, resulting in loss of function. Begins as an asymptomatic cystic degeneration of the lower temporal retinal periphery. Usually an aging change that does not affect vision.

congenital: same as JUVENILE (below).

juvenile: a splitting of the retina into inner and outer layers, usually involving the macular area. Congenital. Hereditary, X-linked. Also called congenital retinoschisis.

retinoscope (RET-in-oh-skohp). *Instrument*. Hand-held device for measuring an eye's refractive error with no response required from the patient. Light is projected into the eye, and the movements of the light reflection from the eye are neutralized (eliminated) with lenses.

spot r: projects a spot of light; movement of the spot is neutralized with lenses.

streak r: projects a rotatable line of light; movement of the line is neutralized with lenses.

retinoscopy (ret-in-AHS-kuh-pee), **skiascopy**. *Test.* Measuring an eye's refractive error by using a retinoscope.

retinotomy (ret-in-AHT-uh-mee). *Surgical procedure.* Retinal incision for internal fluid drainage, relaxing scars or gaining access to subretinal membranes.

retraction syndrome (Duane's), Duane's co-contraction syndrome, Duane's (or) Stilling-Turk-Duane retraction syndrome. *Congenital defect.* Eye muscle abnormality often accompanied by an inward eye deviation (esotropia). Characterized by inability to move one eye outward past the midline (abduction) and retraction of that eye into the orbit with narrowing of the eyelid fissure on attempted movement of that eye toward the nose (adduction).

retractor (ree-TRAK-tur). *Surgical instrument.* For holding tissues or organs away from the field of operation.

retrobulbar (ret-roh-BUL-bar). *Location.* Behind the eyeball, within the orbit.

retrobulbar injection. *Procedure.* Injection (of a drug) behind the eyeball, into the center of the muscle cone. Usually for anesthesia and akinesia (immobilization) of an eye.

retrobulbar neuritis (nu-RI-tis), **retrobulbar optic neuritis**. *Pathologic condition.* Optic nerve inflammation behind the optic disc (within the orbit), which hides early disc changes. Visual acuity is markedly reduced. Frequently in patients with multiple sclerosis. See also OPTIC NEURITIS.

retrobulbar optic neuritis. See RETROBULBUR NEURITIS.

retroequatorial myopexy (RET-roh-ee-kwuh-TOR-ee-ul MI-oh-pek-see), **Faden procedure, posterior fixation suture**. *Surgical procedure.* Method of weakening a rectus muscle (medial, lateral, superior or inferior) by suturing it to the sclera 10–16 mm behind its insertion, restricting its action.

retro-illumination. *Lighting from behind, usually from a slit lamp (biomicroscope), to sillouette a lesion (e.g., to make a corneal opacity more apparent).*

retrolental (ret-roh-LEN-tul). *Location.* Behind the crystalline lens, within the globe (eyeball).

retrolental fibroplasia (RLF) (fi-broh-PLAY-zhuh). Obsolete term for RETINOPATHY OF PREMATURITY.

retropulsion. *Technique.* Pushing back of tissue.

retropulsion of the eyeball. *Clinical test.* For evaluating resilience of orbital tissues or presence of masses behind the eye; examiner notes restance to pushing the eye into its socket.

reverse bobbing. *Clinical sign.* Disordered, spontaneous, fast upward jerk of both eyes, followed by a slow downward drift to straight-ahead (primary) position. Related to advanced disease of the brainstem, usually in a comatose patient. See also OCULAR BOBBING.

reverse Mustarde flap (mus-TAR-day). *Surgical procedure.* For reconstructing the outer half or entire upper eyelid. Skin tissue is dissected from the cheek, lined with a mucous membrane and cartilage graft, and rotated to form a new upper eyelid. See also MUSTARDE FLAP, ROTATION FLAP, TENZEL FLAP.

reversible amblyopia (am-blee-OH-pee-uh), **functional amblyopia**. *Functional defect.* Vision deficiency in one eye with no detectable anatomic damage to the visual pathways. Four types: strabismic, deprivation, anisometropic, ametropic. See also NEUTRAL DENSITY FILTER.

rhabdomyosarcoma (RAB-doh-mi-oh-sahr-KOH-muh). *Pathologic condition.* Highly malignant tumor of striated muscle in children; can affect orbital area.

rhegmatogenous retinal detachment (reg-muh-TAH-jen-us, RET-ih-nul). *Pathologic condition.* Retinal detachment caused by a retinal tear.

rheumatoid arthritis. *Pathologic condition.* Connective tissue disease. Eye findings include scleral and uveal inflammation, scleral thinning, recurrent red eyes and dry eyes.

juvenile: often associated with inflammation of the iris and ciliary body (uveitis) and a band-shaped calcium deposit on the cornea (band keratopathy). Uncommon. Also called Still's disease.

rhinitis (ri-NI-tus). Inflammation of the nasal mucous membrane; runny nose.

rhinosporidium (ri-noh-spoh-RID-ee-um). *Microorganism.* May cause conjunctival inflammation. Many characteristics of a fungus; never been cultured.

rhodopsin (roh-DAHP-sin), **visual purple**. *Chemical.* Primary photopigment of rods; one of four photosensitive pigments in the retina. Composed of vitamin A aldehyde plus the protein opsin. As light strikes the photopigment, it bleaches and begins a chain of electrical impulses that travel along the optic nerve to the brain. See also CHLOROLABE, CYANOLABE, ERYTHROLABE.

Riddoch phenomenon. *Function.* Ability to perceive a moving object in an area of the visual field where a non-moving object is not perceived.

Rieger's anomaly (REE-gurz), **mesodermal dysgenesis of iris**. *Pathologic condition.* Genetic defect occurring in the 5th or 6th week of fetal development. Eye findings include glaucoma, underdeveloped iris, deformed pupil, prominent Schwalbe's ring, corneal defects, and astigmatism.

right beating nystagmus (ni-STAG-mus). *Functional defect.* Rhythmic side-to-side eye movements, with the fast phase to the right.

right deorsumvergence, left sursumvergence, negative vertical vergence *(or)* **divergence**. *Function.* Downward movement of the left eye relative to the right eye, usually to maintain single binocular vision, e.g., when increasing amounts of base-up prism are placed over the left eye.

right gaze. Eye position to the right of straight-ahead, as the head remains stationary. Eyes are moved by contraction of the lateral rectus muscle of the right eye and the medial rectus of the left eye.

    r. g. verticals: extraocular muscles (right inferior rectus, right superior rectus, left inferior oblique, left superior oblique) that move an eye up or down when it is in right gaze.

right sursumvergence, left deorsumvergence, negative vertical vergence *(or)* **divergence**. *Function.* Upward movement of the left eye relative to the right eye, usually to maintain single binocular vision, e.g., when increasing amounts of base-down prism are placed over the left eye.

rigid gas permeable lens (RGP), gas permeable lens. *Optical device.* Rigid plastic contact lens that allows oxygen and carbon dioxide penetration. See also HARD CONTACT LENS, SOFT CONTACT LENS.

Riley-Day syndrome, familial autonomic dysfunction. *Pathologic condition.* Nervous system disorder characterized by reduced tear production (alacrima), decreased corneal sensation, outward eye deviation (exotropia), nearsightedness (myopia), excessive sweating, lack of pain sensitivity, excessive sensitivity to touch, incoordination, recurrent respiratory infections, absence of taste buds, and sudden, unexplained death. Hereditary; found only in Ashkenazic Jews.

rimexolone. *Drug.* Anti-inflammatory steroid suspension used for treating inflammation following ocular surgery or anterior uvetitis. Trade name: Vexol.

riMLF (rostral interstitial nucleus of the medial longitudinal fasciculus). *Anatomy.* Vertical gaze center for downgaze. Structure in upper part of the midbrain that integrates signals from the occipital and frontal cortex.

ring scotoma (skuh-TOH-muh), **annular scotoma**. *Functional defect.* Ring-shaped blind area in the visual field, usually located 20°-40° from central fixation. Associated with some retinal degenerations, e.g., retinitis pigmentosa; can also occur as an optical phenomenon with high plus-powered eyeglasses.

Riolan (muscle of), pars ciliaris. *Anatomy.* Part of the orbicularis oculi muscle, located in the eyelid behind the eyelash follicles. Helps the inner lid margin hug close to the eyeball.

rising eye syndrome. *Pathologic condition*. In an inferior oblique palsy, refers to the higher, non-fixing, non-paretic eye that cannot move downward completely. Occurs years later, when the paretic eye is habitually used for fixation. See also INHIBITIONAL PALSY OF THE CONTRALATERAL ANTAGONIST, FALLEN EYE SYNDROME.

Risley prism, rotary prism. *Instrument*. Used for measuring eye deviations and fusional amplitudes. Two prisms mounted front-to-back are rotated in opposite directions to allow a gradual, continuous change in prism power.

Riter's syndrome. Incorrect spelling of REITER'S SYNDROME.

RK (radial keratotomy). *Surgical procedure*. Series of spoke-like (radial) cuts (usually 4–8) made in the corneal periphery to allow the central cornea to flatten, reducing its optical power and thereby correcting nearsightedness.

river blindness, ocular onchoceriasis. *Pathologic condition*. Infection caused by the microfilarial stage of a worm that invades the eye, primarily the cornea. Most common cause of blindness in Africa, Central and South America.

Rochon-Duvigneaud (bouquet of) (roh-SHAHN du-vee-NOHD). *Anatomy*. 2,500 thin cones comprising the most central zone of the retinal foveal pit.

rod. *Anatomy*. Light-sensitive, specialized retinal receptor cell that works at low light levels (night vision). A normal retina contains 150 million rods. See also CONE, RHODOPSIN.

rod-cone degeneration. See ROD DEGENERATION.

rod degeneration, retinitis pigmentosa, rod-cone degeneration. *Pathologic condition*. Progressive retinal degeneration in both eyes. Night blindness, usually in childhood, is followed by loss of peripheral vision (initially as a ring-shaped defect), progressing over many years to tunnel vision and finally blindness. Hereditary. See also LAURENCE-MOON-BIEDL SYNDROME, REFSUM'S DISEASE.

rod monochromacy, typical monochromacy. *Congenital defect*. Rare inability to distinguish colors as a result of absent or nonfunctioning retinal cones. Associated with light sensitivity (photophobia), involuntary eye oscillations (nystagmus) and poor vision. Nonprogressive. See also CONE MONOCHROMACY.

rosacea (roh-ZAY-shuh). *Pathologic condition*. Skin disease accompanied by chronic staphylococcal infections of the cheeks and eyelids (blepharitis) and, rarely, corneal, scleral or iris inflammations. Cause unknown.

    r. keratitis (kehr-uh-TI-tis): recurrent, progressive punctate corneal inflammations associated with rosacea. Cause unknown.

rose bengal. *Chemical*. Reddish-purple dye used for detecting damaged superficial corneal and conjunctival cells (e.g., in dry eye syndrome).

rosettes. *Pathologic change*. Microscopic ring-like arrangement of retinoblastoma (malignant tumor) cells.

    Flexner-Wintersteiner: when abundant and well-formed, believed to indicate a lower degree of malignancy.

    Homer-Wright: have less differentiation than Flexner-Wintersteiner rosettes; the form is indistinguishable from the rosettes in neuroblastoma and medulloblastoma.

rostral. *Location*. Situated in the direction of the face.

rostral interstitial nucleus of the medial longitudinal fasciculus. See riMLF.

rotary nystagmus (ni-STAG-mus). *Functional defect*. Involuntary, rhythmic, twitching eye movements in a clockwise or counterclockwise rotation. Frequent in brain damaged children.

rotary prism. See RISLEY PRISM.

rotation flap. *Surgical procedure*. Tongue-shaped section of skin and subcutaneous tissue that has been cut to maintain its blood supply; used for covering a defect (from trauma or surgical removal of a tumor or scar) in an adjacent area. See also Z PLASTY.

rotation nystagmus (ni-STAG-mus). *Functional defect.* Involuntary, rhythmic eye movements that occur normally after quick turns of the head or spinning the body around.

Roth-Bielschowsky syndrome (beel-SHAH/OW-skee). *Pathologic condition.* Paralysis of horizontal eye movements, both voluntary and involuntary, caused by loss of both saccadic and pursuit pathways in the upper brainstem.

Rothmund syndrome, Bloch-Stauffer *(or)* **Thomson syndrome**. *Congenital disorder.* Characterized by cataracts and skin pigmentation abnormalities. Hereditary.

Roth's spots. *Clinical sign.* Retinal hemorrhages that have a pale or white central zone. Found in subacute bacterial endocarditis, severe anemia, and leukemia.

roto-extraction. *Surgical procedure.* Cataract or vitreous removal by means of an instrument that uses suction, a rotating tissue cutter, and fluid injection (rinsing). Rarely used.

round top. *Optical device.* Bifocal segment that has a rounded upper edge separating it from main part of the lens. See also FLAT TOP.

rubella (ru-BEL-uh), **German measles**. *Pathologic condition.* Common systemic viral disease. Mild in children, but when contracted during the 1st trimester of pregnancy can generate fetal abnormalities, such as mental retardation, heart disease, hearing defects, and eye defects, e.g., cataracts, glaucoma, retinal changes and eye deviations.

rubeotic glaucoma. See NEOVASCULAR GLAUCOMA.

Rubenstein-Taybi syndrome. *Pathologic condition.* Mental retardation, cardiac and genitourinary abnormalities, short stature, broad thumbs and toes. Eye signs include strabismus, cataract, epicanthus, ptosis, hypertrichosis (excessive hair growth). Hereditary.

rubeola (ru-bee-OH-luh), **measles**. *Pathologic condition.* Common systemic viral disease that may be accompanied by an acute conjunctivitis or superficial corneal inflammation. See also KOPLIK'S SPOTS.

rubeosis iridis (ru-bee-OH-sis IR-id-iss). *Pathologic condition.* Formation of abnormal new blood vessels (neovascularization) and connective tissue on the iris surface; may give it a reddish cast. Commonly associated with late stages of diabetic retinopathy and central vein occlusion. May cause a hard-to-manage form of glaucoma. See also NEOVASCULAR GLAUCOMA.

ruby lens. Incorrect spelling of HRUBY LENS.

running sutures, continuous sutures. *Surgical technique.* Stitches that are not tied separately. See also INTERRUPTED SUTURES.

rust ring. *Clinical sign.* Small brownish stain in the cornea as a residue from an iron-containing foreign body.

S

Sabin-Feldman dye test. *Lab test.* Antibody titer test for diagnosis of toxoplasmosis. Requires live toxo organisms. Now rarely performed.

Sabouraud's dextrose agar (sab-oo-ROHDZ). Laboratory culture medium
used for growing and identifying fungi, e.g., from corneal and conjunctival
scrapings or from fluid removed from inside the eye.

sac. *Anatomy.* Soft-walled cavity usually having a narrow opening or none at
all and often containing fluid.

> **conjunctival**: loose pocket of conjunctiva between the upper eyelid
> and the eyeball, and the lower eyelid and the eyeball; permits the eye to
> rotate freely. Also called cul-de-sac, fornix.

> **lacrimal**: structure that collects tears. Located under the skin near the
> bridge of the nose. Tears enter from the common canaliculus and leave
> through the lacrimal duct into the nose.

> **tear**: same as LACRIMAL SAC (above).

saccades (suh-KAHDZ), **voluntary eye movements**. *Function.* Quick movements of both eyes in same direction. Mechanism for fixation, refixation,
rapid eye movements, and fast phase of optokinetic nystagmus. Initiated
by the frontal lobe of the brain (Brodmann area 8).

saccadic velocity test (suh-KAH-dik). Record of electrical activity produced
by voluntary rapid eye movements. Used for distinguishing between a
mechanical restriction of eyeball movement and a weakness (paresis or
paralysis) of an extraocular muscle.

safety lens. *Optical device.* Eyeglass lens treated (with heat, chemicals, or
lamination) to resist breakage and splintering from a direct blow.

sagittal axis of Fick (SAJ-ih-tul), **anteroposterior** *(or)* **longitudinal** *(or)* **y
axis of Fick**. Imaginary line running through the eye's center of rotation,
connecting the geometric center of the cornea (anterior pole) with the geometric center of the back of the eye (posterior pole). Tilting (torsional) eye
rotations occur around this axis.

sagittal depth. *Measurement.* Distance from the back of a contact lens, at the
center, to the front of the cornea.

salmon patch. *Clinical sign.* Oval-shaped, pale retinal hemorrhage that occurs
in patients with sickle cell disease. See also BLACK SUNBURST.

salt tablets. *Chemical.* Sodium chloride in tablet form. Can be dissolved in dis-
tilled water to produce a saline solution for storage of soft contact lenses.

Salus sign (SAL-us). *Clinical sign.* Retinal vein deflection at a crossing of an
artery and vein. Associated with hardened or stiff retinal arterioles, often
as result of high blood pressure (hypertension).

Salzmann's degeneration. *Pathologic condition.* Non-inflammatory corneal
degeneration. Raised pearly gray nodules are circularly arranged in the
central cornea between the epithelium and Bowman's membrane.

Sandhoff's disease. *Pathologic condition.* Metabolic disorder of the enzymes
hexosaminidase A and B; variant of Tay-Sachs disease. Characterized
by listlessness, slow development, startle reaction to sounds, whitish macula with cherry red spot, and progressive retinal and nervous system degeneration. Hereditary; fatal. See also GANGLIOSIDOSIS, SPHINGOLIPIDOSES.

San Filippo disorder. *Pathologic condition.* Metabolic connective tissue disorder characterized by severe mental and neurological signs and atypical
retinitis pigmentosa. Caused by deficiency of alpha acetyl glucosaminidase
or heparan sulfate sulfatase. See also MUCOPOLYSACCHAROIDOSIS.

sarcoid (SAHR-koyd), **Boeck's sarcoid, sarcoidosis**. *Pathologic condition.* Inflammatory disorder of unknown origin affecting almost all systems of the body. Characterized by microscopic nodule formation. Most common eye findings are large mutton fat keratic precipitates, iritis with iris adhesions to the lens, and heavy vitreous deposits. See also "CANDLEWAX DRIPPINGS," MIKULICZ'S SYNDROME, "SNOW-BALLS," "STRING OF PEARLS."

sarcoidosis. See SARCOID.

sarcoma. *Pathologic condition.* Malignant tumor (cancer) derived from connective tissue (e.g., fibrosarcoma) or supporting cells.

satellite lesion. *Pathologic condition.* Small area of acute infection that occurs near an older infection site. Typical of fungal corneal infections or toxoplasmic retinochoroiditis.

Sattler's layer. *Anatomy.* Central layer of choroid that contains medium-size blood vessels.

Sattler's veil, corneal bedewing. *Pathologic condition.* Swelling and clouding of superficial layers of the cornea, causing loss of surface smoothness, which reduces its image-forming properties. Frequently caused by prolonged increase in intraocular pressure or by contact lens overwear. See also OVERWEAR SYNDROME.

sc (without [sin] correction). Signifies that the patient was not wearing corrective eyeglasses or contact lenses while vision was tested.

scanning electron microscope (SEM). *Instrument.* Type of electron microscope designed to allow extremely high magnification. Used for examinating the surfaces of a fixed tissue or other material.

scaphoid (SKAY-foyd) *Description.* Boat-shaped. Usually refers to a preretinal hemorrhage that has a flattened upper border.

Scheie procedure (shay), **thermal sclerostomy**. *Surgical procedure.* Type of filtering surgery used for treating narrow and open angle glaucoma. Combines a peripheral hole in the iris (iridectomy) with a filtration channel for the aqueous to exit (filtering bleb).

Scheie syndrome. *Pathologic condition.* Systemic disease characterized by slight skeletal abnormalities, heart problems, severe corneal clouding, and sometimes slight mental retardation. Form of mucopolysaccharoidosis (type I-S) with enzyme L-iduronidase deficiency. Hereditary.

Scheiner principle (SHI-nur). *Optics.* When viewing a distant light source through two closely placed pinholes, an eye with an uncorrected refractive error will see two spots of light. If the eye has no refractive error or a corrected refractive error, only one spot of light will be seen. Principle of double images when out-of-focus condition exists; applies to any optical system.

schematic eye (skee-MAT-ik). *Instrument.* Simplified optical and mechanical model of the eye used in teaching retinoscopy and optical fundamentals. See also REDUCED EYE.

Schering lens. Incorrect spelling of SHEARING LENS.

Schilder's disease (SHIL-durz). *Pathologic condition.* Rare disorder of young children. Widespread demyelinization of white matter in the brain causes an acute onset of cortical blindness (destruction of visual cortex).

Schiotz tonometer (SHEE-ahtz). *Instrument.* Mechanical device for measuring tension inside the eye (intraocular pressure) by indenting the anesthetized cornea with a weighted metal plunger. See also INDENTATION TONOMETER, TONOMETRY.

Schirmer test (SHUR-mur). For measuring tear production. Filter paper strips are placed in lower fornix. If topical anesthetic is used, the test measures basic secretion of the accessory glands; if not, tearing comes from lacrimal

SCHIRMER TEST

glands (reflex tearing). See also BASIC SECRETION TEST.

schisis (SKEE-sis), **retinoschisis**. *Degenerative change.* Abnormal splitting of the retinal sensory layers, usually in the outer plexiform layer, resulting in loss of function. Begins as an asymptomatic cystic degeneration of the lower temporal retinal periphery. Usually an aging change that does not affect vision. See also JUVENILE RETINOSCHISIS.

Schlemm's canal (shlemz). *Anatomy.* Circular channel deep in corneoscleral junction (limbus) that carries aqueous fluid from the anterior chamber of the eye to the bloodstream.

Schnabel's atrophy, cavernous atrophy. *Pathologic condition.* Form of glaucomatous optic atrophy characterized histologically by lacunae (pods of liquefaction) in the nerve, posterior to the lamina cribosa.

Schnyder's central crystalline dystrophy (SHNI-durz). *Pathologic condition.* Anterior corneal stromal opacities characterized by a ring-shaped deposition of multicolored cholesterol crystals; may cause decreased vision. Hereditary (dominant).

"school myopia," pseudomyopia. *Functional defect.* Temporary blurring of distance vision brought about by ciliary muscle spasm (causing increased lens convexity, providing too much optical power). Occurs after prolonged near work or accompanying emotional disturbance. See also ACCOMMODATIVE SPASM.

Schwalbe's line (SHWAHL-beez). *Anatomy.* Peripheral edge of Descemet's membrane in the cornea.

Schweigger hand perimeter (SHWI-gur). *Test instrument.* Lightweight portable device for testing the visual field.

scimitar scotoma (SIM-ih-tahr skuh-TOH-muh), **arcuate scotoma, Bjerrum scotoma, comet scotoma**. *Functional defect.* Arc-shaped blind area in the visual field caused by damage to retinal nerve fiber bundles. Common in patients with glaucoma. See also SEIDEL SCOTOMA.

scintigraphy (sin-TIG-ruh-fee), **dacryoscintigraphy**. *Test.* Photographing and measuring a radioactive tracer in the tear film as it travels through the tear drainage system.

scintillating scotoma (SIN-tuh-lay-ting skuh-TOH-muh). *Symptom.* Formless visual hallucination: flickering flashes and expanding circles of light that are seen in occipital lobe disorders. Associated with migraine.

scissors motion. *Clinical sign.* In retinoscopy, confusing moving images that appear as crossing bands of light. Indicates irregular refractive error.

sclera (SKLEH-ruh), **tunica fibrosa oculi**. *Anatomy.* Opaque, fibrous, protective outer layer of the eye ("white of the eye") that is directly continuous with the cornea in front and with the sheath covering optic nerve behind. Contains collagen and elastic fibers. Plural: sclerae.

scleral buckle (SKLEH-rul). *Surgical procedure.* Used in repairing a retinal detachment. The sclera is indented or "buckled" inward, usually by attaching a piece of preserved sclera or silicone rubber to its surface.

scleral depressor. *Instrument.* Rounded rod used in a retinal examination; sometimes mounted on a thimble. Used for pressing on the sclera so the ora serrata can be viewed with an ophthalmoscope.

scleral flap. *Surgical procedure.* Section of sclera that has been dissected on two or three sides. Used for exposing the deeper sclera or inside of eye. Part of trabeculectomy procedure for glaucoma, iridocyclectomy for removing a small intraocular tumor, and (seldom) for retinal detachment surgery.

scleral lens. *Optical device.* Large rigid contact lens used for correcting refractive errors and for protecting some types of diseased corneas. May be molded to fit patient's own cornea and sclera. Rarely used.

scleral plexus (PLEKS-us). *Anatomy.* Capillary network in the sclera that encircles the canal of Schlemm.

scleral rigidity. Relative stiffness of eye's outer layer. Introduces a potential error when measuring intraocular pressure with the indentation method (Schiotz). See also APPLANATION TONOMETRY.

scleral ring. *Surgical instrument.* Single or double ring, temporarily attached to the sclera during eye surgery requiring a wide opening, to provide mechanical support and prevent collapse of the eyeball (globe). See also FLIERINGA RING.

scleral spur. *Anatomy.* Mass of scleral fibers bordered in front by the canal of Schlemm and the trabecular meshwork, and behind by the forward attachment of ciliary muscle fibers.

scleral trabeculae (truh-BEK-yu-lee), **cribiform ligament, ligamentum pectinatum iridis, trabecular meshwork**. *Anatomy.* Mesh-like structure inside the eye at the iris-scleral junction of the anterior chamber angle. Filters aqueous fluid and controls its flow into the canal of Schlemm, prior to its leaving the eye.

sclerectomy. *Surgical procedure.* Removal of a segment of sclera.
> **posterior**: removal of sclera from the rear of the eyeball (globe).

scleritis (sklehr-I-tis). *Pathologic condition.* Inflammation of the sclera.

scleroderma (sklehr-uh-DUR-muh), **systemic sclerosis**. *Pathologic condition.* Autoimmune collagen disease affecting connective tissue of skin, mucous membranes, bone, muscles and internal organs. Characterized by areas of tight leathery skin on limbs and lids, cotton-wool retinal deposits and, sometimes, iritis and cataracts.

sclerokeratoplasty (skler-oh-KEHR-uh-toh-plas-tee). *Surgical procedure.* Removal and replacement of the entire corneal width including a rim of sclera that extends 2–3 mm beyond the corneoscleral junction (limbus).

scleromalacia (skler-oh-muh-LAY-shuh). *Pathologic condition.* Softening and thinning of the sclera. May be associated with rheumatoid arthritis.

sclerosing keratitis (sklehr-OH-sing kehr-uh-TI-tis). *Pathologic condition.* Corneal inflammation of unknown cause; the cornea becomes white and opaque, resembling the sclera.

sclerostomy (sklehr-AHS-tuh-mee). *Surgical procedure.* Opening made into the sclera. May be left permanently, such as for fluid drainage.

sclerotic scatter (sklehr-AH-tik). *Optics.* Method of illuminating the eye with a slit lamp that allows light reflected from the sclera to highlight opacities in the anterior optical media that are not otherwise readily visible.

sclerotomy (sklehr-AH-tuh-mee). *Surgical procedure.* Incision into the sclera.

sclopetaria (retinitis). Severe contusion lesion of the retina from the shock wave generated from a shotgun pellet or BB striking the orbit or eyelid.

scopolamine (skuh-PAH-luh-meen). *Drug.* Eyedrop that blocks the parasympathetic nerves, causing paralysis of iris sphincter (dilation) and ciliary body (cycloplegia) for 2–3 days. For treating anterior uveitis. Trade names: Hyoscine, Isopto Hyoscine.

scotoma (skuh-TOH-muh), **blind spot**. *Functional defect.* Non-seeing area within the visual field that may occur with damage to the visual pathways or retina. A physiologic blind spot ("the blind spot," blind spot of Mariotte) exists normally and marks the site of the optic nerve. Plural: scotomata. See also ALTITUDINAL HEMIANOPSIA, BARING OF THE BLIND SPOT, BITEMPORAL HEMIANOPSIA, HOMONYMOUS HEMIANOPSIA, NASAL STEP, QUADRANTANOPSIA.
> **angioscotoma**: caused by the shadow of a retinal blood vessel.
> **absolute**: any target is invisible, regardless of size or brightness.
> **arcuate**: arc-shaped; caused by damage to the retinal nerve fiber bundles. Common in glaucoma.

Bjerrum: same as ARCUATE (above).

central: loss of the central 5° of the visual field.

centrocecal: loss of central vision, including fixation point and physiologic blind spot. Characteristic of toxic damage to the optic nerve.

comet: same as ARCUATE (above).

eclipse: blind area in central field caused by watching a solar eclipse.

junction: loss of central vision in one eye and the outer half of the visual field in the other eye. Caused by a chiasmal lesion that interrupts lower nasal fibers from one eye and macular fibers of the other eye, just after crossing the chiasm.

negative: scotoma that the patient is not normally aware of.

positive: patient is aware of a black or dark area somewhere in the visual field.

relative: can be detected with small or dim test objects but not with larger or brighter stimuli.

ring: ring-shaped; usually located 20°–40° from central fixation; associated with some retinal degenerations. Also, an optical phenomenon with high plus-powered spectacles.

scimitar: same as ARCUATE (above).

Seidel: comma-shaped extension of the physiologic blind spot; becomes an arcuate scotoma as it enlarges.

scotopic adaptation (skoh-TAHP-ik). *Pathologic condition.* Adaptation to low levels of light at which only rod vision is operative.

scotopic vision, night vision, rod vision. *Function.* Refers to vision at low light levels; primarily a function of (retinal) rods. Maximum sensitivity is usually after 30 minutes in the dark. See also DARK ADAPTATION, MESOPIC VISION, PHOTOPIC VISION.

screen + cover test, alternate prism + cover *(or)* **prism + alternate cover test.** For measuring inward, outward, upward or downward eye deviations. As the target is viewed, a prism is placed over one eye and a cover over the other eye; the cover is moved from eye to eye. Eye movement is noted as prism power is changed. The power used when movement stops is the deviation measurement. See also SIMULTANEOUS PRISM & ALTERNATE COVER TEST.

screen (tangent). *Test instrument.* Screen used for quantifying visual field defects within 30° of a fixation point. Testing is carried out 1 or 2 meters from the eye. See also PERIMETRY.

scurvy (SKUR-vee). *Pathologic condition.* Caused by vitamin C deficiency. Eye findings are related to bleeding tendency: orbital hemorrhage, bulging eyeballs, and hemorrhages in the eyelids, anterior chamber, vitreous and conjunctiva.

"sea-fans." *Clinical sign.* Abnormal new blood vessels (neovascularization) in the peripheral retina. Associated with sickle cell disease.

sebaceous gland (suh-BAY-shus). *Anatomy.* Group of cells in the skin that excrete a greasy lubricant; usually open into hair follicles. See also MEIBOMIAN GLAND, ZEISS GLAND.

sebaceous gland carcinoma. *Pathologic condition.* Malignant eyelid tumor arising from a meibomian or Zeiss gland. May be mistaken for a chalazion.

seborrhea. (seb-ur-EE-uh). *Pathologic condition.* Chronic skin disorder with redness, swelling, itching and scaly skin patches.

seborrheic blepharitis (blef-ur-I-tis). *Pathologic condition.* Chronic dandruff-like inflammation of the eyelid margin that may accompany generalized seborrhea.

secluded pupil, seclusio pupillae. *Pathologic conditon.* Complete (360°) posterior synechiae that prevent aqueous from leaving the posterior chamber. See OCCLUDED PUPIL.

secocentral scotoma. Incorrect for CENTROCECAL SCOTOMA.

secondary cataract, after-cataract. *Pathologic condition.* Remnants of the opaque lens remaining in the eye or opacities forming after extracapsular cataract removal. See also ELSCHNIG PEARLS.

secondary deviation. *Measurement* Amount of deviation measured when an eye with a weak or paralyzed extraocular muscle fixates. Greater than primary deviation.

secondary exotropia (eks-oh-TROH-pee-uh). *Functional defect.* Outward (away from nose) deviation that gradually develops in an eye that originally deviated inward (esotropia). See also CONSECUTIVE EXOTROPIA.

secondary focal point. *Optics.* Point on the lens axis where parallel light rays from a distant object are brought to focus after refraction by the lens. See FOCAL POINT.

secondary glaucoma (glaw-KOH-muh). *Pathologic condition.* Increased intraocular pressure that results from a known cause, e.g., inflammation, degeneration, trauma, or tumor growths within the eye. See also PIGMENT DISPERSION GLAUCOMA, POSNER-SCHLOSSMAN DISEASE, RUBEOSIS.

secondary implant. *Optical device.* Intraocular lens implanted into an eye (to replace an extracted cataract), done as a second surgical procedure at a later date than the original surgery.

secondary positions. *Function.* Four positions (right, left, up, down) to which the eyes move in parallel in a vertical or horizontal direction. See also CARDINAL MOVEMENTS, TERTIARY POSITIONS.

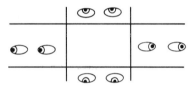

secondary vitreous (VIT-ree-us). *Anatomy.* Second stage of embryologic vitreous formation, beginning in 2nd month of fetal life. Fibrils from the neuroectoderm form around the primary vitreous. See also TERTIARY VITREOUS.

second cranial nerve (N II), optic nerve. *Anatomy.* Largest sensory nerve of the eye; carries impulses for sight from the retina to the brain. Composed of retinal nerve fibers that leave the eyeball through the optic disc and leave the orbit through the optic foramen.

second grade fusion. *Function.* Perceptual blending of similar images into one as the images move off the fovea, allowed by vergence movements. See also CENTRAL FUSION, PERIPHERAL FUSION.

sector defect. *Functional defect.* Missing wedge-shaped portion of the iris, choroid or retina, or of the visual field.

sector iridectomy (ir-ih-DEK-toh-mee). *Surgical procedure.* Removal of a wedge-shaped section of iris from the pupil margin to the iris root, leaving a keyhole-shaped pupil. See also PERIPHERAL IRIDECTOMY.

sedimentation rate. See SED RATE.

sed rate, sedimentation *(or)* **erythrocyte sedimentation rate**. *Lab test.* Rate (in mm per hour) at which red blood cells settle to the bottom of a tube of unclotted blood. Non-specific test used for measuring the progress of various systemic inflammatory diseases.

see-saw nystagmus (ni-STAG-mus). *Pathologic condition.* Involuntary, pendular, torsional eye movements with superimposed vertical eye movements in opposite directions; the intorting eye rises as the extorting eye falls, and vice versa. Occurs with brainstem disease.

segmental syndrome. *Pathologic condition.* Paralysis of half the body, and disordered eye movements. Associated with pontine lesions in the brainstem.

segment (anterior). *Anatomy.* Front third of eyeball; includes structures located between the front surface of the cornea and the vitreous. See also POSTERIOR SEGMENT.

Seidel scotoma (si-DEL skuh-TOH-muh). *Functional defect.* Comma-shaped extension of the normal physiologic blind spot. Becomes an arcuate scotoma as it enlarges.

Seidel sign. *Test.* Application of fluorescein dye to the cornea to locate the site of an abnormal aqueous leak from the anterior chamber. "Positive Seidel" indicated by a bright green flow of liquid.

sella turcica (SEL-uh TUR-sih-kuh). *Anatomy.* Bony pocket in the base of the skull, centered between and behind the orbits. Supports the pituitary gland (hypophysis).

semilunar fold (sem-ee-LU-nur), **plica semilunaris.** *Anatomy.* Crescent-shaped fleshy mound of conjunctival tissue in the nasal corner of each eye.

senile ectropion, involutional ectropion. *Functional defect.* Eyelid that sags away from normal contact with the eyeball because some portions have become stretched or weakened. Usually in the elderly.

senile enophthalmus (en-ahf-THAL-mus). *Degenerative change.* Sinking back of the eyes into the orbits. Usually due to loss of orbital fat with aging.

senile entropion, involutional entropion. *Functional defect.* Eyelid that turns inward against the eyeball because of anatomic changes associated with aging.

senile macular degeneration (SMD) (MAK-yu-lur), **age-related macular degeneration.** *Pathologic condition.* Group of conditions that include deterioration of the macula resulting in a loss of sharp central vision. Two general types: "dry," which is usually evident as a disturbance of macular pigmentation and deposits of yellowish material under the pigment epithelial layer in the central retinal zone; and "wet," (sometimes called Kuhnt-Junius disease) in which abnormal new blood vessels grow under the retina and leak fluid and blood, further disturbing macular function. Most common cause of decreased vision after age 60.

sensory esotropia (ee-soh-TROH-pee-uh). *Functional defect.* Inward (toward nose) deviation of an eye following loss of vision in that eye.

sensory exotropia (eks-oh-TROH-pee-uh). *Functional defect.* Outward (away from nose) deviation of an eye following loss of vision in that eye.

sensory fusion. *Function.* Mental integration of signals from both eyes into a single perception.

sensory nerve, afferent *(or)* **input nerve.** *Anatomy.* Any nerve that carries sensory information (impulses) toward the brain or spinal cord, e.g., the 2nd (optic) cranial nerve. See also MOTOR NERVE.

sensory nystagmus (ni-STAG-mus), **amaurotic nystagmus.** *Pathologic condition.* Involuntary, rhythmic eye movements in both eyes caused by severe visual loss in early childhood. See also ALBINISM, ANIRIDIA, CONGENITAL CATARACT.

sensory receptors, photoreceptors, retinal elements *(or)* **visual cells.** *Anatomy.* Rods and cones; retinal cells that convert light into electrical impulses for transmission of messages to the brain.

sensory retina. *Anatomy.* All retinal layers except the retinal pigment epithelium.

sensory visual pathway, visual pathway. *Anatomy.* The complete course of nerve fibers originating from the retinal visual cells as they travel to the occipital cortex in the brain.

> **anterior**: comprised of nerve fibers from the retina, in the optic nerve, optic chiasm, to the lateral geniculate nucleus in the midbrain.

> **posterior**: comprised of fibers from the lateral geniculate nucleus,

through the parietal and temporal lobes of the brain (optic radiations) and ending in the occipital cortex.

separation difficulty, crowding phenomenon. *Functional defect.* Inability to read an entire line of letters despite the ability to read a single isolated letter of the same size. Characteristic of functional amblyopia.

separation of retina. See RETINAL DETACHMENT.

sepsis (SEP-sis). *Pathologic condition.* Toxic condition that results from the spread of bacteria or their toxic products from a focus of infection somewhere in the body.

septicemia. *Pathologic condition.* "Blood poisoning"; having pathogenic or septic products of bacteria in the bloodstream.

septic retinitis (ret-ih-NI-tis), **metastatic retinitis**. *Pathologic condition.* Infection of the retina caused by microorganisms that reach it through the bloodstream.

septum orbitale (or-bih-TAL-ee), **orbital septum, palpebral fascia**. *Anatomy.* Sheet-like fibrous membrane that forms a protective barrier between the eyelid and the bony orbit; located between the orbital rim of the bone and the tarsal plate of the lid. Supports the eyelid structure, prevents orbital fat from bulging into the eyelids, and prevents eyelid inflammations from entering the orbit.

sequelae (suh-KWEL-ee). After-effects (usually an abnormality) of disease, injury, procedure or treatment.

serology. *Lab test.* Study of blood serum for specific immunological actions or reactions for specific diseases, e.g., tuberculosis. See also PPD.

serous chorioretinopathy (SIH-rus KOR-ee-oh-ret-in-AH-puh-thee) **central serous chorioretinopathy**. *Pathologic condition.* Blister-like elevation of sensory retina in the macula (area of central vision), with localized detachment from the pigment epithelium. Results in a reduction and/or distortion of vision that usually recovers within a few months.

serous detachment. *Pathologic condition.* Any detachment by the clear fluid that separates intraocular layers, e.g., retinal (fluid between retina and retinal pigment epithelium) or choroidal (fluid between choroid and sclera).

serpiginous (sur-PIJ-ih-nus). *Description.* Serpent-like; creeping like a snake from one area to another, e.g., a retinal or corneal lesion.

serpiginous choroidopathy, geographic *(or)* helicoid choroidopathy. *Pathologic condition.* Type of progressive, bilateral choroidal inflammation and degeneration that begins around the optic nerve head (peripapillary) and slowly (over months) extends in a creeping fashion.

Serratia marcescens (seh-RAY-shuh mah-SEZ-senz). *Microorganism.* Gram-negative rod-shaped bacteria; may cause corneal or conjunctival infections.

"setting sun" phenomenon. *Clinical sign.* Down-gaze eye position with upper eyelid retraction, exposing the upper white part of the eye (sclera); creates a staring expression. Associated with congenital hydrocephalus.

seventh cranial nerve (N VII), facial nerve. *Anatomy.* Supplies motor impulses to the muscles of the scalp and face, including the orbicularis oculi surrounding the eye and the tear (lacrimal) glands; also supplies taste sensation for the front two-thirds of the tongue.

sewdotumor. Incorrect spelling of PSEUDOTUMOR.

SF₆, sulfur hexafluoride. *Gas.* Injected into the eye to produce a nontoxic, expansive gas bubble to tamponade (push) dislocated parts into place. See also PNEUMATIC RETINOPEXY, PERFLUOROPROPANE.

shadow-graph. *Instrument.* Magnifies a hard contact lens, measures its size, and checks lens profile for proper blending of peripheral curves.

Shafer's sign. *Clinical sign.* Pigment granules floating in the front part of the vitreous. Can indicate a retinal tear.

skaken baby syndrome, whiplash head shaking syndrome. *Pathologic condition.* Physical damage to the head, retina or brain of an infant or young child caused by violent shaking.

shalazion. Incorrect spelling of CHALAZION.

shallow angle. *Anatomic variation.* Shallower-than-normal space between the iris and cornea. Increases potential for restricting drainage of aqueous fluid drainage through the trabecular meshwork. See also ANGLE, ACUTE ANGLE CLOSURE GLAUCOMA.

sheath syndrome, Brown's *(or)* **superior oblique tendon sheath syndrome.** *Pathologic condition.* Sheath of superior oblique muscle that does not, or cannot, relax when the eye attempts to look upward and inward; mimics an inferior oblique palsy. Unilateral. May be congenital or acquired. See also RESTRICTIVE SYNDROMES.

shell, prosthesis. Cosmetic "false eye" replacement for a removed (enucleated) eye. Plexiglas shell painted to resemble a natural eye fits into the conjunctival sac under the eyelids and over a buried implant.

Sheridan-Gardner. *Test.* Reversible symbols for measuring visual acuity in preschool children. Child points to H, O, T, V, U, A, or X on a test card to match the letter shown in the test booklet. See also HOTV, STYCAR.

Shemer test. Incorrect spelling of SCHIRMER TEST.

Sherrington's law, reciprocal innervation. *Function.* As one extraocular muscle receives an impulse from the brain to contract, its opposing muscle (direct antagonist) in the same eye receives an impulse to relax. See also HERING'S LAW, H_2S.

shingles, herpes zoster. *Pathologic condition.* Extremely painful, blisterlike skin lesions on the face, sometimes with inflammation of the cornea, sclera, ciliary body and optic nerve; affects the 1st division (ophthalmic nerve) of the 5th (trigeminal) cranial nerve. Caused by the chickenpox virus.

Shirmer test. Incorrect spelling of SCHIRMER TEST.

Shiotz tonometer. Incorrect spelling of SCHIOTZ TONOMETER.

short ciliary nerves (SIL-ee eh-ree). *Anatomy.* Motor and sensory nerves in the eye; three to six nerves that originate in ciliary ganglion and branch into approximately 20 as they enter the eye around the optic nerve. Carry parasympathetic fibers to the choroid, ciliary muscle and iris, and sensory fibers back from the eye; these supply sensation to the iris, ciliary body and cornea.

short posterior ciliary arteries. *Anatomy.* Six to 20 blood vessels that enter the eye around the optic nerve and supply blood to the optic nerve head and choroid. See also CILIARY ARTERIES.

Shotts tonometer. Incorrect spelling of SCHIOTZ TONOMETER.

sicca (keratitis) (SIK-uh), **dry eye syndrome, keratoconjunctivitis sicca.** *Pathologic condition.* Corneal and conjunctival dryness due to deficient tear production, mostly in menopausal and post-menopausal women. Causes foreign body sensation, burning eyes, filamentary keratitis, and erosion of conjunctival and corneal epithelium.See also SJÖGREN'S SYNDROME.

sickle cell disease. *Pathologic condition.* Blood (hemoglobin) disorder that causes systemic problems relating to localized clumping of blood cells. In the eye, results in comma-shaped capillaries in the conjunctiva, and retinal changes (retinopathy), e.g., abnormal formation of new vessels (neovascularization) into "sea-fans," arterial blockage, capillary closure, angioid streaks, and iridescent, refractile, glistening retinal deposits. Hereditary; affects blacks predominantly. See also BLACK SUNBURST, SALMON PATCH.

siderosis bulbi (sid-ur-OH-sis BUL-bi). *Pathologic condition.* Degenerative eye toxicity caused by an iron foreign body remaining in the eye.

siderosis lentis (LEN-tis). *Anatomic change.* Rust-brown or yellow lens opacity produced by the toxic effect of an iron foreign body in the eye.

siedel scotoma, siedel sign. Incorrect spelling of SEIDEL SCOTOMA, SEIDEL SIGN.

side vision. *Function.* Peripheral vision; vision elicited by stimuli falling on areas of the retina distant from the macula.

Siegrist's spots. *Clinical sign.* Chains of pigmented spots along a hardened (sclerosed) choroidal vessel, visible with an ophthalmoscope; sometimes found as a sequela of hypertension or choroiditis.

siliary. Incorrect spelling of CILIARY.

silicone (SIH-lih-kohn). Plastic-like material. Available in solid or liquid form.

silicone lens. *Optical device.* Oxygen-permeable contact lens that is soft, flexible, and maintains its size and shape whether or not it is kept in a solution.

silicone oil. Viscous fluids of various densities. Injected into the vitreous cavity after vitreous surgery to help repair a retinal detachment.

"silver wiring." *Clinical sign.* Whitish appearance of opacified retinal arteriolar walls. Commonly associated with arteriosclerosis and hypertension. Advanced form of "copper wiring."

sillinder. Incorrect spelling of CYLINDER.

simple hyperopic astigmatism (hi-pur-AHP-ik uh-STIG-muh-tizm). *Refractive error.* Optical defect in which light rays entering the eye are bent unequally in different meridians, preventing formation of a sharp focus on the retina. Instead, rays form one focal line on the retina, while in the meridian 90° away they strike the retina before forming another focal line. Corrected by a plus cylinder lens.

simple myopic astigmatism (mi-AHP-ik). *Refractive error.* Optical defect in which light rays entering the eye are bent unequally in different meridians, preventing formation of a sharp focus on the retina. Instead, rays form one focal line on the retina, while in the meridian 90° away they form another focal line in the vitreous, in front of the retina. Corrected by a minus cylinder.

simultaneous perception. *Function.* Perception of two images simultaneously (one formed on each retina) that are not necessarily superimposed.

> **foveal (SFP)** (FOH-vee-ul): one image is formed on each fovea.

> **macular (SMP)** (MAK-yu-lur): one image is formed on each macula.

simultaneous prism and cover test (SPCT). Quantifies the constant component of an eye deviation (tropia). A prism held in front of a deviating eye eliminates any refixation movement as the straight, fixating eye is simultaneously covered. See also PRISM + ALTERNATE COVER TEST.

single binocular vision (SBV). *Function.* Blending of the separate images seen by each eye into one composite image. See also BINOCULARITY, FUSION.

Sinskey lens. *Optical device.* Trade name of plastic intraocular lens used as replacement for an extracted cataract. Implanted into the posterior chamber against the posterior lens capsule.

sinus. *Anatomy.* A cavity or hollow space in bone or other tissue, or a confluence of blood channels. Plural: sinuses.

> **cavernous**: intracranial collector channel of venous blood (from the superior and inferior ophthalmic veins of eye) located behind the orbit. The 3rd (oculomotor), 4th (trochlear), 5th (trigeminal) and 6th (abducens) cranial nerves, with sympathetic nerves, travel through it toward the eye. The ophthalmic branch of the internal carotid artery also courses through this network of vessels.

> **ethmoid**: mucus-lined air cavity within the ethmoid bones; one of the nasal sinuses that drains into the nose.

> **frontal**: mucus-lined air cavity within the frontal bones; one of the nasal sinuses that drains into the nose.

>   **maxillary**: mucus-lined air cavity within the maxillary bones; one of the nasal sinuses that drains into the nose.

>   **sphenoid**: mucus-lined air cavity within the sphenoid bones (under the pituitary body, behind the nose); drains into the nose.

sixth cranial nerve (N VI), abducens nerve. *Anatomy.* Motor nerve that innervates the lateral rectus muscle, enabling each eye to rotate outward (away from nose). Originates in the lower pons area of the brainstem; enters the orbit through the superior orbital fissure.

sixth nerve palsy, abducens *(or)* **lateral rectus palsy.** *Pathologic condition.* Partial or total loss of function of the 6th (abducens) cranial nerve, causing the affected eye to deviate inward (esotropia) and have defective ability to turn out beyond the midline (abduct); thus the deviation becomes more apparent when both eyes rotate toward the affected side.

6/6, 20/20. Normal visual acuity. Upper number indicates that a patient can see standardized symbols on a chart 6 meters (20 ft.) away; lower number indicates the same symbols can be seen at 6 meters by an eye with a normal optical system. See also SNELLEN CHART.

Sjögren's syndrome (SHO-grinz). *Pathologic condition.* Chronic connective tissue disease characterized by dry eyes, dry mouth and arthritis. See also KERATOCONJUNCTIVITIS SICCA.

skew deviation (skyu). *Clinical sign.* Vertical eye deviation that has no typical form and which does not fall into a standard category. Caused by a supranuclear disturbance in the midbrain.

skiascopy (skee-AHS-kuh-pee), **retinoscopy.** *Test.* Using a retinoscope to measure an eye's refractive error.

skiascopy bar. *Instrument.* Hand-held rack of graded plus and minus lenses. To measure refractive error, the bar is held in front of the eye and moved from lens to lens while light reflexes are viewed through a retinoscope. See also RETINOSCOPE.

skin flap. *Surgical procedure.* Tongue-shaped section of skin that has been cut so as to keep its blood supply intact. Often used to cover or fill a skin defect, e.g., after removal of a tumor or scar.

skisis. Incorrect spelling of SCHISIS.

slab-off. *Optical device.* Grinding the lower part of a spectacle lens to help compensate for lens-induced vertical prism power, as when the eyes have unequal refractive errors.

sliding flap. *Surgical procedure.* Flap of skin or conjunctiva that is dissected on three sides and stretched or slid over to cover an adjacent area. Common technique used in reconstructive surgery.

slit lamp, biomicroscope. *Instrument.* Table-top microscope used for examining the eye; allows cornea, lens and otherwise clear fluids and membranes to be seen in layer-by-layer detail. Has a low magnifying power (6x to 40x) with a light source that projects a rectangular beam that can be changed in size and focus. One of the most important ophthalmic instruments.

sloping margins. *Description.* Gradual slope of the borders of a visual field depression or relative visual field defect depending on the isopter tested. Absolute defects do not have sloping margins.

slow eye movements (SEM). *Function.* Smooth simultaneous movements of both eyes, in the same or opposite direction, of less than 50°/second. See also BRODMANN AREA 19, FAST EYE MOVEMENTS, PURSUIT MECHANISM, VERGENCE, VERSION, VESTIBULAR SYSTEM.

small angle strabismus, monofixation syndrome, microstrabismus, microtropia. *Functional defect.* Eye misalignment with small, usually inward, deviation and some fusion ability. Deviation usually increases with disruption of fusion (as with covering one eye). Affected eye may be amblyopic and/or anisometropic, usually with a small central suppression scotoma. See also FOUR-PRISM-DIOPTER TEST.

Smith modification of Kuhnt-Szymanowski procedure. *Surgical procedure.* Horizontal eyelid shortening technique for repair of a lower eyelid that does not rest against the eyeball (ectropion). See also SENILE ECTROPION.

Snellen chart. *Test chart.* For assessing visual acuity. Contains rows of letters, numbers, or symbols in standardized graded sizes, with a designated distance at which each row should be legible to a normal eye. Usually tested at 6 m (20 ft.).

Snellen letter. *Test standard.* Letter constructed so as to subtend an angle of 5 minutes of arc at a specified distance from the eye. Each portion of the letter subtends an angle of 1 minute of arc.

Snellen sutures, Feldman suture plication. *Surgical procedure.* Repair of a senile entropion by tightening the inferior obicularis muscle in the lower eyelid with several horizontal stitches.

Snell's law. *Formula.* Relationship between the angle at which a light ray enters a transparent substance and how much it is bent (refracted) within that substance. Ratio determines index of refraction.

"snowballs." *Clinical sign.* Coarse cell clumps within the vitreous; associated with posterior uveitis. Seen typically in sarcoid.

snow blindness. *Functional defect.* Inability to open the eyes due to severe, painful irritation of the cornea and conjunctiva. Secondary to ultraviolet burns by sunlight rays reflected from snow (usually at high altitudes).

soaking solution. Liquid for soaking hard or soft contact lenses to maintain optimal water content and surface wettability.

sodium chloride (hypertonic). *Drug.* Used for topical application to help reduce corneal swelling and clouding. Trade name: Absorbonac.

sodium hyaluronate. *Drug.* Thick elastic gel used during eye surgery to help stabilize structures in their normal positions and protectively coat them. Trade names: Amvisc, Healon. See also VISCOELASTIC AGENT.

Soemmering's ring. *Pathologic condition.* Lens remnants contained within the capsular bag; usually peripherally and arranged as a ring. Sometimes seen after extracapsular cataract extraction.

soft contact lens (SCL). *Optical device.* Water-absorbing (hydrophilic) small plastic disc used for correcting refractive error or protecting a damaged corneal surface. Rests on the cornea; often more comfortable and easier to tolerate than a hard contact lens. See also BANDAGE LENS.

soft exudates (EKS-ih-dayts), **cotton-wool spots**. *Clinical sign.* "Fluffy looking" (like tufts of cotton) white deposits within the retinal nerve fiber layer; represent small patches of retina that have lost their blood supply from vessel obstruction. Often associated with hypertensive or diabetic retinopathy and certain collagen vascular diseases. Gradually disappear without treatment, leaving some functional loss.

solar keratosis, actinic keratosis. *Pathologic condition.* Flat, scaly precancerous skin lesion(s) that appear on skin that is dry and wrinkled from years of sun exposure, usually in fair-skinned persons. May occur on eyelids. See also CUTANEOUS HORN.

solar maculopathy (mak-yu-LAH-puh-thee), **eclipse blindness**. *Pathologic condition.* Macular damage from staring at the sun without proper protective filters, usually during a solar eclipse. A dazzling light sensation soon changes to a central blind spot (scotoma), usually with some permanent reduction in central vision caused by intense radiant energy absorbed in the retina and pigment epithelium. See also ECLIPSE SCOTOMA.

SoluMedrol. *Drug*. Trade name of methylprednisolone, anti-inflammatory steroid for subconjunctival or retrobulbar injection.

Soothe. *Drug*. Trade name of tetrahydrozoline; decongestant for "whitening" the eye.

spasm (lid), blepharospasm. *Functional defect*. Sudden, involuntary spasm of the orbicularis oculi muscle, producing uncontrolled blinking and lid squeezing. See also BLEPHAROCLONUS.

spasmus nutans (SPAZ-mus NU-tanz). *Functional defect*. Fine, rapid eye oscillations (nystagmus) and head nodding, often with a head tilt. Appears in 1st or 2nd year of life, then gradually subsides. Usually harmless.

spastic entropion (en-TROH-pee-un). *Functional defect*. Inward turning of an eyelid against the eyeball that follows acute lid infection or long-term patching of the eye (acute spastic entropian), or is caused by loss of elasticity of eyelid structures with overactivity of the marginal muscle of Riolan (chronic spastic entropion).

spatial localization. *Function*. Perception of an object's position in space. Determined by which retinal elements are stimulated: nasal elements localize in temporal space, temporal elements in nasal space, and the fovea straight ahead. See also VISUAL DIRECTION.

spectacle blur. *Symptom*. Temporary decrease in vision noted with eyeglasses immediately after removing contact lenses. Caused by a temporary shift in refractive error. If prolonged, can be a sign the contacts do not fit properly.

spectacles. *Optical device*. Eyeglasses.

specular endothelial microscopy (SPEK-yu-lur en-doh-THEE-lee-ul mi-KRAHS-kuh-pee), **specular microscopy**. *Test*. Magnified visualization of corneal endothelial cells (pattern and density) by a technique that uses light reflection from the endothelium. Non-contact method: a modified slit lamp focuses light on the epithelium and produces an illuminated specular reflex on it. Contact method: the instrument touches the corneal surface.

specular microscope, endothelial camera. *Instrument*. Used for examining and photographing the size and regularity of endothelial cells that line the undersurface of the cornea. Particularly useful in determining risk to the cornea from cataract extraction.

specular photography. Taking pictures of the corneal endothelium with a specular microscope (endothelial camera).

specular reflection. *Test*. Illumination from a light source placed so its light is reflected directly from the object of regard into the observer's eyes, purposely producing glare. Created with a slit lamp; used for observing corneal endothelial cells. See also PACHOMETER.

speculum (SPEK-yu-lum). *Instrument*. Holds the eyelids apart, to give better access to the eyeball during a surgical procedure.

sphenoidal fissure (sfee-NOY-dul). See SUPERIOR ORBITAL FISSURE.

sphenoid bone. *Anatomy*. One of seven bones of the orbit (eye socket). Forms the back part of the lateral and medial orbital walls.

sphenoid sinus. *Anatomy*. Mucus-lined air cavity within the sphenoid bones (under the pituitary body, behind the nose); drains into the nose. Others include the maxillary, ethmoid and frontal sinuses.

spherical aberration. *Optics*. Type of image blur caused by light rays (from an object point) striking the lens periphery where they are bent too much (overrefracted), compared with rays coming through the center of the lens.

spherical equivalent. *Optical measurement*. "Average" power of a toric lens, equal to the sum of the spherical power plus half the cylindrical power. Represented by the dioptric power of a spherical lens that positions the circle of least confusion.

spherical lens. *Optical device*. Lens with smooth spherical surfaces that bend light rays equally in all meridians.

sphero-cylindrical lens (SFIR-oh sih-LIN-druh-kul), **toric lens**. *Optical device*. Any lens with a cylindrical component. Used for correcting an astigmatic refractive error. Most eyeglasses are of this type.

spheroid degeneration, climatic droplet keratopathy, Labrador keratopathy. *Pathologic condition*. Corneal disorder caused by chronic inflammation and by exposure to ultraviolet light. Characterized by amber fatty-like protein droplets from collagen degeneration in the cornea. Seen in older patients who have led an outdoor life.

sphincterotomy. *Surgical procedure*. Cut made through the iris sphincter muscle.

sphincter pupillae (SFINK-tur pyu-PIL-ee), **iris sphincter**. *Anatomy*. Circle of iris muscle that surrounds the pupillary margin. Receives innervation from parasympathetic nerves to contract pupil size (miosis) in response to bright light.

sphingolipidoses (SFING-oh-lip-ih-DOH-seez). *Pathologic condition*. Numerous hereditary metabolic disorders characterized by excess fatty substance accumulation in various tissues, causing abnormalities of the nervous system, eyes, and other organs. Includes Fabry's, Gaucher's, Krabbe's, Neimann Pick, Sandhoff's, and Tay-Sachs disease; gangliosidosis; generalized, juvenile Gm_1 and Gm_2 gangliosidosis; sulfatide lipidosis.

sphingomyelin lipidosis (sfing-oh-MI-uh-lin lip-uh-DOH-sis), **Niemann Pick disease**. *Pathologic condition*. Defect of fat (lipid) metabolism caused by deficiency of the enzyme sphingomyelinase. Fatty deposits accumulate in many organs, nervous tissue and eyes. Retinal changes may include cherry red spots or a grayish haze. Life span is about 20 years. Hereditary. See also SPHINGOLIPISOSES.

spinal tap. *Test*. Removal of cerebrospinal fluid through a needle inserted into the lumbar area of the spinal canal. See also LUMBAR PUNCTURE.

spin-cast lens. *Optical device*. Soft contact lens manufactured by whirling liquid plastic in a revolving mold at high speed.

spiral field. *Functional defect*. Abnormal visual field that becomes progressively smaller as a light stimulus is presented in serial meridians; plotted as an inward spiral. Characteristic of an hysterical patient. See also FUNCTIONAL DEFECT, STAR-SHAPED FIELD.

spiral of Tillaux (til-OH). Imaginary line connecting the insertions of the medial, inferior, lateral and superior rectus muscles on the eyeball. Spiral is formed from their successive distances from the limbus.

Spirilla (spih-RIL-uh). *Microorganism*. Filamentous or spiral-shaped spirochete bacteria. May cause eye infection.

spot retinoscope (RET-in-uh-skohp). *Instrument*. Determines refractive error by projecting a spot of light into the eye, then neutralizing the light's movement with lenses. See also STREAK RETINOSCOPE.

squamous cell carcinoma (SKWAY-mus). *Pathologic condition*. Type of skin cancer that can occur on any skin surface, including the eyelids. Arises from epithelial surface cells. Malignant; can metastasize.

"squashed tomato." *Clinical sign*. Slang description of hemorrhagic retinopathy. Describes appearance of the retina following a hemorrhagic central retinal vein occlusion.

Squid. *Instrument*. Trade name of computerized apparatus for mapping visual field defects. See also PERIMETER.

squint, deviation, heterotropia, strabismus, tropia. *Functional defect*. Eye misalignment caused by extraocular muscle imbalance: one fovea is not directed at the same object as the other. Present even when both eyes are uncovered. See also PHORIA.

SRK formula. *Measurement.* One of several formulas for calculating the proper power for an intraocular lens prior to cataract surgery. See also BINKHORST EQUATION.

Staphylococcus epidermidis (staf-il-oh-KAH-kus ep-ih-DUR-mid-is). *Microorganism.* Gram-positive round bacteria found normally in the skin around the eye.

Staphylococcus aureus (OR-ee-us). *Microorganism.* Common, round, gram-positive bacteria; causes infections, including corneal ulcers. See also AERUGINOSA, PNEUMO, PSEUDOMONAS.

staphyloma (staf-ih-LOH-muh). *Pathologic condition.* Bulging of the eye surface that includes part of the uvea (e.g., iris, ciliary body) into an area of thin, stretched sclera. If no uveal tissue is included in the stretched area, the condition is called an ectasia.

Stargardt's disease (STAHR-gahrtz). *Pathologic condition.* Macular degeneration characterized by central vision loss with minimal ophthalmoscopic changes. Later, the macula may show pigment clumping surrounded by a hammered-metal appearance. Occurs between ages 6–20. Hereditary.

star-shaped field. *Functional defect.* Peculiar visual field that shows erratic responses; characteristic of a malingering or hysterical patient. See also FUNCTIONAL DEFECT, SPIRAL FIELD.

stasis (STAY-sis). *Pathologic condition.* Slowing or stoppage of normal flow of blood or bodily fluid.

static perimetry (puh-RIM-ih-tree). *Test.* Visual field test using nonmoving (static) targets that are gradually increased in light intensity until perceived. See also KINETIC PERIMETRY.

> **suprathreshold**: for identifying minimum target threshold intensity that can be seen just within a kinetic isopter.

steamy cornea, corneal edema. *Clinical sign.* Hazy, swollen cornea.

steepest meridian. *Measurement.* Direction (meridian), in degrees, of an astigmatic surface (e.g., cornea) having the greatest amount of curvature and thus greatest plus-power. Measured with a keratometer. See also FLATTEST MERIDIAN, K-READINGS.

stellate (STEL-ayt). *Description.* Star-shaped.

stenopaic slit, stenopeic slit (sten-oh-PAY-ik). *Instrument.* Opaque disc with a long slit-like opening; rotated to different positions to determine presence of an astigmatic refractive error.

stenosis (sten-OH-sis). *Abnormal condition.* Abnormal narrowing, especially of a channel or opening.

stent. *Surgical device.* Supporting structure for keeping a channel open or a graft immobilized until healed.

stereo acuity. *Measurement.* Ability to see stereoscopically. Graded by small differences in binocular parallax. See also RANDOT TEST, TITMUS CHART.

stereogram. Two pictures or drawings representing right- and left-eye views of an image, placed on a card for viewing (e.g., with a stereoscope). Used for binocular exercises or recreational viewing.

stereopsis (stehr-ee-AHP-sis), **binocular depth perception, stereoscopic vision, 3rd grade fusion.** *Function.* Visual blending of two similar (not identical) images, one falling on each retina, into one, with visual perception of solidity and depth.

stereoscope (STEH-ree-uh-skohp). *Instrument.* Device for viewing a stereogram; image intended for each eye is kept optically separate. Used for developing fusional amplitudes or for recreational viewing.

stereoscopic vision (steh-ree-uh-SKAHP-ik). See STEREOPSIS.

stereotactic surgery (steh-ree-oh-TAK-tik). *Surgical procedure.* Neurosurgical technique for treating internal structures of the head without removing skull bones. Includes x-ray localization and rigid stabilization of the skull with clamps, which serve to prevent movement and provide reference points for accurate localization of instruments or radiation treatment.

steroid, corticosteroid. *Drug.* Cortisone derivative. For treating inflammatory and allergic diseases. Serious side effects, e.g., osteoporosis, immunosuppression, cataracts and glaucoma can result from long-term use. See also DEXAMETHASONE, METHYLPREDNISOLONE, PREDNISONE, PREDNISOLONE, RIMEXOLONE.

Stevens-Johnson syndrome. *Pathologic condition.* Severe conjunctival disease; inflammation that may result in adhesions binding lower eyelids and conjunctiva to the eyeball (symblepharon), eyelid scarring, dry eyes, and closure of the tear ducts. Occurs in about one-half the patients with erythema multiforme, an allergic skin disease.

Stickler's syndrome. *Pathologic condition.* Progressive connective tissue disease that causes joint problems (enlargement, degeneration, arthritis). Associated with midfacial flattening, cleft palate and hearing loss. Ocular findings include high myopia, cataracts, and vitreoretinal degeneration. Hereditary. See also MARFAN'S SYNDROME, PIERRE ROBIN SYNDROME, WAGNER'S DISEASE.

stigmata (stig-MAH-tuh). *Clinical sign.* Distinguishing marks or signs that identify a bodily condition or disease. Singular: stigma.

Stiles-Crawford effect. *Optics.* Light passing through the center of the pupil is more effective in evoking the sensation of brightness than the same amount of light passing through an equal area near the edge of the pupil. Caused by the directional sensitivity of the retinal cones, i.e., they are less sensitive to light striking them obliquely.

Stilling-Turk-Duane retraction syndrome, Duane's co-contraction *(or)* **retraction syndrome**. *Congenital defect.* Eye muscle abnormality often accompanied by an inward eye deviation (esotropia). Characterized by inability to move one eye outward past midline (abduction) and retraction of that eye into the orbit, with narrowing of eyelid fissure on attempted movement of that eye toward the nose (adduction).

Still's disease, juvenile rheumatoid arthritis. *Pathologic condition.* Uncommon childhood connective tissue disease. Often associated with inflammation of the iris and ciliary body (uveitis) and a band-shaped calcium deposit on the cornea (band keratopathy).

stimulus. Anything that can elicit or evoke action (response) or augmenting action in a muscle, nerve, gland, sensory organ, or other excitable tissue. Plural: stimuli.

Stocker line. *Clinical sign.* Pigmented line sometimes seen in the cornea in front of the advancing edge of a pterygium.

Stock-Spielmeyer-Vogt syndrome (SPEEL-mi-ur voht), **Batten-Mayou** *(or)* **Vogt Spielmeyer syndrome**. *Pathologic condition.* Childhood form of hereditary amaurotic familial idiocy. Characterized by diffuse nervous system disease, macular lesions, and optic nerve degeneration.

Stoxil (STAHKS-il). *Drug.* Trade name for idoxuridine, an anti-viral agent for treating herpetic corneal infections.

strabismic amblyopia (struh-BIZ-mik am-blee-OH-pee-uh). *Functional defect.* Type of amblyopia associated with a continuous eye deviation (usually inward) that begins before a child's visual acuity stabilizes. Can usually be reversed during the first 9 years of life by total occlusion of the non-affected eye (often for months). See also HEIMANN-BIELSCHOWSKY PHENOMENON.

strabismus (struh-BIZ-mus), **deviation, heterotropia, squint, tropia**. *Functional defect.* Eye misalignment caused by extraocular muscle imbalance: one fovea is not directed at the same object as the other. Present even when both eyes are uncovered. See also PHORIA.

alternating: continuous changing between a deviating right eye and straight left eye, and a deviating left eye and straight right eye.

antipodean: one eye turns in; when it straightens, other eye turns out.

comitant: the degree of misalignment is the same in all directions of gaze, and there is no ocular muscle paralysis.

horizontal: one eye deviates inward or outward.

incomitant: degree of misalignment changes in different positions of gaze because an extraocular muscle is paretic, paralytic or restricted.

noncomitant. same as INCOMITANT (above).

vertical: one eye is higher or lower than the other.

strabismus fixus. *Congenital defect.* Eye(s) are fixed in an extreme position due to tightened medial or lateral recti muscles. Results in the eyes deviating either inward (esotropia) or outward (exotropia).

streak retinoscope (RET-in-uh-skohp). *Instrument.* Determines refractive error by projecting a rotatable line of light into the eye that is neutralized with lenses. See SPOT RETINOSCOPE.

Streptococcus pneumoniae (strep-tuh-KAHK-us nu-MOH-nee-ee), **pneumo**. *Microorganism.* One of the most common gram-positive bacteria causing eye infections, especially corneal ulcers. Bacteria grow in pairs. See also PSEUDOMONAS AERUGINOSA, STAPHYLOCOCCUS AUREUS.

streptomycin. *Drug.* Antibiotic agent for treating eye infections.

striae (STREE-uh). *Anatomic defect.* Wrinkles or folds anywhere in the body, e.g., in the choroid or cornea, as caused by abnormal pressure or distortion of tissue.

striate area (STRI-ayt), **Brodmann area 17, visual *(or)* primary visual cortex**. *Anatomy.* Area (cerebral end of sensory visual pathways that begin at the retina) in occipital lobes of brain, where initial conscious registration of visual information takes place. See also OCCIPITAL CORTEX.

string of pearls. *Clinical sign.* Concentration of inflammatory cells in the vitreous; resembles a pearl necklace. Typical of sarcoid.

stroke, cerebrovascular accident. *Pathologic condition.* Sudden loss of specific brain functions (e.g., speech, specific movement), resulting from interrupted blood supply, as by an embolus, thrombosis or hemorrhage; usually from cerebral blood vessel disease (atherosclerosis).

stroma. *Anatomy.* Framework, usually of connective tissue or an organ, gland or other structure.

corneal: middle tissue layer that forms 90% of cornea; composed of layered collagen fibrils and cells. Also called subtantia propria.

iris: primary substance of the iris; contains pigment cells that determine eye color, and two non-striated muscles: the ring-shaped sphincter and the radially fibered dilator.

Sturge-Weber syndrome, encephalofacial angiomatosis. *Congenital anomaly.* Characterized by reddish pigmentation (port wine stain) usually on one side of the face, prominent in area supplied by the 5th (trigeminal) cranial nerve. Associated with high intraocular pressure, large eye, and hemangiomas in the skin, choroid, and brain; if in the brain may result in seizures and mental retardation. Hereditary.

Sturm's conoid (KOH-noyd). *Optics.* Somewhat cone-shaped image of a point created by a cylindrical (astigmatic) lens. Lies between the two focal line images (interval of Sturm) and contains the circle of least confusion.

Sturm's interval. *Optics.* Space lying between the two focal line images formed by a cylindrical (astigmatic) lens.

sty. See STYE.

STYCAR. *Test.* Acronym: Screening Test for Young Children And Retardates.

Distance-vision test using the letters H, O, T, V, U. See also HOTV, SHERIDAN-GARDINER TEST.

stye, sty, external hordeolum. *Pathologic condition.* Acute pustular infection of the oil glands of Zeis, located in an eyelash follicle at the eyelid margin.

subacute sclerosing panencephalitis (SSPE) (skler-OH-sing pan-en-cef-uh-LI-tis). *Pathologic condition.* Late complication from a childhood viral disease (e.g., measles) that affects brain and retinal tissue, with macular or perimacular inflammation, retinal swelling (edema) and hemorrhage. Begins with personality changes and seizures; death occurs within a few months. No known treatment.

subconjunctival hemorrhage (sub-kahn-junk-TI-vul HEM-uh-rij). *Clinical sign.* Bleeding from a small blood vessel under the conjunctiva; often spontaneous or from coughing. Creates appearance of bright-red blood over the sclera. Harmless; blood absorbs in about one week without treatment.

subconjunctival injection. *Treatment.* Injection (of ocular drugs) between the conjunctiva and Tenon's capsule.

subcutaneous (sub-kyu-TAY-nee-us). *Location.* Under the skin.

subhyaloid hemorrhage (sub-HI-uh-loyd HEM-uh-rij). *Clinical sign.* Bleeding between the sensory retina and vitreous body. The upper edge of the blood is often flattened, giving it a boat-shaped (scaphoid) appearance.

subjective test. Examination requiring responses from the patient.

subluxation (sub-luks-AY-shun). *Pathologic condition.* Partial displacement of the crystalline lens from its normal position. Caused by broken or absent zonules. See also DISLOCATED LENS, ECTOPIC LENS, HOMOCYSTINURIA, LUXATION, MARCHESANI'S SYNDROME, MARFAN'S SYNDROME.

subretinal neovascularization (SRNV) (sub-REH-tih-nul nee-oh-VAS-kyu-lur-ih-ZAY-shun). *Pathologic condition.* Abnormal formation of new blood vessels between the retinal pigment epithelium and the choroid. May cause fluid leakage and bleeding under the retina with eventual destruction of the overlying retinal function. Occurs in some forms of macular degeneration. See also SUBRETINAL NEOVASCULAR MEMBRANE.

substantia propria (sub-STAN-shuh PROH-pree-uh). See CORNEAL STROMA.

sudotumor. Incorrect spelling of PSEUDOTUMOR.

sulcus fixation. *Surgical technique.* One way an intraocular lens is held in place when the posterior capsule is torn. The footplates (haptics) of a posterior chamber IOL are set into the natural groove (ciliary sulcus). See also CAPSULAR FIXATION.

sulfur hexafluoride. See SF$_6$.

sulfatide lipidosis (SUL-fuh-tide lip-ih-DOH-sis), **metachromatic leukodystrophy**. *Pathologic condition.* Group of genetic defects in fat (lipid) metabolism that produce disruption in nerve tissue. Characterized by weakness, mental retardation, eye muscle palsies, optic nerve degeneration, and blindness. Affects young children; death occurs within a few years. See also SPHINGOLIPIDOSES.

"sunburst" dial, clock dial, Lancaster Regan dial #1. *Test chart.* Radial arrangement of black lines used during refraction to subjectively refine the axis of an astigmatic refractive error. See also ASTIGMATIC CLOCK, FAN DIAL, LANCASTER-REGAN DIAL #2.

"sunflower" cataract. *Pathologic condition.* Lens opacity caused by metallic copper deposits under the lens capsule. May have minimal effect on vision. See also WILSON'S DISEASE.

sunglasses, absorptive lenses. *Optical device.* Spectacles whose lenses absorb a high percentage of light, thus reducing the amount of light transmitted to the eye. Worn in bright sunlight for comfort and for protection from light damage.

sunrise symptom. *Surgical complication*. Upward malposition of a posterior chamber intraocular lens. May be a late complication from asymmetric implantation of vertical lens haptics.

sunset symptom. *Surgical complication*. Dislocation (downward into vitreous) of a posterior chamber intraocular lens. May be a late complication from rupture of zonules below the lens.

superficial punctate keratitis (SPK) (PUNK-tayt kehr-uh-TI-tus), **punctate *(or)* Thygeson's superficial punctate keratitis**. *Pathologic condition*. Corneal disease characterized by small superficial corneal lesions. Symptoms include foreign body sensation and sensitivity to bright light. Cause unknown; sometimes recurs after spontaneous remission.

superimposition (SU-pur-im-puh-ZIH-shun), **1st grade fusion**. *Function*. Perception of two dissimilar images, one formed on each retina, as one composite image.

superior. *Location*. On or near the upper part of an organ or the body. See also INFERIOR.

superior arcade. *Anatomy*. Arch of superior temporal retinal arterioles and venules, leading from the optic disc and extending above the fovea to the retinal periphery. See also INFERIOR ARCADE.

superior canaliculus (kan-uh-LIK-yu-lus), **upper canaliculus**. *Anatomy*. Part of tear drainage system. Thin elastic duct within the upper eyelid on the nasal side, connecting the upper punctum to the common canaliculus.

superior cervical ganglion (SUR-vih-kul GANG-lee-un). *Anatomy*. Large clump (one of a pair) of neural interconnections (ganglia) in the neck, beside the spine and internal carotid artery. Contains sympathetic nerve fibers from cervical and thoracic spinal nerves that supply the eye and orbit.

superior colliculus. *Anatomy*. One of a pair of mounds on the roof of the midbrain. Contains centers for coordination of eye movements. Plural: colliculi. See also COLLICULAR PLATE, CORPORA QUADRAGEMINA, INFERIOR COLLICULUS.

superior limbic keratoconjunctivitis (LIM-bik KEHR-uh-toh-kun-junk-tih-VI-tis). *Pathologic condition*. Inflammation involving the upper tarsus, bulbar conjunctiva and corneal limbus. Cause unknown.

superior nasal artery. *Anatomy*. One of four main branches of the central retinal artery; nourishes the upper inner retinal quadrant from the optic disc to the ora serrata.

superior nasal vein. *Anatomy*. One of four main branches of the central retinal vein; drains the upper inner retinal quadrant from the ora serrata to the optic disc.

superior oblique (SO) (oh-BLEEK or oh-BLIKE). *Anatomy*. Extraocular muscle attached to the upper, outer side of the eyeball behind the equator. Three functions: intorsion (rotates top of eye toward the nose, which increases as eye turns outward); depression (which increases as eye turns inward), and abduction (movement of eye outward from midline). Innervated by the 4th (trochlear) cranial nerve.

superior oblique palsy, 4th nerve palsy. *Pathologic condition*. Head tilt and upward eye deviation (hypertropia) caused by partial or total loss of function of the 4th (trochlear) cranial nerve, with reduced effectiveness of the superior oblique muscle.

superior oblique tendon sheath syndrome, Brown's *(or)* sheath syndrome. *Pathologic condition*. Sheath of superior oblique muscle that does not, or cannot, relax when the eye attempts to look upward and inward; mimics an inferior oblique palsy. Unilateral; may be congenital or acquired. See also RESTRICTIVE SYNDROMES.

superior ophthalmic vein (ahf-THAL-mik). *Anatomy*. Major vein that drains the orbit. Joined by many branches (anterior and posterior ethmoidal, muscular, lacrimal, central retinal, anterior ciliary, inferior ophthalmic, and both superior vortex veins).

superior orbital fissure (SOF), sphenoidal fissure. *Anatomy*. Opening in the back of the orbit, between the lesser and greater wings of the sphenoid bone. Entry site to the orbit for the 3rd (oculomotor), 4th (trochlear) and 6th (abducens) cranial nerves, and the lacrimal and nasociliary nerves, and exit site of the superior ophthalmic vein.

superior orbital fissure syndrome, orbital fissure syndrome. *Pathologic condition*. Characterized by a droopy eyelid, decreased corneal and eyelid sensation, numbness, and the eye positioned downward and outward. Disease involvement of structures passing through the superior orbital fissure causes large pupil, paralysis of 3rd (oculomotor), 4th (trochlear), ophthalmic division of 5th (trigeminal) and 6th (abducens) cranial nerves and sympathetic nerves, with no engorged veins. See also CAVERNOUS SINUS SYNDROME, ORBITAL APEX SYNDROME, TOLOSA-HUNT SYNDROME.

superior palpebral furrow, lid fold. *Anatomy*. Fold in the upper eyelid when the eye is open.

superior punctum, upper punctum. *Anatomy*. Tiny opening in upper eyelid margin near the nose; upper entrance to the eye's tear drainage (lacrimal) system. See also INFERIOR PUNCTUM, SUPERIOR CANALICULUS.

superior quadrantanopia (kwahd-ran-tuh-NOH-pee-uh), **"pie in the sky" defect**. *Functional defect*. Upper quadrant visual field defect on the same side in each eye, caused by damage to the inferior fibers of the optic radiations in the brain's temporal lobe (in Meyer's temporal loop).

superior rectus (SR). *Anatomy*. Extraocular muscle attached to the upper side of the eyeball (globe). Three functions: elevation of the eyeball (which increases as eye moves outward), intorsion (rotates top of eye toward the nose, which increases as eye turns inward); and adduction (movement of the eye inward toward the nose. Innervated by the 3rd (oculomotor) cranial nerve.

superior temporal artery. *Anatomy*. One of four main branches of the central retinal artery. Nourishes the upper outer retinal quadrant from the optic disc to the ora serrata.

superior temporal vein. *Anatomy*. One of four main branches of the central retinal vein. Drains the upper outer retinal quadrant from the ora serrata to the optic disc.

superonasal (suh-PEHR-oh-NAY-zul). *Location*. Situated above a reference position (e.g., the eyeball or optic disc) and toward the nose. See also INFERONASAL.

superotemporal (suh-PEHR-oh-TEM-pur-ul). *Location*. Situated above a reference position (e.g., the eyeball or optic disc) and toward the ear. See also INFEROTEMPORAL.

suprachoroidal hemorrhage. *Pathologic condition*. Bleeding in the outer layers of the choroid that can occur as a rare complication during intraocular surgery (e.g., cataract extraction). Can result in an expulsive hemorrhage (with extrusion of intraocular contents).

suppression. *Functional defect*. Subconscious inhibition of an eye's retinal image. Usually occurs in strabismus when a deviated eye's image interferes with that received from the straight eye. Unconscious mechanism to avoid double vision (diplopia). See also AMBLYOPIA.

    obligatory: continues when the straight eye is covered; associated with amblyopia.

    facultative: image is seen when the straight eye is covered and the deviated eye is forced to fixate.

suppression amblyopia (am-blee-OH-pee-uh). *Functional defect*. Decreased vision in one eye without detectable anatomic damage in eye or visual pathways. Thought to result from a physiologic process in which the retinal image transmitted by that eye is ignored. Occurs in children whose eyes have a marked difference in refractive errors (anisometropia) or have a deviation of one eye.

suppurate (SUP-yur-ayt). To form or discharge pus.

suppuration (sup-yur-AY-shun). *Pathologic condition.* Forming or discharging pus.

suprachoroid (su-pruh-KOR-oyd), **lamina fusca sclerae, lamina suprachoroidea**. *Anatomy.* Thin, brown, outermost layer of choroid that lies against the sclera.

supraduction (su-pruh-DUK-shun), **sursumduction**. *Function.* Upward movement of one eye from the straight-ahead position. See also ELEVATION, SURSUMVERSION.

supranuclear pathways (su-pruh-NU-klee-ur). *Anatomy.* Nerve fiber bundles that connect the brain cortex or cerebellum with cranial nerve nuclei in the brainstem. Usually refers to higher brain pathways that control coordination of eye movements. See also INFRANUCLEAR PATHWAYS.

supraorbital artery (su-pruh-OR-bih-tul). *Anatomy.* Branch of the ophthalmic artery that supplies blood to the upper eyelid, scalp, and levator muscle; runs along the orbital roof and through the supraorbital notch.

supraorbital nerve. *Anatomy.* Larger of the two branches of the frontal nerve (largest branch of the ophthalmic division of the 5th, trigeminal, cranial nerve), which supplies sensation to conjunctiva, upper eyelid, forehead and scalp. Enters the orbit above the levator muscle and passes through the supraorbital notch in the upper orbital margin.

supraorbital notch. *Anatomy.* Indentation in the orbital rim of the frontal bone near the nose.

supratentorial. *Location.* Above the (cerebellar) tentorium (sheet-like tissue lying above the cerebellum); often used for referring to the position of the cerebral hemisphere. Also slang for brain functioning.

suprathreshold static perimetry. *Test.* Visual field test using nonmoving (static) targets to identify minimum target threshold light intensity that can be seen just within a kinetic isopter.

supratrochlear artery (su-pruh-TROH-klee-ur). *Anatomy.* Branch of ophthalmic artery that crosses the orbital roof and supplies blood to the central part of the forehead.

supratrochlear nerve. *Anatomy.* Smaller of the two branches of the frontal nerve (largest branch of the ophthalmic division of the 5th, trigeminal, cranial nerve) after it divides near the front of the orbit. Passes above the superior oblique pulley to supply sensation to the upper eyelid, upper conjunctiva, and forehead skin.

supraversion (su-pruh-VUR-zhun). See SURSUMVERSION.

sursumduction (sur-sum-DUK-shun). See SUPRADUCTION.

sursumvergence (sur-sum-VUR-junss). *Function.* Upward movement of one eye relative to the other, usually to maintain single binocular vision, as when increasing amounts of base-down prism are placed in front of that eye. See also DEORSUMVERGENCE.

sursumversion (sur-sum-VUR-zhun), **supraversion**. *Function.* Upward movement of both eyes. See also ELEVATION, SUPRADUCTION.

suture. 1. *Anatomy.* Irregular junction between immovable bones. In the crystalline lens, the Y-shaped junction zone of the lens fiber tips. 2. *Surgical procedure.* To sew together. Also refers to the stitch itself. 3. *Material.* The "thread" used for surgical sutures. See also BRIDLE SUTURE, INTERRUPTED SUTURES, RUNNING SUTURES.

suture plication, Feldstein suture plication, Snellen sutures. *Surgical procedure*. Repair of a senile entropion by tightening the inferior obicularis muscle in the lower eyelid with several horizontal stitches.

Swan incision. *Surgical procedure*. A cut made through the conjunctiva and Tenon's capsule over the belly of an extraocular muscle to be repositioned; for correcting an eye deviation.

Swan syndrome, blind spot mechanism *(or)* syndrome. *Functional defect*. Adaptive mechanism for avoiding double vision that may accompany an inward eye deviation (esotropia). Deviation increases until the image falls on the optic disc of the deviated eye, which eliminates double vision. Controversial concept; may not be clinically significant.

Sweet's technique. *Diagnostic method*. Radiologic localization of an intraocular foreign body. Based on a triangulation principle using a radiopaque marker (in a contact lens) placed a known distance in front of the eyes.

swinging flashlight test. Comparison of the eyes' pupillary response to light in dim illumination; unequal decrease in pupil size indicates a Marcus-Gunn pupil, an important sign of optic nerve disease. See also CONSENSUAL LIGHT RESPONSE.

Sylvian aqueduct syndrome (SIL-vee-un AK-wih-dukt), **dorsal midbrain *(or)* Parinaud's *(or)* pretectal *(or)* tectal midbrain syndrome**. *Pathologic condition*. Decreased ability to move the eyes up or down. Attributed to a brainstem lesion near the vertical gaze center. Sometimes associated with inability to converge and poor pupil responses to light. See also ARGYLL-ROBERTSON PUPILS.

symblepharon (sim-BLEF-uh-rahn). *Pathologic condition*. Abnormal adhesion of eyelid (palpebral) conjunctiva to eyeball (bulbar) conjunctiva.

symmetric surgery. *Surgical procedure*. Weakening or strengthening procedure performed on the same muscle in both eyes, to correct an eye misalignment.

sympathetic nervous system. *Anatomy*. Part of the autonomic nervous system responsible for "flight or fight" response. Innervates the iris dilator muscle in the eye, Müller's muscle in the eyelid, causes secretion by the ciliary epithelium, and controls size (diameter) of the blood vessels in the eye.

sympathetic ophthalmia (off-THAL-mee-uh), **sympathetic uveitis**. *Pathologic condition*. Granulomatous inflammation of the uvea (choroid, ciliary body, and iris) as a late complication of a penetrating injury. Dangerous because a similar uveitis may also occur (within several months) in the other (sympathizing) eye. Rare. See also DALEN-FUCHS NODULES, POLIOSIS.

sympathetic uveitis (yu-vee-I-tis). See SYMPATHETIC OPHTHALMIA.

sympatholytic drug (sim-path-oh-LIT-ik), **beta blocker, adrenergic blocking agent**. *Drug*. 1. Used topically to treat glaucoma. Blocks action of sympathetic nerve fibers by blocking beta adrenergic receptor sites for nerve impulse transmission; sometimes causes pupillary constriction. Betaxolol is a beta-one blocker; carteolol, levobunolol, metipranolol, timolol are beta-one and beta-two blockers. 2. Used systemically as a heart medication to treat rapid arrhythmia and hypertension. Discontinuation may decrease intraocular pressure control.

sympathomimetic drug (sim-path-oh-mim-ET-ik), **adrenergic stimulating agent**. *Drug*. Mimics action of sympathetic nerves. Used (1) to control glaucoma by opening the anterior chamber angle to increase aqueous outflow, decrease aqueous secretion and help nerve transmission (beta-two receptors); examples: aproclonidine, dipivefrin, epinephrine, isoproterenol; (2) to dilate the pupil without affecting accommodation; examples: hydroxyamphetamine, phenylephrine; (3) to "whiten" the eye by constricting dilated conjunctival blood vessels; examples: naphazoline, phenylephrine, tetrahydrozaline.

synchysis scintillans (sin-KEE-sis SIN-tih-lanz). *Degenerative change.* Formation of asymptomatic floating white cholesterol crystals in the vitreous. See also ASTEROID HYALOSIS.

syncope (SIN-kuh-pee). *Clinical sign.* Brief loss of consciousness. Fainting.

syndrome. Group of signs and symptoms that tend to occur together and characterize a particular abnormality.

synechia (sin-EEK-ee-uh). *Pathologic condition.* Adhesion(s) that bind the iris to any adjacent structures. Plural: synechiae.

    anterior: between iris and cornea.

    peripheral anterior: between iris periphery and cornea. Occurs with unrelieved attacks of angle-closure glaucoma; may occur following injury or surgery.

    posterior: between iris and lens. Occurs commonly in uveitis.

synechiolysis (sin-EE-kee-oh-LI-sis). *Procedure.* Breaking of abnormal adhesions (synechiae) between the iris and the lens or the iris and the cornea, usually by surgery.

synephris (SIN-ih-frus). *Anatomic defect.* Eyebrows that continue across the bridge of the nose.

syneresis (sin-ur-EE-sus). *Degenerative change.* Shrinkage, sometimes with collapse, of the gel-like vitreous following liquefication. Occurs with age and precedes posterior vitreous detachment.

synergist (SIN-ur-jist). *Function.* Extraocular muscle that assists the primary muscle in that eye for making a particular eye movement.

synergistic divergence. *Functional defect.* Eye muscle abnormality characterized by decreased ability to move an eye inward toward the nose (adduction). Simultaneous outward movement of both eyes occurs when inward movement is attempted. Often the affected eye also deviates outward when the other eye looks straight ahead.

synkinesis (sin-kin-EE-sis). Occurrence of two simultaneous movements associated with one another; e.g., closing the eyes while sneezing.

synkinetic near reflex (sin-kin-EH-tik). *Function.* Three associated reactions of the eyes that occur with near visual tasks: convergence (turning inward), accommodation (change in lens curvature to maintain a clear image), and miosis (decrease in pupil size).

synophthalmia (sin-ahf-THAL-mee-uh). *Congenital anomaly.* Two incomplete eyes joined in the center of the forehead as one eyeball. Incompatible with life. See also CYCLOPS

synoptophore (sin-AHP-tuh-for), **troposcope**. *Instrument.* Type of major amblyoscope used in evaluation and treatment of binocularity problems. See also HAPLOSCOPE.

syphilis (SIF-ih-lus), **lues**. *Pathologic conditon.* A venereal disease. In the late stages may affect the optic nerves (producing visual field loss) and cause Argyll-Robertson pupils, interstitial keratitis, uveitis, vitritis, retinal vasculitis and choroiditis.

systemic (sis-TEH-mik). *Description.* Affecting the body generally, rather than a specific (local) area.

systemic lupus erythematosus (LU-pus ehr-ih-thee-muh-TOH-sus), **lupus erythematosus**. *Pathologic condition.* Autoimmune collagen disease characterized by fever, facial rash in a "butterfly" pattern, and heart and kidney problems. May be associated with double or decreased vision, nystagmus, swollen and puffy eyelids, dry eyes, cotton-wool retinal deposits and, rarely, optic nerve degeneration, retinal hemorrhages and retinal blood vessel blockage.

systemic sclerosis (skluh-ROH-sis), **scleroderma**. *Pathologic condition.* Auto-immune collagen disease that affects connective tissue of the skin, mucous membranes, bones, muscles, and internal organs. Characterized by areas of tight, leathery skin on limbs and eyelids, cotton-wool retinal deposits and, sometimes, iritis and cataracts.

systolic blood pressure. *Function.* Highest pressure (measured in mm of mercury) during the cardiac cycle. Occurs during heart contraction. See also DIASTOLIC BLOOD PRESSURE.

T

tachycardia (tak-ih-KAHR-dee-uh). *Clinical sign.* Unusually rapid heart rate. May be physiological, as after exercise, or pathological.

taco test. For determining front from back of a soft contact lens. Lens is flexed between thumb and forefinger; the slant of the outer edge in same direction that the lens is flexed indicates the side that is worn away from the eye.

Tagamet. *Drug.* Trade name of cimetidine; for treating gastric ulcer.

Takayasu's disease (tah-kuh-YAH-shuz), **idiopathic arteritis of Takayasu, pulseless disease.** *Pathologic condtion.* Inflammatory disorder of large arteries caused by obstruction. Characterized by insufficient blood flow reaching the brain, upper extremities and eyes. Most frequently affects children and young people.

tamponade (tam-puh-NAHD). *Treatment.* Closure or blockage of a wound or body cavity (e.g., to stop bleeding) by pressing on or plugging.

tangent screen, campimeter. *Test instrument.* Screen used for quantifying visual field defects within 30° of a fixation point. Testing is carried out 1 or 2 meters from the eye. See also PERIMETRY.

Tangier disease, familial lipoprotein deficiency. *Pathologic condition.* Congenital defect of fat (lipid) metabolism characterized by orange cholesterol deposits in the tonsils and tiny corneal deposits seen only by slit lamp. Does not affect vision.

tapetoretinopathy (tuh-PEE-toh-reh-tin-AH-puh-thee). *Pathologic condition.* General term for group of hereditary degenerations of the retinal pigment epithelium and sensory retina.

tapetum (tuh-PEE-tum), **tapetum lucidum.** *Anatomy.* Reflectile layer associated with the retinal pigment epithelium. Found in many animals, but not in man.

tarsalconjunctival resection below the punctum. See TARSAL CONJUNCTIVAL SPINDLE EXCISION.

tarsalconjunctival spindle excision, diamond conjunctival resection, tarsalconjunctival resection below the punctum. *Surgical procedure.* Removal of a spindle- or diamond-shaped section of conjunctival tissue from inside the lower lid parallel to the lid margin, to invert a malpositioned punctum and reposition the lower lid against the eyeball. See also ECTROPION.

tarsal gland (TAR-sul), **meibomian gland.** *Anatomy.* Oil gland (one of a series) within eyelid tissue (tarsus) whose duct opens onto the eyelid margin just behind the gray line. Secretions supply outer portion of the tear film, which prevents rapid tear evaporation and tear overflow and provides tight eyelid closure. See also CHALAZION.

tarsal plate. See TARSUS.

tarsectomy (tar-SEK-tuh-mee). *Surgical procedure.* Removal of the tarsal plate (part or all) in the upper or lower eyelid.

tarsoconjunctival resection, internal tarsal-orbicularis resection. *Surgical procedure.* For repair of an inward turning eyelid due to aging. Part of the tarsus and the underlying orbicularis muscle are removed. See also SENILE ENTROPION.

tarsorrhaphy (tar-SOR-uh-fee). *Surgical procedure.* Stitching upper and lower eyelids together, partially or completely, usually to provide temporary protection to the eye. Plural: tarsorrhaphies.

tarsus (TAHR-sus), **tarsal plate.** *Anatomy.* Dense plate-like framework within the upper and lower eyelids that provides stiffness and shape. Plural: tarsi.

tatik, tautic. Incorrect spelllig of PTOTIC.

Tay-Sachs disease. *Pathologic condition.* Fat (lipid) metabolism disorder that occurs predominantly in Ashkenazic Jewish children. Eye signs include an opaque central retina due to lipid-filled ganglion cells; fovea that appears as a cherry red spot; pale, degenerated optic nerve. Leads to increasing mental deterioration, spastic paralysis, and blindness, with death by age 3. Hereditary. See also AMAUROTIC FAMILIAL IDIOCY, GANGLIOSIDOSIS, SPHINGO-LIPIDOSES.

T-cell. Type of lymphocyte (white blood cell) produced in the thymus gland. Part of the body's immune system.

teaching mirror. *Instrument.* Mirror that attaches to an indirect ophthalmoscope, allowing visualization of the retina by two observers.

tear breakup time (BUT). *Measurement.* Test for tear function. Time interval between a blink and the development of a dry spot in the pre-corneal tear film; less than 10 seconds is abnormal. Spot is visible after fluorescein staining, especially with the cobalt blue beam on the slit lamp.

tear drainage system, lacrimal apparatus. *Anatomy.* Orbital structures for tear production and drainage. Tears (produced in lacrimal gland above eyeball) flow across the corneal surface, drain into the upper and lower puncta (openings at inner eyelid margins), through the upper and lower canaliculi to the common canaliculus, into the tear sac, then through the nasolacrimal duct into the nose.

tear duct, lacrimal *(or)* **nasolacrimal duct**. *Anatomy.* Tear drainage channel that extends from the lacrimal sac to an opening in the mucous membrane of the nose.

tear film, pre-corneal tear film. *Anatomy.* Liquid that bathes the cornea and conjunctiva. Composed of three layers: outer oily layer secreted by the meibomian glands, middle aqueous layer secreted by the lacrimal glands, inner mucin layer produced by the conjunctival goblet cells.

tearing. *Function.* Secretion of fluid by the lacrimal system by means of which the conjunctiva and cornea are kept moist. See also SCHIRMER TEST.

> **basal**: tear secretion (mainly from tiny glands in the conjunctiva) that maintains a normal moisture level in the tear film to keep the conjunctiva and cornea moist. Reduced in dry eyes (keratoconjunctivitis sicca).

> **reflex**: tears produced by the lacrimal glands in response to a corneal or conjunctival surface irritant.

tears. Fluid secreted by the lacrimal glands by means of which the conjunctiva and cornea are kept moist.

> **artificial**: eyedrops that approximate the consistency of normal tears, such as weak methylcellulose solution or polyvinyl alcohol. Alleviates dry eye symptoms; some products used for treating recurrent corneal erosion. See also TEAR FILM BREAKUP TIME.

> **crocodile**: tears and excessive saliva produced while eating. Occurs with paralysis of the 7th (facial) cranial nerve, after salivary gland nerve fibers regenerate abnormally and grow into the lacrimal gland. See also ABERRANT REGENERATION.

Tearisol (TIR-uh-sol). *Drug.* Trade name of methylcellulose eyedrops; for treating dry eyes.

tear sac, lacrimal sac. *Anatomy.* Tear collecting structure lying under the skin near the bridge of the nose. Tears enter from the common canaliculus and leave from the lacrimal duct into the nose.

Tears Naturale. Trade name of methylcellulose eyedrops; for treating dry eyes.

Tears Plus. Trade name of polyvinyl alcohol eyedrops; for treating dry eyes.

tectal midbrain syndrome (TEK-tul), **dorsal midbrain** *(or)* **Parinaud's** *(or)* **pretectal** *(or)* **Sylvian aqueduct syndrome**. *Pathologic condition.* Decreased ability to move the eyes up or down. Attributed to a brainstem lesion near the vertical gaze center. Sometimes associated with inability to converge and poor pupil responses to light. See also ARGYLL-ROBERTSON PUPILS, SEGMENTAL SYNDROME.

teichopsia (ti-KAHP-see-uh). *Symptom.* Scintillating aura that accompanies a migraine attack.

telangiectasia (tee-lan-jee-ek-TAY-zhuh). *Abnormal condition.* Abnormal dilation of groups of capillaries and small blood vessels.

telebinocular (tel-uh-bi-NAHK-yu-lur). *Test instrument.* Screening tool for binocular ability; tests fusion and stereopsis.

telecanthus (tel-uh-KAN-thus). *Anatomic defect.* Wider-than-normal space between the eyes (intercanthal distance), with normal space between the pupils (interpupillary distance). See also HYPERTELORISM.

Teller acuity cards (TAC). *Test.* Measures visual acuity in young non-verbal children by testing their ability to detect alternating black and white stripes of varying widths (spatial frequencies).

temple length. *Measurement.* 1. Distance from the outermost edge of an eye to the ear on the same side. 2. Length of the temple piece on an eyeglass frame.

temporal. *Location.* Relating to the side of head (temple); the direction away from the nose (toward the ear), or the half of the visual field from the midline toward the temple. See also NASAL.

temporal arcades. *Anatomic description.* Normal pattern of retinal blood vessels as they leave the optic nerve head and arch around the macula.

temporal arteritis (ahr-tur-RI-tus), **cranial *(or)* giant cell arteritis**. *Pathologic condition.* Inflammation of many of the arteries supplying the head and eyes. Often accompanied by severe headache, fever, weight loss, stroke and heart attack. Eye involvement includes sudden vision loss and optic nerve inflammation (caused by the closing off of the central retinal artery or one of its branches), double vision, or droopy lids. Usually affects people over age 60.

temporal crescent. 1. *Anatomic variation.* Rim of sclera that is visible at the temporal edge of optic nerve head with ophthalmoscopy. 2. *Function.* The portion of the far peripheral temporal monocular visual field that is located beyond the binocular field.

temporal lobe. *Anatomy.* In the brain, the area at the side of each cerebral hemisphere. Contains the major portion of the optic radiations, the vision-conducting pathway to the occipital lobe. See also FRONTAL LOBE, OCCIPITAL CORTEX, PARIETAL LOBE.

temporal loop, Meyer's temporal loop. *Anatomy.* Portion of optic radiations in the temporal lobe of the brain that circles the lateral ventricles before continuing to the occipital lobe. See also "PIE IN THE SKY" DEFECT.

temporal pallor. *Clinical sign.* Loss of normal pinkish color of the temporal part of the optic disc. Usually signifies some degree of optic nerve damage.

tendon. *Anatomy.* Strong fibrous band of tissue that attaches a muscle to another part of the body, e.g., an extraocular muscle to sclera.

tenectomy (teh-NEK-tuh-mee). *Surgical procedure.* Removal of part of a tendon; weakens action of the muscle to which it is attached.

Tenon's capsule, fascia bulbi. *Anatomy.* Thin, fibrous, somewhat elastic membrane that envelops the eyeball from the limbus (edge of the cornea) to the optic nerve; attaches loosely to the sclera and to extraocular muscle tendons. See also INTERMUSCULAR MEMBRANE, MUSCLE SHEATH.

Tenormin. *Drug.* Trade name of atenolol, which controls high blood pressure (hypertension).

tenotomy (ten-AH-tuh-mee). *Surgical procedure.* Cutting a tendon without actually removing any severed tissue. Weakens action of the muscle to which it is attached.

    free: cutting an extraocular muscle from its place of insertion on the eyeball, allowing it to retract. Rarely used.

    intrasheath: weakening a superior oblique muscle by dissecting and then severing its tendon from the sheath.

Tensilon (TEN-sil-on). *Drug.* Trade name of edrophonium chloride; used in testing for myasthenia gravis.

tension (intraocular) (TN), intraocular pressure. 1. *Function.* Fluid pressure inside the eye. 2. *Test.* Assessment of pressure inside the eye with a tonometer. See also GLAUCOMA, HYPOTONY, TONOMETRY.

tension by applanation (TA, TAP) (ap-lan-AY-shun), **applanation tonometry**. *Test.* Determination of intraocular pressure by measuring the force required to flatten a specific amount of central cornea. See also TONOMETRY.

Tenzel flap. *Surgical procedure.* For reconstructing a central eyelid (upper or lower). Skin tissue is dissected from cheek and the flap rotated nasally. Similar to Mustarde flap, but does not require a mucous membrane graft.

teratogen (TEHR-uh-tuh-gen). Any agent (e.g., drug, virus) that produces a functional or anatomic abnormality while an embryo or fetus is developing.

teratoma. *Pathologic condition.* Congenital benign tumor mass containing tissue representative of all three germ layers. See also CHORISTOMA.

terigium. Incorrect spelling of PTERYGIUM.

Terrien's ulcer (TEHR-ee-inz). *Pathologic condition.* Thinning of cornea at the corneal margin (limbus), sometimes with vascularization and fat (lipid) deposits. Results in progressive astigmatism and the potential for leaking and perforation.

Terson's syndrome. *Pathologic condition.* Vitreous and retinal hemorrhages caused by increased ocular venous pressure secondary to increased intracranial pressure from a subdural or subarachnoid hemorrhage. Usually clears spontaneously.

tertiary positions (TUR-shee-ehr-ee). *Function.* Four positions (up/right, up/ left, down/right, down/left) to which the eyes move in parallel. Useful for testing how well the four pairs of vertically-acting yoke muscles move and for determining the extraocular muscle

causing an eye deviation. See also DIAGNOSTIC POSITIONS OF GAZE, PRIMARY POSITIONS, SECONDARY POSITIONS.

tertiary vitreous (VIT-ree-us). *Anatomy.* Develops in the lens zonules from fine vitreous fibrils, beginning in the 3rd month of fetal life. See also PRIMARY VITREOUS, SECONDARY VITREOUS.

tetracaine. *Drug.* Anesthetic eyedrop. Trade name: Pontocaine.

Tetracon. *Drug.* Trade name of tetrahydrozoline; decongestant for "whitening" the eye.

tetracycline. *Drug.* Antibiotic agent for treating eye infections.

tetrahydrozoline (TEH-truh-hi-DRAH-zoh-leen). *Drug.* Decongestant sympathomimetic eyedrop that constricts conjunctival blood vessels to "whiten" the eye. Trade names: Murine Plus, Soothe, Tetracon, Visine.

TFT, F₃T. See TRIFLUOROTHYMIDINE.

thermal burns. *Injury.* Burns caused by heat.

thermal sclerostomy (skler-AHS-toh-mee), **Scheie procedure**. *Surgical procedure.* Type of filtering surgery used in the treatment of narrow angle and open angle glaucoma. Combines a peripheral hole in the iris (iridectomy) with a filtration channel for aqueous exit (filtering bleb).

thermal sclerotomy (sklehr-AH-tuh-mee). *Surgical procedure.* Use of heat cautery to burn through the sclera. Shrinks tissue to produce a triangular hole, permitting permanent drainage of aqueous fluid; for control of glaucoma. See also PERIPHERAL IRIDECTOMY, TRABECULECTOMY.

thermoplasty. *Surgical procedure.* Type of refractive surgery in which heat is applied to the cornea to shrink the stroma, which alters its curvature.

thimerosal (thi-MEHR-uh-sol). *Chemical.* Preservative used in many eyedrops and contact lens wetting and cleaning solutions.

thioglycollate broth (thi-oh-GLI-koh-layt). Laboratory culture medium designed to foster growth of anerobic (not needing oxygen) bacteria.

third cranial nerve (N III), oculomotor nerve. *Anatomy.* Primary motor nerve to the eye. Originates in front of the cerebral aqueduct in mid-brain area of the brainstem; runs through the cavernous sinus to enter the orbit through the superior orbital fissure, where it divides. The superior division innervates the superior rectus and eyelid levator muscles. The inferior division innervates the medial rectus, inferior rectus and inferior oblique muscles, and carries parasympathetic fibers to the pupil sphincter and ciliary body muscles.

third grade fusion, binocular depth perception, stereopsis, stereoscopic vision. *Function.* Visual blending of two similar (not identical) images, one falling on each retina, into one, with visual perception of solidity and depth.

third nerve (N III) palsy. *Pathologic condition.* Weakness of the muscles innervated by the 3rd (oculomotor) cranial nerve: includes the eyelid levator, inferior oblique, medial rectus, inferior rectus and superior rectus muscles, and sometimes the pupillary sphincter and ciliary muscles. The involved eye usually deviates outward and slightly downward and has an extremely droopy (ptotic) upper eyelid without its lid fold; sometimes the pupil is dilated and accommodation is reduced. See also OCULOMOTOR PALSIES.

thisis bulbi. Incorrect spelling of PHTHISIS BULBI.

Thomson syndrome, Bloch-Stauffer *(or)* **Rothmund syndrome**. *Congenital disorder.* Characterized by cataracts and skin pigmentation abnormalities. Hereditary.

Thorazine. *Drug.* Trade name for a type of phenothiazine; tranquilizing agent used also to prevent vomiting.

three-mirror lens. *Instrument.* Large diagnostic contact lens that has three embedded mirrors inclined at different angles; allows examiner to visualize the equatorial and peripheral retina, ciliary body and anterior chamber angle structures with a slit lamp. See also GOLDMANN LENS, GONIOLENS.

three-step test. For determining which extraocular muscle is underacting, causing a vertical eye deviation (hypertropia) in the absence of any mechanical restriction of the eyeball. See also BIELSCHOWSKY HEAD TILT TEST.

three-suture operation (Quickert), lid-bracing sutures. *Surgical procedure.* For repair of an inturned lower eyelid (ectropion). Three horizontal stitches are placed just below the tarsal edge to penetrate the lower eyelid at its inner, central and outer portions. See also SENILE ENTROPION.

threshold stimulus. *Test target.* Weakest size or intensity of a target that can be detected by an individual.

thromboendarterectomy. *Surgical procedure.* Removal of a clot from the inner lining of a blood vessel.

thrombophlebitis (thrahm-boh-fluh-BI-tus), **phlebitis**. *Pathologic condition.* Inflammation of a vein.

thrombus (THRAHM-bus). *Pathologic condition.* Clot of blood formed within a blood vessel and remaining attached there, sometimes blocking all flow. Can result from slowed circulation, abnormal blood, or abnormal blood vessel walls. Plural: thrombi.

Thygeson's superficial punctate keratitis (SPK) (TI-guh-sunz). *Pathologic condition.* Corneal disease characterized by small superficial corneal lesions. Symptoms include foreign body sensation and sensitivity to bright light. Sometimes recurs after spontaneous remission. Cause unknown.

thyroid eye disease, Basedow's *(or)* **Graves' disease, endocrine exophthalmos** *(or)* **ophthalmopathy, thyrotoxic** *(or)* **thyrotrophic exophthalmos**. *Pathologic condition.* Eye signs that may occur in patients with excessive thyroid-related hormone concentration. Includes eyelid retraction, eyelid lag on downward gaze, corneal drying, eye bulging (proptosis), fibrotic extraocular muscles, and optic nerve inflammation. See also DALRYMPLE'S SIGN, HYPERTHYROIDISM, STELLWAG'S SIGN, VON GRAEFE'S SIGN.

thyrotoxic exophthalmos (thi-roh-TAHK-sik eks-ahf-THAL-mus). See THYROID EYE DISEASE.

thyrotrophic exophthalmos (thi-roh-TROH-fik). See THYROID EYE DISEASE.

tic douloureux (doh-luh-RU), **trigeminal neuralgia**. *Pathologic condition.* Repeated, excruciating, stabbing pain in the face in the areas supplied by branches of the 5th (trigeminal) cranial nerve.

timolol (TIM-uh-lol). *Drug.* 1. Beta-one and beta-two adrenergic-blocking agent that reduces aqueous secretion. Used as eyedrop for treating glaucoma. Has no effect on the pupil or on accommodation. Trade names: Betimol, Timoptic. 2. Medication that controls high blood pressure (hypertension) by its action as a beta-blocker. Trade name: Blocardren. See also BETAXOLOL, CARTEOLOL, LEVOBUNOLOL, METIPRANOLOL, SYMPATHOLYTIC DRUGS.

Timoptic, Timoptic-XE (tim-AHP-tik). *Drug.* Trade name of timolol eyedrops; for treating glaucoma.

tinnitus (TIN-uh-tus). *Symptom.* Sensation of ringing or buzzing in the ears.

tisis. *Incorrect spelling of* PHTHISIS.

tissue adhesive. *Surgical material.* Plastic substance that can attach tissues to each other, e.g., isobutyl 2-cyanacrylate.

Titmus chart (TIT-mus). *Test.* Stereo-acuity test for near, based on retinal image disparity. Wearing polarized filters, the patient views a vectograph composed of a series of nine diamond-shaped figures, each with four dots, of which one should appear closer to the eye than the others. See also RANDOT TEST, TNO TEST.

TNO stereo test. For measurement of stereo acuity. With a red filter placed over one eye and a green filter over the other, the patient views patterns that will be seen as three-dimensional only when both eyes are working together. See also RANDOT TEST, TITMUS CHART.

tobacco amblyopia (am-blee-OH-pee-uh). *Functional loss.* Decreased vision in both eyes, presumably caused by excessive use of tobacco but may actually be due to poor nutrition, especially lack of B vitamins. Results in a central visual field defect extending to the blind spot (centrocecal scotoma). May be reversible with proper nutrition. See also NUTRITIONAL AMBLYOPIA.

"tobacco dust." *Clinical sign.* Descriptive term for clumps of pigment in the vitreous. Can accompany a retinal tear, retinitis pigmentosa or other problem.

TobraDex. *Drug.* Trade name of a combination of tobramycin (antibiotic) and dexamethasone (steroid).

tobramycin (toh-bruh-MI-sin). *Drug.* Wide spectrum antibiotic eyedrop used for treating external eye infections. Trade name: Tobrex.

Tobrex. *Drug.* Trade name for tobramycin eyedrops; for treating external eye infections.

tolazamide. *Drug.* For controlling blood sugar levels in diabetics. Trade name: Tolinase. See also GLIPIZIDE, GLYBURIDE, TOLBUTAMIDE.

tolazoline (toh-LAZ-oh-leen). *Drug.* Stimulates sympathetic nerves. May be injected behind the eyeball in an attempt to increase blood flow and unblock a blocked central retinal artery. Trade name: Priscoline.

tolbutamide. *Drug.* For controlling blood sugar levels in diabetics. Trade name:

Orinase. See also GLIPIZIDE, GLYBURIDE, TOLAZAMIDE.

Tolinase. *Drug.* Trade name of tolazamide; for treating diabetes.

Tolosa-Hunt syndrome (tuh-LOH-suh), **painful ophthalmoplegia.** *Pathologic condition.* Inflammatory condition characterized by severe pain and restricted eye movement due to palsy of the 3rd (oculomotor), 4th (trochlear), 5th (trigeminal) and 6th (abducens) cranial nerves; sympathetic nerve fibers and optic nerve may be involved. No optic disc swelling (papilledema); affects one eye; occurs in 4th or 5th decade of life. See also CAVERNOUS SINUS SYNDROME, ORBITAL APEX SYNDROME, SUPERIOR ORBITAL FISSURE SYNDROME.

tomogram (TOH-moh-gram). *Test.* X-ray image of thin "slices" of tissue that does not show the structures in front and behind. See also COMPUTERIZED TOMOGRAPHY.

tomography (tuh-MAH-gruh-fee), **polytomography.** *Test.* X-ray imaging technique that utilizes moving film plate and x-ray tube. Displays thin "slices" of tissue (structures in front and behind are blurred out and do not show).

    computerized: low dosage x-rays coupled with computers to generate a film showing fine tissue detail. Also called CT scan.

tonic convergence. *Function.* Portion of convergence ability that occurs by changing from the sleeping to the awake state.

tonic pupil, Adie's pupil, pupillotonia. *Pathologic condition.* Characterized by defective, slow pupillary constriction to light with sluggish redilation and decreased focusing ability (accommodation) for near. Unilateral; at first, the affected pupil is larger, later smaller than in the fellow eye. Seen with diseases of, or injury to, the ciliary ganglion. See also MECHOLYL TEST.

tonography (tuh-NAH-gruh-fee). *Test.* Determination of how intraocular pressure responds to pressure on the eye, based on how easily fluid can be forced out of the eye by pressing on the cornea with a fixed weight. Eye pressure decrease is graphed electronically over a 4-minute period; is slower than normal in glaucoma. See also INDENTATION TONOMETER.

tonometer (tuh-NAH-mih-tur). *Instrument.* Device that measures intraocular pressure. See also TONOPEN.

    applanation: measures the force required to flatten a small area of central cornea. Does not indent the eyeball, so actual intraocular pressure is not distorted. Usually attaches to slit lamp. Examples: Goldmann, Draeger.

    indentation: measures amount the cornea is indented by a fixed weight that artificially raises the pressure. Somewhat less accurate than applanation. Example: Schiotz.

    pneumo-, pneumatic: blows puff of air against the cornea and flattens it slightly. Gas pressurized; does not require contact with the eye.

tonometry (tuh-NAH-mih-tree). *Test.* Measurement of intraocular pressure in millimeters of mercury. See also TONOMETER.

Tonopen. *Instrument.* Trade name of compact electronic tonometer that provides a digital reading of intraocular pressure.

topical. *Description.* Refers to local application to or action on the surface of a body part.

topography. Process of creating a map that describes the shapes of surfaces. Shows relative elevations connected by contour lines.

    corneal: map of the variations in front surface curvature of the cornea. See also PHOTOKERATOSCOPY, PLACIDO DISK.

TORCH. Acronym (TOxoplasmosis, Rubella, Cytomegalovirus, Herpes) for organisms that cause intrauterine infection of the mother and can cross the placenta to infect the infant. Example: optic atrophy.

toric lens (TOR-ik), **sphero-cylindrical lens.** *Optical device.* Lens that has a cylindrical component; used for correcting an astigmatic refractive error. Most eyeglasses are of this type.

torsion, wheel rotation. *Function.* Rotation of an eye around its antero-posterior axis so that it tilts either inward (toward nose) or outward. See also CYCLODUCTION, CYCLOVERSION, Y AXIS OF FICK.

torticollis (tor-tih-KAHL-is). *Abnormal function.* Twisted neck that results in an abnormal head position. May be related to an extraocular muscle problem or to an orthopedic neck or spine problem.

tortuous. *Description.* Having repeated bends and twists; usually refers to blood vessels.

tosis. Incorrect spelling of PTOSIS.

total astigmatism (uh-STIG-muh-tizm). *Refractive error.* Sum of corneal and lenticular astigmatism; used in determining a contact lens prescription. See also K-READINGS.

touton giant cell (TOO-tahn) (*Pathologic change*). A multinucleated cell with the nuclei distributed regularly around the periphery with a rim of foamy cytoplasm. Seen in juvenile xanthogranuloma (JXG).

toxic amblyopia (am-blee-OH-pee-uh). *Functional defect.* Reduced vision and accompanying visual field defects with no obvious ocular abnormality; usually in both eyes. Caused by excessive consumption of tobacco, alcohol, or a poisonous substance. See also CENTROCECAL SCOTOMA.

toxin. Noxious or poisonous substance derived from a living organism.

Toxocara canis (tahks-uh-KEHR-uh KAY-nus). *Organism.* Worm larva (ascarid) that develops from eggs carried in the gastrointestinal tract of puppies. Infects humans (usually children) who accidentally eat fecal material, causing visceral larva migrans. Larva may enter the retina from the bloodstream and lead to localized inflammation; later may cause an elevated retinal or vitreous mass, sometimes with violent vitreous reaction. See also "WIPE-OUT" SYNDROME.

toxocariasis (tahks-oh-kehr-I-uh-sis). *Pathologic condition.* Infection by the larva of the *Toxocara canis* worm, which can invade the eye and retina.

toxoplasmosis (tahks-oh-plaz-MOH-sus). *Pathologic condition.* Infection from the protozoan *Toxoplasma gondii*. Affects many body tissues, especially lungs, liver and brain. When retina is involved, an acute retino-choroidal inflammation is produced; when healed, results in a dense scar surrounded by pigment. Reactivations may occur adjacent to the primary scar and create satellite lesions.

T-PRK (tracker-assisted laser). *Surgical procedure.* Photorefractive keratoplasty using a small (1 mm) excimer laser beam and scanning technology coupled with a sophistocated eye tracker.

trabecular meshwork (truh-BEK-yu-lur), **cribiform ligament, ligamentum pectinatum iridis, scleral trabeculae, trabeculum**. *Anatomy.* Mesh-like structure inside the eye at the iris-scleral junction of the anterior chamber angle. Filters aqueous fluid and controls its flow into the canal of Schlemm, prior to its leaving the anterior chamber.

trabeculectomy (truh-bek-yu-LEK-tuh-mee). *Surgical procedure.* Removal of part of the trabecular meshwork to increase outflow of aqueous from the eye; type of filtering procedure used in treatment of glaucoma.

    excimer (partial): unroofing Schlemm's canal with an excimer laser, then creating a conjunctival flap to cover the opening, forming a filtering bleb. Decreases outflow resistance for glaucoma control.

trabeculoplasty (laser) (truh-BEK-yu-loh-plas-tee). *Surgical procedure.* Application of a laser beam to selectively burn the trabecular meshwork area, to lower intraocular pressure. Used for treating open angle glaucoma.

trabeculotomy (truh-bek-yu-LAH-tuh-mee). *Surgical procedure.* Incision into the trabeculum to increase aqueous drainage from an eye with glaucoma.

    t. ab externo: cutting from outside the eye inward to reach Schlemm's canal, the trabecular meshwork, and the anterior chamber; treatment for congenital glaucoma, especially when there is a cloudy cornea.

partial excimer t: unroofing Schlemm's canal with an excimer laser, then forming a conjunctival flap to cover the opening to form a filtering bleb. Decreases outflow resistance for glaucoma control.

trabeculum. See TRABECULAR MESHWORK.

trachoma (truh-KOH-muh). *Pathologic condition*. Severe, chronic, contagious conjunctival eyelid and corneal infection caused by a virus (chlamydial microorganisms); leads to corneal blood vessel formation, corneal clouding, conjunctival and eyelid scarring, and dry eyes. Leading cause of blindness in the world.

trachoma inclusion conjunctivitis virus family (TRIC) (kun-junk-tih-VI-tus). *Microorganism*. Group of chlamydial microorganisms that cause conjunctivitis-producing follicles and microscopic intracellular inclusion bodies.

traction detachment. *Pathologic condition*. Separation of the sensory retina from the pigment epithelium, caused by fibrovascular scars that pull and hold the retina. May result from eye inflammation or trauma that has caused new blood vessel formation on the surface of the retina and into the vitreous. See also PROLIFERATIVE RETINOPATHY.

traction sutures. *Surgical technique*. Stitches attached to a muscle or the sclera to permit temporary immobilization of the eyeball.

traction test, forced ductions, passive forced duction test. Forcibly moving the eyeball into different positions by grasping the anesthetized conjunctiva and episclera with forceps at the corneo-scleral junction (limbus). For determining if there are any mechanical restrictions to movement.

transient ischemic attack (TIA) (is-KEE-mik), **"ministroke."** *Pathologic condition*. Temporary interruption of blood supply to the small blood vessels of the brain, producing temporary (less than an hour) loss of vision. See also AMAUROSIS FUGAX.

transient obscuration of vision (TOV). *Symptom*. Temporary vision loss in both eyes upon standing or sneezing, sometimes in association with papilledema and increased intracranial pressure. Lasts minutes; recovery usually complete. See also PSEUDOTUMOR CEREBRI.

transillumination. *Test*. Use of an intense light beam (e.g., slit lamp or small flashlight) to shine through translucent eye tissue to better visualize ocular tumors, cysts or hemorrhages in sillhouette.

transposition. 1. *Surgical procedure*. Repositioning a normal extraocular muscle beside a non-functioning muscle to correct an eye deviation. 2. *Mathematical formula*. Converting a prescription for a sphero-cylindrical lens from plus-cylinder form into equivalent minus-cylinder form, or vice versa.

transposition flap, pedicle flap. *Surgical procedure*. Tongue-shaped section of skin and its subcutaneous tissue, cut to maintain its blood supply. Used for covering a defect (from trauma or surgical removal of a tumor or scar) from an adjacent or nonadjacent area. Variation of a rotation flap.

transverse axis of Fick, x axis of Fick. Imaginary horizontal line passing through the center of each eye as an axle around which the eye rotates for up and down movements.

transverse blepharotomy with lid marginal rotation, Wies procedure. *Surgical procedure*. For repair of an inward turning eyelid (entropion) due to scarring. See also CICATRICIAL ENTROPION.

transverse keratotomy. *Surgical procedure*. Incision into the cornea parallel to the limbus; usually to reduce astigmatism after corneal surgery. See also REFRACTIVE SURGERY.

Trantas dots (TRAN-tus). *Clinical sign*. Clumps of inflammatory cells in tissues at the corneo-scleral junction (limbus); appears with vernal conjunctivitis.

trauma. Injury.

traumatic cataract. *Pathologic condition*. Cloudiness of the crystalline lens caused by injury. Penetration of the lens capsule results in total opacity within hours.

Treacher-Collins syndrome, Franceschetti syndrome, mandibulofacial dysostosis. *Congenital anomaly*. Bony deformity of skull and face characterized by a bird-like appearance (small jaw, "parrotbeak" nose), indistinct orbital margins, notching of lower eyelids (coloboma), and an anti-mongoloid eyelid slant. Rare; hereditary. See also HALLERMANN-STREIFF SYNDROME.

trephine (TREE-fine). 1. *Surgical instrument*. Cutting tool that makes a circular hole in tissue, e.g., corneal "button" for a corneal transplant. 2. *Surgical procedure*. Small hole through the sclera at the limbus, for treatment of glaucoma; obsolete.

Treponema pallidum immobilization test (TPI) (trep-oh-NEE-muh PAL-ih-dum). *Lab test*. Blood test to detect previous syphilis infection.

trial frame. *Instrument*. Lens holder with adjustable parts for fitting the face and holding lenses, used in refraction. Resembles a spectacle frame.

trial lenses. *Test instrument*. Set of lenses in graded powers that are used with a trial frame for refining refractions.

TRIC. *Microorganism*. Acronym for TRachoma and Inclusion Conjunctivitis. See TRACHOMA INCLUSION CONJUNCTIVITIS VIRUS FAMILY.

trichiasis (trih-KI-uh-sus). *Pathological condition*. Misdirected upper or lower eyelashes that turn inward toward the eyeball; may scratch the cornea. Usually follows severe eyelid inflammation or scarring. See also ENTROPION.

trichromatism (tri-KROH-muh-tizm). *Function*. Color vision status of an individual whose retinal cones contain three photopigments.

> **normal**: normal proportion of color cones and cone pigments.

> **anomalous**: abnormal proportion of color cones or cone pigments, resulting in the most common types of "color blindness."

trifluorothymidine (F$_3$T, TFT) (tri-flor-oh-THI-mih-deen). *Drug*. Antiviral eyedrop used for treating herpetic corneal infections. Trade name: Viroptic.

trifocal (TRI-foh-kul). *Optical device*. Eyeglass lens that incorporates three lenses of different powers. The main portion is usually focused for distance (20 ft.), the center segment for about 2 ft., and the lower segment for near (14 in.). See also MULTIFOCAL LENS.

trigeminal nerve (tri-JEM-in-ul). *Anatomy*. Fifth cranial nerve. Large three-branched cranial nerve originating in the pons area of brainstem. The 1st branch (ophthalmic nerve) carries sensory impulses to the brain from the eyeballs, conjunctiva, eyelids, brow, forehead, and front half of the scalp.

trigeminal neuralgia, tic douloureux. *Pathologic condition*. Repeated, excruciating, stabbing pain in the face in the areas supplied by branches of the 5th (trigeminal) cranial nerve.

triple procedure. *Surgical procedure*. Any group of three surgical procedures performed at the same time, e.g., corneal transplant, cataract extraction, and intraocular lens implantation.

triplopia (trih-PLOH-pee-uh). *Functional defect*. Seeing three images of one object; usually caused by an early cataract. May be monocular (visible with one eye) or binocular. See also DIPLOPIA, POLYOPIA.

trisomy 13 syndrome (tri-SOH-mee), **D-trisomy** *(or)* **Patau's syndrome**. *Congenital anomaly*. Multiple defects in brain, face, and eyes caused by an extra chromosome. Fatal.

trisomy 21, Down's syndrome, mongolism. *Congenital defect*. Mental retardation associated with an extra chromosome (#21). Eye signs include lower eyelid margins that slant upward toward the lateral canthi (mongoloid slant), Brushfield spots in iris, cataracts, inward deviation (esotropia), nearsightedness (myopia), blepharitis, keratoconus.

tritanomaly (tri-tuh-NAHM-uh-lee). *Functional defect.* Color vision deficiency that affects blue-yellow hue discrimination. Rare; hereditary. See also DEUTERANOMALY, PROTANOMALY.

tritanopia (tri-tan-OH-pee-uh). *Functional defect.* Color vision disturbance; form of dichromatism in which there are only two cone pigments and total absence of blue retinal receptors. Rare.

trochlea (TROH-klee-uh). *Anatomy.* Ring-like cartilage attached nasally to the frontal bone along the upper orbital rim. Acts as a pulley for the tendon of the superior oblique muscle.

trochlear nerve (TROH-klee-ur). *Anatomy.* Fourth cranial nerve. Motor nerve that innervates the superior oblique muscle of the eye. Originates in the lower midbrain; enters the orbit through the superior orbital fissure.

tropia (TROH-pee-uh), **deviation, heterotropia, squint, strabismus**. *Functional defect.* Eye misalignment caused by extraocular muscle imbalance: one fovea is not directed at same object as the other. Present even with both eyes uncovered. See also PHORIA.

tropicamide (truh-PIK-uh-mide). *Drug.* Short-acting cycloplegic eyedrop. Trade name: Mydriacyl.

troposcope (TROH-puh-skohp), **synoptophore**. *Test instrument.* Type of major amblyoscope; used in the evaluation and treatment of binocularity problems. See also HAPLOSCOPE.

true exfoliation. *Pathologic condition.* Peeling of the superficial layers of the lens capsule. Usually accompanies exposure to extreme heat (e.g., molten glass). See also PSEUDOEXFOLIATION.

true image. In diplopia, the image received by the non-deviating eye.

Trusopt. *Drug.* Trade name of dorzolamide eyedrops; for treating glaucoma.

tuberculosis. *Pathologic condition.* Communicable disease caused by the tubercle bacillus; affects the entire body but especially the lungs. Eye findings include blurred vision, "mutton fat" keratic precipitates, "cell and flare," iris nodules, and gray isolated masses (tubercles) in the choroid.

tuberous sclerosis (TU-bur-us sklehr-OH-sis), **Bourneville's disease**. *Pathologic condition.* Characterized by seizures, mental retardation, behavior disorders and skin tumors. Eyes may show benign retinal tumors (resembling tapioca or mulberries). Hereditary.

tubular visual fields. See TUNNEL VISION.

tuberculin skin test, PPD (purified protein derivative). Skin test for tuberculosis.

tuck. *Surgical procedure.* Folding and stitching a muscle tendon into a loop, to shorten it. Used to strengthen a weak eyelid muscle (as in ptosis surgery) or extraocular muscle.

tucking of the levator aponeurosis. *Surgical procedure.* For repair of a slight-to-moderately drooping eyelid (ptosis). An incision into the upper eyelid in the lid crease is extended through the orbicularis muscle. Thin or torn levator aponeurosis is brought forward and stitched to the tarsus.

tuck of the eyelid retractors, tuck of the inferior aponeurosis. *Surgical procedure.* For repair of an inward turning lower eyelid (entropion). A horizontal incision is made below the lid to remove the orbicularis muscle and restore the lid to its normal position. See also SENILE ENTROPION.

tuck of the inferior aponeurosis. See TUCK OF THE EYELID RETRACTORS.

tumbling E, illiterate E. *Test.* The letter E presented in different sizes and rotated to different directions; used for testing visual acuity in illiterates and children who do not know the alphabet.

tunica fibrosa oculi (TU-nih-kuh fi-BROH-suh AHK-yu-li), **sclera**. *Anatomy.* Opaque, fibrous, protective outer layer

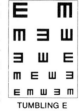

TUMBLING E

265

of the eye ("white of the eye"), continuous with the cornea in front and with the sheath covering the optic nerve behind. Contains collagen and elastic fibers.

tunica nervosa oculi (nur-VOH-suh), **retina**. *Anatomy.* Part of the eye (embryologically part of brain) that converts images from the eye's optical system into electrical impulses that are sent along the optic nerve for transmission to the brain. Forms a thin membranous lining of the rear two-thirds of the globe. Consists of layers that include rods and cones; bipolar, amacrine, ganglion, horizontal and Müller cells; and all interconnecting nerve fibers. See also EXTERNAL LIMITING MEMBRANE, INNER NUCLEAR LAYER, INNER PLEXIFORM LAYER, INTERNAL LIMITING MEMBRANE, NERVE FIBER BUNDLE LAYER, OUTER NUCLEAR LAYER, OUTER PLEXIFORM LAYER.

tunica vascularis oculi (vas-kyu-LEHR-is), **uvea**. *Anatomy.* Pigmented layers of the eye (iris, ciliary body, choroid) that contain most of the intraocular blood vessels.

tunica vasculosa lentis (vas-kyu-LOH-suh LEN-tis). *Anatomy.* Embryonic blood vessel network covering the back of the lens until the 5th month of fetal life.

tunnel vision, tubular field. *Functional loss.* Loss of peripheral visual field with retention of some central field. Typical of the end stage of glaucoma and retinitis pigmentosa. Tubular field sometimes refers to the narrowed field of a malingerer, which remains of constant size at any testing distance.

turijium. Incorrect spelling of PTERYGIUM.

Turkish saddle, sella turcica. *Anatomy.* Bony pocket in the base of the skull, between and behind the orbits. Supports the pituitary gland.

Turner's syndrome. *Pathologic condition.* X-chromosome abnormality (female with one of the two X chromosomes missing). May be associated with widely set eyes, vertical skin folds over the epicanthus, and droopy eyelids (ptosis).

20/20, 6/6. Normal visual acuity. Upper number indicates that a patient can see standardized symbols on a chart 20 ft. (6 m) away; lower number indicates that the same symbols can be seen at 20 ft. by an eye with a normal optical system. See also SNELLEN CHART.

two-snip *(or)* **one-snip operation**. *Surgical procedure.* Technique(s) for opening a constricted punctum to the lacrimal canaliculus.

two-stitch *(or)* **one-stitch** *(or)* **no-stitch surgery**. *Surgical procedure.* Cataract extraction technique using minimal size incision into the eye, with lens fragmentation and removal by phacoemulsification. See also EXTRACAPSULAR CATARACT EXTRACTION.

tylosis ciliaris. *Abnormal condition.* Thickening of the eyelid margins, often as a consequence of chronic blepharitis.

Tyndall effect (TIN-dul), **aqueous flare**. *Clinical sign.* Scattering of a slit lamp light beam directed into the anterior chamber; occurs when aqueous has increased protein content. Sign of iris and/or ciliary body inflammation (iritis).

typical monochromacy, rod monochromacy. *Congenital defect.* Rare inability to distinguish colors as a result of absent or nonfunctioning retinal cones. Associated with light sensitivity (photophobia), involuntary eye oscillations (nystagmus) and poor vision. Nonprogressive. See also CONE MONOCHROMACY.

tysis. Incorrect spelling of PHTHISIS.

U

UGH syndrome. *Pathologic condition*. Acronym (Uveitis, Glaucoma, Hyphema) for complications that occur secondary to intraocular lens implantation in the anterior chamber. Caused by rubbing of the lens loops (haptics).

Uhtoff's sign. *Clinical sign*. Temporary decrease in vision, double vision, or nystagmus when body temperature rises. Seen in patients with multiple sclerosis.

ulcer (corneal). *Pathologic condition*. Area of epithelial tissue loss from the corneal surface; associated with inflammatory cells in the cornea and anterior chamber. Usually caused by a bacterial, fungal or viral infection.

ultrasonography. See ULTRASOUND

ultrasound, echography, ultrasonography. *Test*. Transmission of high frequency sound waves into the eye, which are reflected by the ocular tissues and displayed on a screen so that internal structures can be visualized. Aids in diagnosis of eye and orbital problems. See also A-SCAN, B-SCAN.

Ultra Tears. *Drug*. Trade name of methylcellulose eyedrops; for treating dry eyes.

ultraviolet. *Optics*. Light with wavelengths between about 250–400 nm (invisible to naked eye).

umbilicated. *Description*. Having a small pit-shaped depression; resembles a navel.

uncrossed diplopia, homonymous diplopia. *Symptom*. Double vision in which the image seen by the right eye appears to the right of the left eye's image. Associated with an inturning eye (esotropia).

undermine. *Surgical technique*. To cut underneath.

unharmonious ARC (abnormal retinal correspondence). *Functional defect*. Binocular adaptation to a long-standing *eye* deviation. Fovea of the straight (non-deviating) eye and a non-foveal point of the deviated eye (but not one that corresponds to the angle of deviation) work together. See also ABNORMAL RETINAL CORRESPONDENCE, HARMONIOUS ARC.

unilateral. *Location*. On one side of the body.

uniocular (yu-nee-AHK-yu-lur). *Description*. Refers to (or affecting) one eye.

up-drawn pupil, ectopic *(or)* **peaked pupil**. *Abnormal condition*. Pupil that is displaced from its normal position. May be from a congenital defect, ocular surgery, or trauma.

up-gaze. *Function*. Upward eye rotation with the head in the straight-ahead position. See also ELEVATION, ELEVATORS.

upbeat nystagmus (ni-STAG-mus). *Functional defect*. Involuntary, rhythmic, upward jerking of both eyes.

upper canaliculus (kan-uh-LIK-yu-lus), **superior canaliculus**. *Anatomy*. Part of the tear drainage system. Thin elastic duct within the upper eyelid on the nasal side; connects the upper punctum to the common canaliculus.

upper punctum, superior punctum. *Anatomy*. Dimple-like opening in the upper eyelid margin near the nose; upper entrance to the tear drainage system. See also SUPERIOR CANALICULUS.

upside down ptosis. *Clinical sign*. Lower eyelid that is higher than normal, giving the appearance of a "sunken" eye. Caused by loss of sympathetic innervation (Horner's syndrome).

urinalysis (U/A) (yur-un-AL-uh-sis). *Lab test*. Chemical analysis of urine, to test for abnormal contents (e.g., albumin, pus, sugar) that may indicate systemic disease.

urticaria. *Clinical sign*. Hives.

Usher's syndrome. *Pathologic condition.* Retinal pigment epithelium degeneration accompanied by congenital nerve deafness. Hereditary. See also COCKAYNE'S SYNDROME.

uvea (YU-vee-uh), **tunica vascularis oculi, uveal tract**. *Anatomy.* Pigmented layers of the eye (iris, ciliary body, choroid) that contain most of the intraocular blood vessels.

uveal tract. See UVEA.

uveitis (yu-vee-I-tis). *Pathologic condition.* Inflammation of any of the structures of the uvea: iris, ciliary body, or choroid. Plural: uveitides.

> **anterior**: inflammation of iris or ciliary body. Also called iridocyclitis.
> **endogenous**: thought to arise from causes within the body.
> **posterior**: inflammation of the choroid.

uveitis-vitiligo-alopecia-poliosis syndrome (vih-til-I-goh al-oh-PEE-shuh poh-lee-OH-sis), **Harada's** *(or)* **Vogt-Koyanagi-Harada syndrome**. *Pathologic condition.* Characterized by headache, hearing defect, hair loss, premature graying, patchy depigmentation of skin, lashes and retina, steamy corneas, vitreous opacities, and diffuse exudative choroiditis. Vision and hearing loss may occur, with incomplete recovery. Progressive, chronic. Rare; tends to affect young Italian or Japanese adults. See also POLIOSIS.

V

valve of Hasner (HAZ-nur), **plica lacrimalis**. *Anatomy.* Mucous membrane fold at the lower end of the nasolacrimal duct. Acts as a valve in preventing air from entering the lacrimal sac when the nose is blown.

vancomycin (van-coh-MI-sin). *Drug.* Antibiotic injected intravenously for treating severe ocular infections.

van der Hoeve's syndrome (VAN-duh-hoovz), **osteogenesis imperfecta**. *Pathologic condition.* Characterized by blue scleras, deafness, and fragile bones. Congenital; hereditary.

van Lint akinesia, van Lint facial nerve block. *Surgical technique.* Injection of an anesthetic under the skin along the edge of the lateral and inferior walls of the orbit, to decrease sensation from the 7th (facial) cranial nerve. See also ATKINSON, NADBATH, AND O'BRIEN FACIAL NERVE BLOCKS.

variable strabismus (struh-BIZ-mus). *Functional defect.* Eye deviation (in, out, up or down) that is constant but degree of misalignment varies.

varix. *Abnormal condition.* Dilated, tortuous blood or lymph vessel, such as a varicose vein. Plural: varices.

varrucous lesion. Incorrect spelling of VERRUCOUS LESION.

vascular. *Description.* Referring to, affecting, or constituting a blood or lymph vessel.

vasculature. *Anatomy.* Arrangement of blood vessels in an organ or part.

vasculitis. *Pathologic condition.* Inflammation of a blood or lymph vessel.

Vasocidin. *Drug.* Trade name of eyedrops containing sulfacetamide and prednisolone; for treating eye infections.

Vasoclear. *Drug.* Trade name of naphazoline eyedrops; for "whitening" the eyes.

Vasocon. *Drug.* Trade name of naphazoline eyedrops; for "whitening" the eyes.

Vasocon A. *Drug.* Trade name of eyedrops containing naphazoline (a decongestant) and antazoline (an antihistamine); for treating allergic conjunctivitis.

vectograph. *Test chart.* Chart or picture composed of two polarized images that can be separated visually when viewed with polarized glasses, allowing each eye to see letters or figures that are invisible to the other. For measuring stereo acuity (e.g., Titmus chart) and testing visual acuity.

vectograph slide (Polaroid). *Test chart.* Visual acuity master slide viewed with polarized glasses, to allow each eye to see letters or figures that are invisible to the other. Useful for measuring stereo acuity and for testing visual acuity in monofixators and malingerers.

vein. *Anatomy.* Blood vessel that carries blood toward the heart. See also ARTERY.

venae vorticosae (VEE-nee vor-tih-KOH-see), **vortex veins**. *Anatomy.* Four veins (2 superior, 2 inferior) that provide main blood outflow from the eyes, exiting near the equator on each side of the superior and inferior recti and draining into the superior and inferior ophthalmic veins.

venous beading (VEE-nus). *Sign.* Pattern of nodular irregularity in the retinal venous blood vessel walls. Found in some retinopathies, e.g., Coats' disease, diabetic retinopathy.

venous phase. *Clinical sign.* Last phase of fluorescein angiography; the veins fill with dye before the fluorescence fades. Follows arterial phase.

venous stasis retinopathy (STAY-sus). *Pathologic condition.* Characterized by engorged retinal veins, splinter hemorrhages in the nerve fiber layer, and optic disc swelling. Caused by occlusion or partial occlusion of the central retinal vein. Retinal findings are less severe and less extensive than in hemorrhagic retinopathy. Vision usually improves over months unless retinal swelling causes irreversible macular changes. Patients are often middle-age or younger. See also AMAUROSIS FUGAX, CYSTOID MACULAR EDEMA.

ventral. *Location*. Nearer to the front of the body. Often same as anterior.

vergence (VUR-junss), **disjunctive** *(or)* **disconjugate** *(or)* **disjugate movement**. *Function*. Movement of both eyes in opposite directions (toward or away from each other, up and down) to obtain or maintain single binocular vision.

verapamil. *Drug*. Heart medication that acts as a calcium channel blocker for heart pain (angina) and high blood pressure (hypertension). Trade name: Calan. See also NIFEDIPINE.

vergence ability, amplitudes, fusional amplitudes. *Measurement*. Amount (in diopters) the eyes can move inward (converge) added to the amount they can move outward (diverge), while maintaining single vision.

vergence power. *Optics*. Expression of optical power (in diopters). Applies to distances (e.g., between an object and a lens plane) or to the refractive power of a lens. Equal to the reciprocal of the distance or the lens focal length in meters, e.g., a lens that has a 1/2 m focal length has 2 D of power. See also CONCAVE LENS, CONVEX LENS.

vergence reflex. *Function*. Movement of both eyes outward (divergence) or inward (convergence) to allow maintenance of similar images on both foveae.

vernal catarrh. See VERNAL CONJUNCTIVITIS.

vernal conjunctivitis, vernal·catarrh. *Pathologic condition*. Allergic conjunctival inflammation, with itching and excess mucous, recurring in children during warm weather. Numerous small lumps (papillae) form on the palpebral conjunctiva. Scrapings exhibit many eosinophils.

vernier acuity (vur-NEER). *Function*. The eye's ability to detect minute misalignments of lines. Physiological basis for stereoscopic acuity. See also LANDOLT RING CHART.

verruca (vuh-RU-kuh), **verrucous lesion**. *Pathologic condition*. Wart caused by a virus infection. Can occur anywhere on the skin, including the eyelid. Plural: verrucae.

verrucous lesion. See VERRUCA.

version, conjunctive *(or)* **conjugate** *(or)* **gaze movement**. *Function*. Parallel movement of both eyes in any direction. See also PURSUIT MECHANISM, SACCADES.

vertex distance. *Measurement*. Distance from the front surface of an eye to the back surface of an eyeglass lens. See also DISTOMETER.

vertex power, back vertex *(or)* **effective power**. *Measurement*. Power of a spectacle or contact lens, measured at the back surface with a lensometer.

vertical axis of Fick, z axis of Fick. Imaginary line passing vertically through the center of each eye. Associated with horizontal eye rotations.

vertical gaze center (VGC). *Anatomy*. Area in the upper brainstem near the superior colliculi that integrates vertical gaze signals from the frontal and occipital cortex. See also riMLF.

vertical meridian. 1. *Anatomy*. Imaginary vertical line that divides the eye into temporal and nasal halves. 2. *Optics*. Imaginary vertical reference line on the cornea (from 12 to 6 o'clock). Denotes the 90° meridian for cylinders. 3. *Visual fields*. Imaginary vertical line passing through fixation; divides the visual field of each eye into temporal and nasal zones.

vertical nystagmus (ni-STAG-mus). *Functional defect*. Involuntary, rhythmic vertical movement of both eyes.

vertical strabismus. *Functional defect.* Eye misalignment in which one eye is higher or lower than the other. See also HYPERTROPIA, HYPOTROPIA.

vertical vergence. *Function.* Ability to maintain binocular vision when the eyes are forced to move vertically in opposite directions, as when increasing base-down or base-up prism is placed before one eye.

> **negative:** downward movement of left eye relative to the right, usually to maintain single binocular vision, e.g., when increasing amounts of base-up prism are placed in front of the left eye. Also called left sursumvergence, right deosumvergence.

> **positive:** upward movement of right eye relative to the left, usually to maintain single binocular vision, e.g., when increasing amounts of base-down prism are placed in front of the right eye. Also called left deorsum-vergence, right sursumvergence.

vertigo. *Symptom.* Dizziness.

vestibular nystagmus, caloric *(or)* **labyrinthine nystagmus.** *Functional defect.* Involuntary, jerky eye movements in any direction caused by a disturbance in normal innervation from the labyrinths in the ears. Unrelated to visual stimuli. See also COWS.

vestibular system. *Function.* Neural reflex system with sensory organs in the inner ear. Governs balance and coordination during body movement; also coordinates eye movements with head movements (e.g., keeping eyes fixed on a non-moving object as the head moves). See also OTOLITH APPARATUS.

vestibulo-ocular reflex (VOR), oculo-cephalic reflex. *Function.* Involuntary rotation of the eyes in the opposite direction from head rotation, to maintain fixation on a non-moving target. Abnormal with some brainstem defects. See also OTOLITH APPARATUS, VESTIBULAR SYSTEM.

Vexol. *Drug.* Trade name of rimexolone, a steroid.

vidarabine (vi-DAR-uh-been). *Drug.* Anti-viral ointment used in treating herpes simplex conjunctivitis. Trade name: Vira A.

videokeratoscope. *Instrument.* Video camera that produces a color-coded, 3- dimensional map of the shape of the cornea, calculated in corneal dioptric power by computer to detect variations in optical power across the corneal surface. See also PHOTOKERATOSCOPY.

Viers rod. *Surgical device.* Serves as a stent (supporting structure for keeping a channel open) for repair of lacrimal canalicular tears.

Vieth-Müller horopter (veeth MYU-lur); also spelled Mueller. Imaginary circular representation of the locus of points in space that are imaged simultaneously on corresponding points in the two retinas.

Vira A (VI-ruh). *Drug.* Trade name of vidarabine eye ointment; for treating herpetic keratitis.

viral conjunctivitis (kun-junk-tih-VI-tis), **"pink eye."** *Pathologic condition.* Virus inflammation of the conjunctiva (mucous membrane that covers white of eye and inner eyelids). Characterized by discharge, grittiness, redness and swelling. Usually contagious.

Viroptic. *Drug.* Trade name of trifluorothymidine; for treating herpes virus eye infections.

virtual image. *Optics.* Image created by light rays diverging from an optical system. Rays do not pass through image points, hence cannot be focused directly onto a screen. See also REAL IMAGE.

VISC. *Instrument.* Trade name (acronym): vitreous infusion suction cutter, used in vitreous surgery. Becoming obsolete.

viscoelastic agent. Thick, elastic protective gel injected into the eyeball during corneal or cataract surgery. Helps maintain ocular structures in their normal position, keeps tissues moist, and protects the back of the cornea (endothelium) from surgical damage. Trades names: Amvisc, Healon, Ocucoat. See also SODIUM HYALURONATE.

viscosity. *Description.* Characteristic of a fluid that denotes its resistant to flow or change in shape; describes the ease with which the fluid can be injected through a small needle.

viscosurgery. *Technique.* Eye surgery performed with the aid of viscoelastic fluids. See also SODIUM HYALURONATE.

visible spectrum. *Optics.* That part of the electromagnetic spectrum (wavelengths between about 400 to 750 nm) that can be seen by the naked eye.

Visine. *Drug.* Trade name of tetrahydrozoline decongestant eyedrops.

vision. *Function.* Ability of the eye to receive, resolve and transmit light images to the occipital lobe in the brain, where the light sensation is interpreted. "Seeing ability" in its broadest sense.

   central: an eye's best vision. Results from stimulation of the fovea and macular area.

   distance: visual acuity measured with the target at 20 ft., the optical equivalent of an "infinite distance."

   near: visual acuity measured with the target at 16 in. (approx. 40 cm), corresponding to normal reading distance.

   night: see scotopic (below).

   peripheral: side vision; vision elicited by stimuli falling on areas of the retina distant from the macula.

   photopic (foh-TAHP-ik): eyesight under daylight conditions. Involves the cone photoreceptors, which function for sharp resolution of detail and color discrimination.

   rod: see scotopic (below).

   scotopic: refers to vision at low light levels; primarily a function of (retinal) rods. Maximum sensitivity is usually after 30 minutes in the dark.

Vistech system. Test for contrast sensitivity; ability to detect detail with subtle gradations in grayness between the test target and the background.

visual acuity. *Measurement.* Assessment of the eye's ability to distinguish object details and shape, using the smallest identifiable object that can be seen at a specified distance (usually 20 ft. or 16 in.).

visual association areas. *Anatomy.* Cortical areas in the brain that surround the primary occipital visual cortex, where visual messages are interpreted, integrated and relayed. See also BRODMANN AREA 17, 18, 19.

visual angle. *Measurement.* Angle that an object or detail subtends at the eye; usually measured in degrees or minutes of arc.

visual axis, line of fixation, primary line of sight, principal line of direction, visual line. Imaginary line connecting a viewed object and the fovea. See also FIXATION.

visual cortex (primary), Brodmann area 17, striate area. *Anatomy.* Area (cerebral end of sensory visual pathways) in the occipital lobes of the brain, where initial conscious registration of visual information takes place. See also OCCIPITAL CORTEX.

visual direction. Eye's ability to determine the location of an object in space. See also SPATIAL LOCALIZATION.

visual evoked response (VER), visual evoked cortical potential. *Test.* Computerized recording of electrical activity in the occipital cortex (back of brain) that results from stimulating the retina with light flashes. Used for detecting defects in the retina-to-brain nerve pathway (which can change brain wave patterns).

visual field, field of vision. Full extent of the area visible to an eye that is fixating straight ahead. Measured in degrees from fixation.

visual line. See VISUAL AXIS.

visual pathway, sensory visual pathway. *Anatomy*. The complete course of nerve fibers originating from the retinal visual cells as they travel to the occipital cortex in the brain.

anterior: comprised of nerve fibers from the retina, in the optic nerve, optic chiasm, to the lateral geniculate nucleus in the midbrain.

posterior: comprised of fibers from the lateral geniculate nucleus, through the parietal and temporal lobes of the brain (optic radiations) and ending in the occipital cortex.

visual perseveration, palinopsia. *Functional defect*. Recurrence of visual sensations after removal of the viewed object. Symptoms may be mistaken for monocular double vision.

visual purple, rhodopsin. *Chemical*. Primary photopigment of the rods; one of four photosensitive pigments in the retina. Consists of retinal (a derivative of vitamin A) and the protein opsin. As light strikes the photopigment, it bleaches and begins a chain of electrical impulses that travel along the optic nerve to the brain. See also CHLOROLABE, CYANOLABE, ERYTHROLABE.

visuosensory cortex. See VISUAL CORTEX.

visuscope (VEEZ-uh-skohp). *Instrument*. Modified ophthalmoscope used for examining the fixation pattern. Patient looks at its star-shaped target while the examiner notes the fixation position relative to the fovea.

vitamin A, retinol. *Chemical*. Vitamin A alcohol. Stored in the liver and perhaps retinal pigment epithelium. Ultimately modified and used by the rods and cones as the photosensitive pigment that initiates the visual process.

vitamin deficiency. *Pathologic condition*. Chronic long-term lack of a specific vitamin.

A: affects the eyes severely; causes conjunctival and corneal dryness (xerosis), corneal softening (keratomalacia), conjunctival dry (Bitot) spots, and night blindness. See also XEROPHTHALMIA.

B$_1$ (thiamine): nervous system and gastrointestinal disturbances usually accompanied by conjunctivitis and/or staphylococcal inflammation of the eyelids. Can lead to optic nerve damage and amblyopia. Also called beriberi. See also WERNICKE'S ENCEPHALOPATHY.

B$_{12}$ (cobalamin): can cause pernicious anemia (worsened by heavy smoking) with, possibly, optic nerve degeneration and atrophy. See also TOBACCO AMBLYOPIA.

C (ascorbic acid): causes generalized tendency to hemorrhage. Eye signs include bleeding in the orbit, which can result in eye bulging (proptosis), the eyelids, conjunctiva, iris, retina, and anterior chamber. See also SCURVY.

D: may cause lamellar cataracts.

vitelliform degeneration (vi-TEL-ih-form), **Best's disease**. *Pathologic condition*. Pigment epithelial degeneration primarily affecting the macular area. Lesion initially has appearance of an egg yolk; in later stages it can resemble a scrambled egg. Hereditary.

vitiligo (vih-tih-LI-goh). *Pathologic condition*. Patches of depigmented skin. See also VOGT-KOYANAGI-HARADA SYNDROME.

vitreal bleed (VIT-ree-ul). See VITREOUS HEMORRHAGE.

vitrectomy (vih-TREK-tuh-mee). *Surgical procedure*. Removal of vitreous, blood, and/or membranes from the eye, usually by entering through the pars plana with a needle-like cutter that is associated with suction and fluid injection capabilities. See also OCUTOME.

anterior: removal of the front portion of vitreous tissue. Used for preventing or treating vitreous loss during cataract or corneal surgery, or to remove misplaced vitreous in conditions such as aphakic pupillary block glaucoma.

"open sky": gaining access to the eye from the front, such as by incising the corneal edge (limbus), or removing a corneal button and extracting the lens.

> **Weck cell**: "open sky" vitrectomy with Weck cell cellulose sponges to hold the vitreous while being cut with scissors.

vitreous (VIT-ree-us), **vitreous body** *(or)* **gel** *(or)* **humor**. *Anatomy.* Transparent, colorless gelatinous mass (fine collagen fibrils and hyaluronic acid) that fills the rear two-thirds of the eyeball, between the lens and the retina.

> **primary**: earliest part to develop. Originates from mesodermal tissue during the 1st month of fetal life and regresses to form zonules and the hyaloid canal.

> **secondary**: second stage of embryologic vitreous formation, beginning in the 2nd month of fetal life. Fibrils from the neuroectoderm form around the primary vitreous.

> **tertiary**: develops the lens zonules from fine vitreous fibrils, beginning in the 3rd month of fetal life.

vitreous base. *Anatomy.* Dense, ribbon-like (2 mm wide) firm attachment of vitreous to the surface of the peripheral retina and ora serrata.

vitreous bulge. Forward protrusion of vitreous gel into the anterior chamber. Common during and following cataract extraction.

vitreous detachment, posterior vitreous detachment. *Pathologic condition.* Separation of vitreous gel from the retinal surface. Frequently occurs with aging as the vitreous liquifies, or in some disease states, e.g., diabetes and high myopia. Usually innocuous but can cause retinal tears, which may lead to retinal detachment.

vitreous face. *Anatomy.* Condensation of the front surface of the vitreous, lying behind the lens, or of the back surface that attaches to the retina's inner limiting membrane. See also ANTERIOR HYALOID MEMBRANE, POSTERIOR HYALOID MEMBRANE.

vitreous floaters. *Pathologic condition.* Particles that float in the vitreous and cast shadows on the retina; seen as spots, cobwebs, spiders, etc. Occur normally with aging or in association with vitreous detachment, retinal tear, or intraocular inflammation.

vitreous gel. See VITREOUS.

vitreous hemorrhage, vitreal bleed. *Pathologic condition.* Blood in the vitreous. May result from blunt eye trauma, blood leakage from abnormal new retinal vessels (neovascularization), vitreous detachment, or retinal tear.

vitreous humor. Less common term for VITREOUS.

vitreous opacities. *Anatomic defect.* Obstructions in the vitreous gel, such as a foreign body, blood, or inflammatory debris.

vitreous tap. *Surgical procedure.* Puncture into the vitreous to remove a small sample, usually for culturing or microscopic study.

vitreous touch. *Pathologic condition.* Contact between the vitreous gel and corneal endothelium, following cataract extraction. Sometimes causes endothelial damage with resultant corneal swelling.

vitritis (vih-TRI-tus), **hyalitis**. *Clinical sign.* Inflammatory intraocular reaction (with clouding and cells) in the vitreous. Often accompanies inflammation of the ciliary body, iris, choroid or retina.

vocational trifocals. Plus lens correction for specific near-vision needs, to compensate for age-related decrease in focusing ability (accommodation). Example: "baseball lens," with bifocal segments at top and bottom, for seeing up close below and above eye level, e.g., by librarians. See also ADD, PRESBYOPIA.

VOD (vision right eye). *Measurement.* Visual acuity tested in the right eye while the left eye is covered.

Vogt-Koyanagi-Harada syndrome (voht koy-ah-NAH-gee huh-RAH-duh),

Harada's *(or)* uveitis-vitiligo-alopecia-poliosis syndrome. *Pathologic condition.* Characterized by headache, hearing defect, hair loss, premature graying, patchy depigmentation of skin, lashes and retina, steamy corneas, vitreous opacities, and diffuse exudative choroiditis. Vision and hearing loss may occur, with incomplete recovery. Progressive; chronic. Rare; tends to affect young Italian or Japanese adults. See also POLIOSIS.

Vogt's line. *Abnormal condition.* Thin vertical stress line in the deeper corneal layers, in patients with keratoconus.

Vogt-Spielmeyer syndrome, Batten-Mayou *(or)* Stock-Spielmeyer-Vogt syndrome. *Pathologic condition.* Childhood form of amaurotic familial idiocy. Characterized by diffuse nervous system disease, macular lesions, and optic nerve degeneration.

voluntary convergence. *Function.* Amount the eyes can voluntarily turn inward (toward each other).

voluntary eye movements, saccades. *Function.* Quick movements of both eyes in the same direction; mechanism for fixation, refixation, rapid eye movements, and the fast phase of optokinetic nystagmus. Initiated by the frontal lobe in the brain (Brodmann area 8).

voluntary nystagmus (ni-STAG-mus). *Function.* Short bursts of rhythmic, horizontal eye movements under voluntary control. Rarely last over 1–2 minutes. Unusual but not pathological.

von Gierke's disease (GHIR-keez). *Pathologic condition.* Metabolic disturbance resulting in short stature, low blood sugar levels, and high blood fat. Retinal changes include flat, round, yellowish flecks in the macular region that do not affect vision. Hereditary.

von Graefe sign (GRAY-fee), **lid lag**. *Clinical sign.* Delay (lag) in downward movement of upper eyelid as it follows the eye into downgaze. Common sign of thyroid eye disease. See also DALRYMPLE'S SIGN, STELLWAG'S SIGN.

von Graefe's syndrome, congenital bulbar paralysis, congenital facial diplegia, Moebius syndrome. *Congenital anomaly.* Bilateral malformation in cranial nuclei of the 6th (abducens) and 7th (facial) cranial nerves, resulting in inability to move either eye outward past the midline or to close the eyelids, large inward eye deviation (esotropia), and a droopy, expressionless facial appearance.

von Hippel-Lindau disease, angiomatosis retinae, Lindau's disease. *Pathologic condition.* One of several hereditary disorders called phakomatoses; characterized by tumors of the retina, central nervous system and visceral organs. Primary eye findings are blood-filled retinal tumors (hemangiomas) fed by large, tortuous blood vessels; may also be associated with exudate leakage into the retina and retinal detachment.

von Recklinghausen's disease, neurofibromatosis, Recklinghausen's disease. *Pathologic condition.* One of several hereditary disorders called phakomatoses; characterized by small tumors under the skin and in the central nervous system, and bony defects in the orbital bones. Common sites for these tumors include the upper eyelid, optic nerve, 8th (acoustic) cranial nerve, and spinal cord.

von Willebrandt's knee (WIL-brandz), **Willebrandt's knee**. *Anatomy.* Group of inferior nasal optic nerve fibers at the front part of the chiasm, that loop forward into the opposite optic nerve before traveling back into the appropriate optic tract. See also JUNCTION SCOTOMA.

vortex dystrophy. *Degenerative change.* Random lines of pigment in the superficial layers of the cornea.

vortex veins, venae vorticosae. *Anatomy.* Four veins (2 superior, 2 inferior) that provide the main blood outflow from the eyes, exiting near the equator on each side of the superior and inferior recti and draining into the superior and inferior ophthalmic veins.

VOS (vision left eye). *Measurement.* Visual acuity tested in the left eye while the right eye is covered.

Vossius' ring (v/WAH-see-us). *Clinical sign.* Temporary ring-shaped deposit of iris pigment granules on the front surface of the lens, found after blunt eye trauma. Larger than and concentric with the pupillary margin.

VOU (vision both eyes). *Measurement.* Visual acuity tested with both eyes open.

V-pattern. *Functional defect.* Horizontal eye misalignment in which an inturning (esotropic) eye deviates more on down-gaze than than on up-gaze, or an outward turning (exotropic) eye deviates more on up-gaze than on down-gaze. See also A-PATTERN.

v-shaped groove. *Instrument.* Used for measuring contact lens diameter.

V-to-Y plasty. *Surgical procedure.* Plastic surgery technique for changing tension between two areas of skin. See also Z-PLASTY, Y-TO-V PLASTY.

W

Waardenburg-Klein syndrome. *Pathologic condition*. Characterized by a different color in each iris (heterochromia), large bridge of the nose with a wider-than-normal distance between the eyes (telecanthus), a white forelock, and deafness.

Wagner's disease. *Pathologic condition*. Syndrome of vitreoretinal degeneration that leads to retinal tears and detachment. Other ocular findings include moderate myopia, strabismus, and cataracts that begin in the teen years. Hereditary. See also JANSEN'S SYNDROME, MARFAN'S SYNDROME, STICKLER'S SYNDROME.

Waldenstrom's macroglobulinemia. *Pathologic condition*. Very large protein globulin molecules in the blood. May cause blockage of blood vessels because of increased viscosity of the blood. Cause unknown.

Wallenberg syndrome, lateral medullary syndrome. *Pathologic condition*. Most common brainstem stroke. Characterized by eye overshoot (dysmetria), Horner's syndrome, rotary nystagmus, and skew deviations on the same side of the body and facial and body weakness on the opposite side.

wall-eyes, divergent strabismus, exotropia, external strabismus. *Functional defect*. Eye misalignment in which one eye deviates outward (away from nose) while the other remains straight and fixates normally. See also EXOPHORIA.

warfarin. *Drug*. Heart medication. Blood "thinner" for preventing blood clot formation. Trade names: Athrombin K, Coumadin.

water drinking test. Patient drinks 1 quart of water, to stress the aqueous drainage mechanism. Intraocular pressure is then measured over the next hour; a rise of 8 mm of mercury suggests the presence of open angle glaucoma. See also PROVOCATIVE TEST.

watt. *Measurement*. Unit of power used in comparing laser burns.

wavelength. *Optics*. Length of one complete cycle of a wave, such as a light wave (e.g., from the crest of one wave to the crest of the next).

Weber-Osler-Rendu syndrome. *Pathologic condition*. Multiple star-shaped clumps of blood vessels (telagiectasias) in the retina, conjunctiva, skin, mucous membranes, gastrointestinal and genito-urinary tract. Can lead to bleeding, e.g., from the nose (epistaxis), gastrointestinal tract (hemoptysis and melena), urinary tract (hematuria). Hereditary.

Weber's law. *Psychophysics*. A constant ratio exists between the intensity of a stimulus and that needed to produce a just-detectable difference ($I \div \Delta I$ = constant). Relates to many types of stimuli: weights, sound, light. See also FECHNER'S LAW, PHOTOMETRY.

Weber's syndrome. *Pathologic condition*. Group of signs and symptoms caused by a small stroke in the cerebral peduncle of the brain. Results in a 3rd (oculomotor) cranial nerve paralysis in one eye with spastic body paralysis and unsteady gait on the opposite side.

Weck cell, Weck sponge. *Surgical material*. Trade name of highly absorbent cellulose sponge used during eye surgery to absorb blood, vitreous, and other fluids.

Weck cell vitrectomy (vih-TREK-tuh-mee). *Surgical procedure*. Removal of vitreous using the "open sky" procedure (front access) with a cellulose sponge that holds the vitreous as it is cut with scissors.

Weck sponge. See WECK CELL.

Wegener's granulomatosis. *Pathologic condition*. Progressive systemic disease that frequently involves the respiratory tract (sinuses and lung) and kidney. Severe inflammatory tumor-like masses (granulomas) develop in and around blood vessels, causing cell death. Characteristic eye findings include uveitis, chemosis, lid swelling, limited eye movement, and proptosis. No known cause.

Weiger's ligament, Egger's line, hyaloideo-capsular ligament. *Anatomy*. A weak line of adherence between the anterior vitreous and the posterior surface of the lens, in the form of a ring 8–9 mm in diameter.

Weill-Marchesani syndrome (wile-mahr-cheh-SAH-nee). *Congenital anomaly*. Characterized by compact stature, short fingers and toes, glaucoma, and a small lens that tends to be dislocated downward.

Werner's syndrome. *Pathologic condition*. Rare genetic abnormality characterized by juvenile cataracts, glaucoma and corneal opacities, with degeneration of the skin on the face, limbs, hands and feet, and graying and thinning of hair beginning between ages 20–30.

Wernicke's encephalopathy (WUR-nih-keez en-sef-uh-LAH-puh-thee). *Pathologic condition*. Extraocular muscle paralysis that causes double vision, gaze palsies, nystagmus, and unsteady gait. Associated with thiamine (vitamin B_1) deficiency and chronic alcoholism.

wetting solution. *Chemical*. Liquid applied to hard a contact lens prior to its insertion on the cornea. Allows smoother flow of tears on the water-repellent plastic surface and helps cushion the lens on the cornea.

wheel rotation, torsion. *Function*. Rotation of an eye around its antero-posterior axis so it tilts either inward or outward. See also CYCLODUCTION, CYCLOVERSION, Y AXIS OF FICK.

whiplash head shaking syndrome, shaken baby syndrome. *Pathologic condition*. Physical damage to the head, retina or brain of an infant or young child caused by violent shaking.

"white of the eye," sclera, tunica fibrosa oculi. *Anatomy*. Opaque, fibrous, protective outer layer of the eye that is directly continuous with the cornea in front and the sheath covering the optic nerve behind. Contains collagen and elastic fibers.

Whitnall's ligament. *Anatomy*. Transverse suspensory ligament extending from the region of the trochlea to the fascia surrounding the lacrimal gland; a condensation of the fascia of the levator muscle and tendon. Clinically important in ptosis surgery.

Wieger's ligament (WEE-gurz). *Anatomy*. Ring-like attachment of the front face of the vitreous to the back surface of the lens.

Wies procedure (wize), **transverse blepharotomy with lid margin rotation**. *Surgical procedure*. For repair of an inward turning eyelid (entropion) due to scarring. See also CICATRICIAL ENTROPION.

Wildervanck syndrome, cervico-oculo-acoustic malformation. *Congenital anomaly*. Consists of neck and cervical spine deformity, Duane's syndrome and hearing loss. See also GOLDENHAR'S SYNDROME, KLIPPEL-FEIL SYNDROME.

Willebrandt's knee. See VON WILLEBRANDT'S KNEE.

Wilson's disease, hepato-lenticular degeneration. *Pathologic condition*. Characterized by abnormal copper accumulation. Causes brain cell and liver degeneration and copper deposits in the eye (Kayser-Fleisher ring in Descemet's membrane and sometimes a "sunflower" cataract. Rare; hereditary.

window defect. *Sign*. Retinal pigment epithelial defect due to cellular loss; especially visible with fluorescein angiography as hyperfluorescent spots.

windshield wiper syndrome. *Surgical complication*. Sideways movement of an intraocular lens as the head or eye moves, as when the lens is too small for a snug fit.

"wipe-out" syndrome, diffuse unilateral subacute neuroretinitis. *Pathologic condition*. Insidious gradual vision loss in one eye, usually in children. Thought to be caused by an intraocular *Toxocara* worm.

Wirt test. For assessing stereoscopic acuity. No longer generally available; replaced by Titmus, TNO, Randot, and Lang stereotests.

with correction (cc). Vision tested with the patient wearing corrective eyeglasses or contact lenses.

"with" motion. *Optics*. Image movement in same direction as movement of the instrument, light or lens that creates it, e.g., light from a retinoscope moves in the same direction as the image seen in the patient's pupil. Can be neutralized with plus lenses. See also "AGAINST" MOTION, RETINOSCOPY.

"with-the-rule" astigmatism (uh-STIG-muh-tizm). *Refractive error*. Optical power that is greater (more plus power) in the vertical meridian of an eye than in the horizontal meridian. Corrected by a plus-cylinder lens with its axis at 90°. See also "AGAINST-THE-RULE" ASTIGMATISM.

without correction (sc). Vision tested without the patient wearing glasses or contact lenses.

Wolfring's glands. *Anatomy*. Accessory lacrimal glands located just above the upper tarsus, and occasionally in the lower lid as well.

Wolf's syndrome. *Congenital anomaly*. Rare genetic disorder associated with skeletal abnormalities, severe mental retardation, small head, round face, ear abnormalities, widely set eyes, epicanthus, anti-mongoloid slant, eye deviations, uveal defects, and bulging eyes.

working distance. *Measurement*. In a refraction, the distance between the patient's eye and the examiner's retinoscope, usually 50 to 70 cm. Dioptric equivalent of this distance (2 to 1.4 diopters) is subtracted from the retinoscopy measurement to determine the refractive error.

Worth 4-dot test (W4D). For evaluating the eyes' capacity to perceive images simultaneously. Patient views four lights (1 red, 1 white, 2 green) through a red filter before one eye and a green filter before the other.

wound dehiscence. *Pathologic condition*. Breaking open or coming apart of the layers of a wound.

wound leak. *Abnormal condition*. Escape of fluid or tissue through a cut or wound. May be a complication of ocular surgery, requiring repair.

W plasty. *Surgical procedure*. Skin incision forming two parallel rows of Ws. Forms a saw-toothed design when triangular points are stitched together.

Wyburn-Mason syndrome. *Congenital abnormality*. Malformed blood vessels that lack capillaries; occur in the brain, face, and retina. Unilateral; nonprogressive. See also VON HIPPEL-LINDAU'S DISEASE.

Wydase. Trade name for hyaluronidase, enzyme added to anesthetic agents to hasten and spread an anesthetic block.

X

Xalatan. Drug. Trade name for latanoprost; used for treating glaucoma.

xanthelasma (zan-thel-AZ-muh). See XANTHOMA.

xanthoma (zan-THOH-muh), **xanthelasma**. *Pathologic condition.* Small yellowish eyelid tumors, usually near the nose, that appear in the elderly or others with high blood fat levels.

xanthopsia (zan-THAHP-see-uh). *Clinical sign.* Vision abnormality in which objects appear to be tinted yellow. Can be caused by the drug digitalis, by jaundice, or by hysteria. See also CYANOPSIA, ERYTHROPSIA.

xenon (ZEE-non). *Chemical.* Inert gas used in some light bulbs and photocoagulators.

xerophthalmia (zir-aff-THAL-mee-uh). *Pathologic condition.* Drying of eye surfaces. Characterized by loss of corneal and conjunctival luster, Bowman's membrane degeneration, and infiltration of the corneal stroma with cells and fluid. Associated with vitamin A deficiency and any condition in which the eyelids do not close completely.

xerosis (zir-OH-sis). *Functional defect.* Conjunctival and corneal dryness caused by deficiency of tears or conjunctival secretions.

xerostomia (zir-uh-STOH-muh). *Clinical sign.* Dry mouth due to insufficient mucous secretions. See also SJOGREN'S SYNDROME.

X-linked. *Description.* Hereditary characteristic carried on the X (female) chromosome.

Xylocaine (ZI-loh-kayn). *Drug.* Trade name of lidocaine, injected for local anesthesia.

Y

YAG laser, Nd:YAG. *Surgical instrument*. Laser that produces short pulsed, high energy light beam to cut, perforate, or fragment tissue. Acronym: Yttrium-Aluminum-Garnet. See also PHOTOCOAGULATION.

y axis of Fick, anteroposterior *(or)* **longitudinal** *(or)* **sagittal axis of Fick**. Imaginary line through an eye's center of rotation, connecting the geometric center of the cornea (anterior pole) with the geometric center of the back of the eye (posterior pole). Tilting (torsional) eye rotations occur around this axis.

yellow spot. *Anatomy*. Refers to the macula lutea of the retina.

yoke muscles, contralateral synergists. *Function*. Extraocular muscles that move the eyes in parallel. Six pairs (one from each eye, e.g., right medial rectus and left lateral rectus). See also DIAGNOSTIC POSITIONS OF GAZE.

youthyscope. Incorrect spelling of EUTHYSCOPE.

Y sutures. *Anatomy*. Junction lines within the lens of the eye; formed by end-to-end contact of the tips of lens fibers. An upright Y is found in front of the fetal nucleus of an adult lens, an inverted Y behind it.

Y-to-V plasty. *Surgical procedure*. For closing defects; a skin incision forming a Y creates a triangular flap that is pulled forward to the bottom of the center line and stitched into place. See also ADVANCEMENT FLAP, GLABELLAR FLAP.

yureeblefarin. Incorrect spelling of EURYBLEPHARON.

Z

zanthopsia. Incorrect spelling of XANTHOPSIA.

z axis of Fick, vertical axis of Fick. Imaginary line that passes vertically through the center of each eye; associated with horizontal eye rotations.

Zeis glands (zice). *Anatomy.* Oil-producing glands that surround the eyelashes. Ducts enter lash follicles near the eyelid margins. See also STYE.

zenon. Incorrect spelling of XENON.

Zephiran. *Preservative.* Trade name for benzalkonium chloride. Commonly used in ophthalmic solutions; causes allergy in some patients.

zerophthalmia. Incorrect spelling of XEROPHTHALMIA.

zerosis. Incorrect spelling of XEROSIS.

zero vergence. *Optics.* Refers to light rays that are parallel and have no converging or diverging optical power.

Ziegler cautery. *Treatment.* Use of cautery applications to the lid for correction of minimal ectropion (conjunctival surface) or entropion (skin surface)

Zinn (annulus of). *Anatomy.* Ring of fibrous tissue surrounding the optic nerve at its entrance to the eye (at the rear of the orbit); consists of the origins of five extraocular muscles (lateral, medial, superior and inferior recti and superior oblique).

"zipped up angle." *Pathologic condition.* Slang for a gradual closure of the anterior chamber angle. See also ANGLE CLOSURE GLAUCOMA.

Z marginal tenotomy (ten-AH-tuh-mee). *Surgical procedure.* Type of cut into a tendon to weaken an extraocular muscle, to correct an eye misalignment. See also MARGINAL MYOTOMY.

Z myotomy (mi-AH-tuh-mee). *Surgical procedure.* Type of cut into an extraocular muscle to weaken it; to correct an eye misalignment. See also MYOTOMY.

Zolyse (ZOH-lize). *Chemical.* Trade name of alphachymotrypsin, an enzyme injected into the eye before intracapsular cataract extraction to loosen and dissolve suspensory zonules. See also CATARASE.

zonular cataract, lamellar cataract. *Pathologic condition.* Form of cataract in which concentric thin layers (lamellae) of opacities are surrounded by zones of clear lens. Usually in both eyes. Vision may remain good.

zonules (ZAHN-yoolz), **zonules of Zinn**. *Anatomy.* Radially arranged fibers that suspend the lens from the ciliary body and hold it in position. See also ACCOMMODATION.

zonules of Zinn. See ZONULES.

zonulysis (zahn-yu-LI-sis). *Surgical procedure.* During cataract extraction, instillation of the enzyme alpha-chymotrypsin into the aqueous to dissolve lens zonules. Facilitates surgical removal of entire lens.

zoster (herpes), shingles. *Pathologic condition.* Extremely painful, blister-like skin lesions on the face, sometimes with inflammation of the cornea, sclera, ciliary body and optic nerve. Affects the 1st division (ophthalmic nerve) of the 5th (trigeminal) cranial nerve. Caused by the chickenpox virus.

Zovirax. *Drug.* Trade name of acyclovir; for treating viral eye infections.

Z-plasty. *Surgical procedure.* Plastic surgery technique to reduce tension along a scar.

zygoma (zi-GOH-muh), **zygomatic bone**. *Anatomy.* Cheek bone; forms part of the orbital floor and most of the lateral wall. One of seven bones of the orbit (eye socket).

zygomatic nerve (zi-goh-MAT-ik). *Anatomy.* Branch of maxillary nerve (2nd division of 5th [trigeminal] cranial nerve) that supplies sensation to facial skin below the lower eyelid and temporal region. Enters the orbit through the inferior orbital fissure, divides into zygomatico-temporal and zygomatico-facial branches, then both exit through canals in the zygoma (cheekbone).

zylocaine. Incorrect spelling of XYLOCAINE.

ORDER FORM

Please send me_____copies DICTIONARY OF EYE TERMINOLOGY, 3rd edition @ $24.95 per copy + shipping and handling (see table).

SHIP TO: NAME _____

ADDRESS _____

CITY/STATE/ZIP _____ PHONE_____

Add 6% sales tax for books sent to Florida addresses.

To charge to Visa or MasterCard:

Cardholder's name_____

Card number_____ Expiration date_____

Fax to 1-800-854-4947 (credit card orders) or mail to Triad Publishing Company P.O. Box 13355, Gainesville, FL 32604

Foreign orders: payable in U.S. funds drawn on a U.S. bank, or by Visa or MasterCard. Fax number 1-352-373-1488.

SHIPPING & HANDLING CHARGES						
DOMESTIC & CANADIAN ADDRESSES				INTERNATIONAL ORDERS		
	CONT. US	AL, HI, US TERR.	CANADA		AIR	SURFACE
Up to $30	$6	$12	$15	Up to $30	$35	$16
$30 to $80	$8	$16	$20	$30 to $80	$50	$23
$80 to $200	$10	$20	$25	$80 to $200	$65	$29

Most shipments to continental U.S. are sent by UPS surface; to Canada by air parcel post; to Alaska, Hawaii and U.S. territories by air mail.

RELATED BOOKS AND SOFTWARE

I would like to receive information about:

☐ Triad's EYE CARE NOTES (Lawrence A. Winograd, MD & Melvin L Rubin, MD). Patient education handouts. Two formats: book and computer software. Updated annually.

☐ EYECHECK: spell-checker with 20,000 ophthalmic words. For PC: Word, any version; WordPerfect, version 5.0, 5.1, 6.0, 6.1; or Mac: Word 5.0, 5.1.

☐ THE FINE ART OF PRESCRIBING GLASSES WITHOUT MAKING A SPECTACLE OF YOURSELF (Benjamin Mllder, MD & Melvin L. Rubin, MD). Practical practice-builder full of case histories and clinical pearls.

☐ OPTICS FOR CLINICIANS (Melvin L. Rubin, MD). The classic text that makes this subject understandable and enjoyable.

☐ A CHILD'S EYES (John W. Simon, MD & Joseph H. Calhoun, MD). The basics of pediatric ophthalmology for primary care physicians.

Prices subject to change without notice.

ORDER FORM

Please send me_____copies DICTIONARY OF EYE TERMINOLOGY,
3rd edition @ $24.95 per copy + shipping and handling (see table).

SHIP TO: NAME _____

ADDRESS _____

CITY/STATE/ZIP _____ PHONE_____

Add 6% sales tax for books sent to Florida addresses.

To charge to Visa or MasterCard:

Cardholder's name_____

Card number _____ Expiration date _____

**Fax to 1-800-854-4947 (credit card orders)
or mail to Triad Publishing Company
P.O. Box 13355, Gainesville, FL 32604**

Foreign orders: payable in U.S. funds drawn on a U.S. bank, or by Visa or
MasterCard. Fax number 1-352-373-1488.

SHIPPING & HANDLING CHARGES						
DOMESTIC & CANADIAN ADDRESSES				INTERNATIONAL ORDERS		
	CONT. US	AL, HI, US TERR.	CANADA		AIR	SURFACE
Up to $30	$6	$12	$15	Up to $30	$35	$16
$30 to $80	$8	$16	$20	$30 to $80	$50	$23
$80 to $200	$10	$20	$25	$80 to $200	$65	$29

Most shipments to continental U.S. are sent by UPS surface; to Canada by air
parcel post; to Alaska, Hawaii and U.S. territories by air mail.

RELATED BOOKS AND SOFTWARE

I would like to receive information about:

☐ Triad's EYE CARE NOTES (Lawrence A. Winograd, MD & Melvin L Rubin,
MD). Patient education handouts. Two formats: book and computer software. Updated annually.

☐ EYECHECK: spell-checker with 20,000 ophthalmic words. For PC: Word,
any version; WordPerfect, version 5.0, 5.1, 6.0, 6.1; or Mac: Word 5.0, 5.1.

☐ THE FINE ART OF PRESCRIBING GLASSES WITHOUT MAKING A
SPECTACLE OF YOURSELF (Benjamin MIlder, MD & Melvin L. Rubin,
MD). Practical practice-builder full of case histories and clinical pearls.

☐ OPTICS FOR CLINICIANS (Melvin L. Rubin, MD). The classic text that
makes this subject understandable and enjoyable.

☐ A CHILD'S EYES (John W. Simon, MD & Joseph H. Calhoun, MD). The
basics of pediatric ophthalmology for primary care physicians.

Prices subject to change without notice.